Pathology and Visual Culture

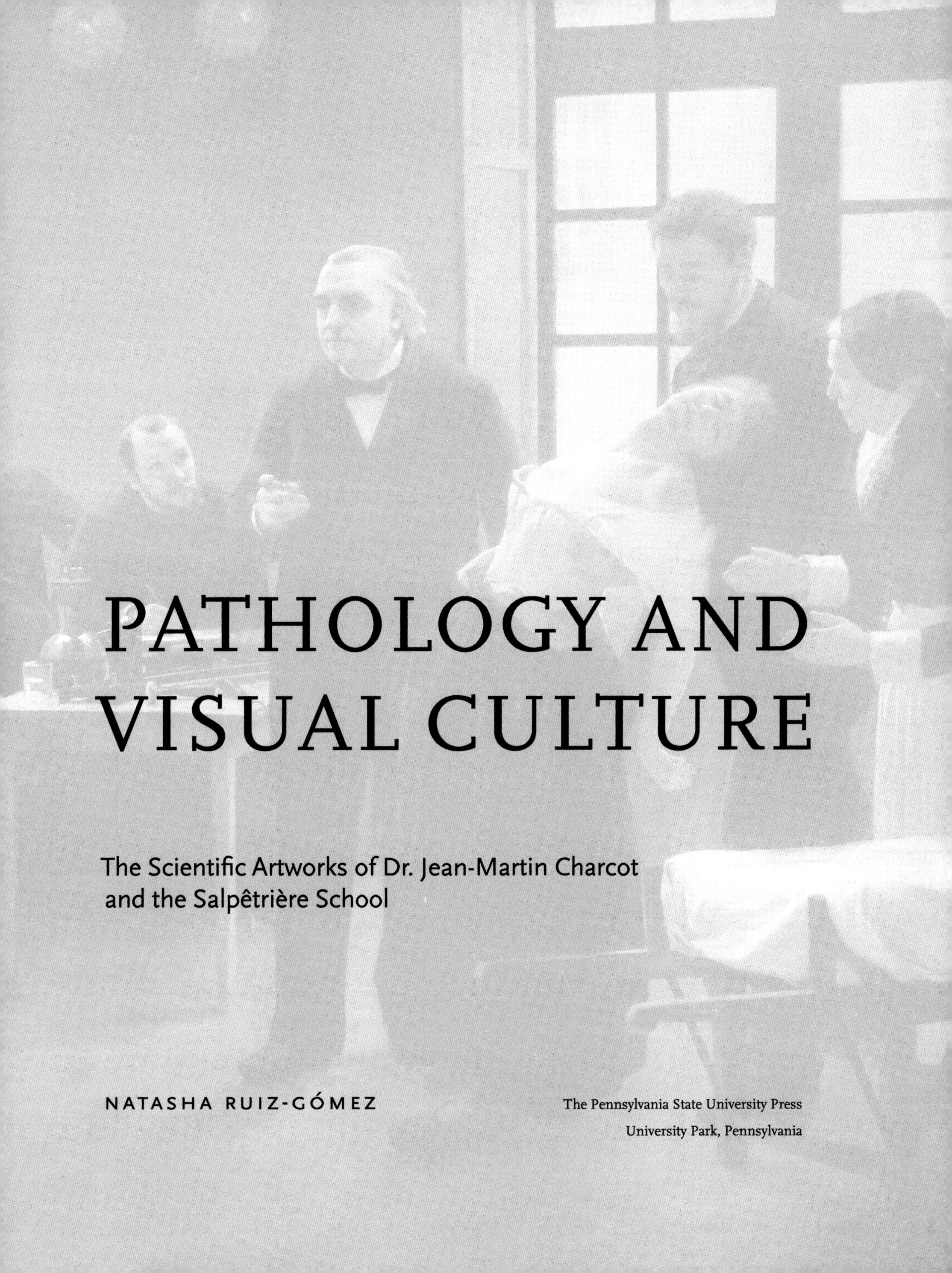

PATHOLOGY AND VISUAL CULTURE

The Scientific Artworks of Dr. Jean-Martin Charcot and the Salpêtrière School

NATASHA RUIZ-GÓMEZ

The Pennsylvania State University Press
University Park, Pennsylvania

Library of Congress Cataloging-in-Publication Data

Names: Ruiz-Gómez, Natasha, author.
Title: Pathology and visual culture : the scientific artworks of Dr. Jean-Martin Charcot and the Salpêtrière School / Natasha Ruiz-Gomez.
Description: University Park, Pennsylvania : The Pennsylvania State University Press, [2024] | Includes bibliographical references and index.
Summary: "Examines the extraordinary drawings, photographs, casts, and sculptures produced by Dr. Jean-Martin Charcot (1825–1893) and the Salpêtrière School that combine medical knowledge and artistic expression"—Provided by publisher.
Identifiers: LCCN 2023052089 | ISBN 9780271096803 (hardback)
Subjects: LCSH: Charcot, J. M. (Jean Martin), 1825-1893. | Salpêtrière (Hospital) | Medicine and art—France—History—19th century. | Pathology—France—History—19th century.
Classification: LCC N8223 .R85 2024 | DDC 700/.4561—dc23/eng/20231117
LC record available at https://lccn.loc.gov/2023052089

Printed in the United States of America
Published by The Pennsylvania State University Press,
University Park, PA 16802–1003

The Pennsylvania State University Press is a member of the Association of University Presses.

It is the policy of The Pennsylvania State University Press to use acid-free paper. Publications on uncoated stock satisfy the minimum requirements of American National Standard for Information Sciences—Permanence of Paper for Printed Library Material, ANSI Z39.48–1992.

I learnt [. . .] to follow the unforgotten advice of my master, Charcot: to look at the same things again and again until they themselves begin to speak.

—SIGMUND FREUD, 1914

Archival research starts off slowly and steadily through banal manual tasks to which one rarely gives much thought. Nonetheless, in doing these tasks, a new object is created, a new form of knowledge takes shape, and a new "archive" emerges. As you work, you are taking the preexisting forms and readjusting them in different ways to make possible a different narration of reality. This is not a question of repetition, but of beginning anew, of dealing the cards over again.

—ARLETTE FARGE, 2013

For My Parents

Contents

Illustrations

Figures

Acknowledgments

I remember the first time I heard Charcot's name: I was in a café in Philadelphia, discussing Auguste Rodin with Christine Poggi. I have her to thank for introducing me to this larger-than-life figure from the history of medicine, and for teaching me how to be an art historian. In these last twenty years, my scholarship has toggled largely between Rodin and Charcot; for the last ten or so, Charcot has enjoyed more of my attention, and I am indebted to many people for their intellectual engagement and support throughout this extended endeavor.

The University of Essex provided periods of research leave that afforded me the time and mental space to write. I am grateful to my colleagues in the School of Philosophy and Art History (SPAH) for picking up the slack that results by definition from a colleague's leave. A Research Fellowship from The Leverhulme Trust provided a crucial term off and funds for many of the images in the book. Travel funds provided by both SPAH and the History of Art Department at the University of Pennsylvania allowed me to conduct the primary research that forms the core of this book. SPAH very generously also covered the subvention for publication, as well as providing funds for images; my thanks to Diana Bullen Presciutti for being in my corner.

I am also grateful to the MA students in my "scientific artworks" seminars at Essex and to the many audiences at talks and conferences in the United States, United Kingdom, France, Belgium, Norway, Spain, and Switzerland who have offered their insights on earlier iterations of my chapters. Previous versions of parts of this book have appeared elsewhere, and my thanks go to their publishers for allowing me to include that work here. Excerpts of chapter 2 appeared in "The Model Patient: Observation and Illustration at the Musée Charcot," *Visualizing the Body in Art, Anatomy, and Medicine since 1800: Models, Modelling*, edited by Andrew Graciano (New York: Routledge, 2019), 203–32. A shorter version of Chapter 5 was published as "The 'Scientific Artworks' of Doctor Paul Richer," *Medical Humanities* [special issue on Patients' Portraits, organized by Ludmilla Jordanova and Keren Hammerschlag] 39, no. 1 (June 2013): 4–10. And portions of the Coda were included in "Shaking the Tyranny of the Cadaver: Doctor Paul Richer and the *Living Écorché*," *Bodies Beyond Borders: Moving Anatomies, 1750–1950*, edited by Kaat Wils, Raf de Bont, and Sokhieng Au (Leuven: University of Leuven Press, 2017), 231–57. All of these editors helped to sharpen and nuance my argument.

This book would not have been possible without the kind and informed assistance of archivists and librarians—the unsung heroes of academic research—at many institutions who facilitated access to sources in the histories of art and medicine that were essential to my work. In the United States, these include the Avery Architectural and Fine Arts Library of Columbia University; the Health Sciences Library, Archives, and Special Collections of the Columbia University Medical Center; the Fisher Fine Arts Library, the Kislik Center for Special Collections, Rare Books and Manuscripts, and the Biomedical Library of the University of Pennsylvania; and the New York Academy of Medicine. In France, I had the good fortune to spend time in the Bibliothèque Charcot at the Salpêtrière, the Archives de l'Assistance Publique-Hôpitaux de Paris, the Bibliothèque nationale de France, the library of the École nationale supérieure des beaux-arts, and the Bibliothèque historique de la Ville de Paris. In the United Kingdom, I am grateful to the staff of the Rare Books and Music Room of the British Library, the National Art Library at the Victoria and Albert Museum, the library of the Wellcome Collection, and the Albert Sloman Library of the University of Essex, especially the Interlibrary Loan team. And for their gracious assistance with images, I would like to thank Isabelle Lacabarats; Jacques Marie; Sylvie Nayral; Philippe Richer; Agnes Virole and Alexane Pasquier of the Musée de l'Assistance Publique-Hôpitaux de Paris; Holly Peel of the Wellcome Collection; and the SPAH administrative team, especially Hannah Whiting.

I am indebted to several people whose generosity changed the course of my research. Véronique Leroux-Hugon, former librarian of the Bibliothèque Charcot, first introduced me to its riches while I was still a student. Jean-François Minot, former keeper of the collections of the Musée de l'Assistance Publique-Hôpitaux de Paris, opened cabinets, unlocked basements, and traveled with me to storage facilities around Paris to show me the now widely scattered material remnants of the Musée Charcot—my direct personal encounter with the *Ataxic Venus* remains one of the most memorable moments of my professional life. His successor, Dominique Plancher-Souveton, similarly granted me extraordinary access to materials, especially the albums of the Musée Charcot. Philippe Comar, Professor of Anatomy at the École des beaux-arts, welcomed me into the galerie Huguier and shared his unparalleled knowledge of Richer, who once held his position. Olivier Walusinski, MD, also an expert on Richer, patiently answered all my questions and shared unpublished manuscripts and photographs. The late Philippe Richer graciously invited me into his home to show me his family's archives and library, immeasurably enriching my knowledge and appreciation of his grandfather's oeuvre; his son, Philippe Richer, has kindly allowed me to publish images I needed for this book. Cornelia Golimbu, MD, generously took the time to review my manuscript to verify my understanding of medical terminology. Of course, all errors are my own.

Given how many years it has taken for this book to enter the world, it would be impossible for me to thank everyone who contributed to its creation. Conversations with Sam Alberti, Felicity Callard, Eleanor Crook, Céline Eidenbenz, Christopher Goetz, Rae Beth Gordon, Fiona Johnstone, Bertrand Marquer, Jonathan Marshall, Ruth Patel, Mike Sappol, Joanna Woodall, and Alfons Zarzoso helped at important moments. Suzannah

Biernoff, Gemma Blackshaw, Fae Brauer, Anthea Callen, Mechthild Fend, Zeynep Devrim Gürsel, Ludmilla Jordanova, Jacky Maggs, Magali Le Mens, Jane Partington, and Elisabeth Schneider have all inspired me in different ways. Susan Sidlauskas's wisdom has proved indispensable at key moments, in both my research and my personal life. Mary Hunter and I are comrades in Charcot; she commented on my introduction when I was still trying to sort out my overall argument. Allison Morehead provided extensive feedback on the manuscript in the final stages which improved it significantly, as did the other peer reviewer. I am elated to have Ellie Goodman as my editor and Penn State University Press as my publisher—they have always been my first choice for this project. My thanks also to Maddie Caso at Penn State for her patience and to Laura Reed-Morrisson for her eagle-eyed copyediting.

I am lucky to have extraordinary people in my life: Juliet Bellow, Meredith Clair, Patricia d'Eça, Patricia Di Iorio, Beck Feibelman, Chin Ru Foo, Ann Fordham, Michaela Giebelhausen, Eusun Kim, Victoria Macdonald, Meredith Malone, Jennifer O'Sullivan Salmon, Jennifer Randall, Freyda Spira, Lisa Temple-Cox, Lisa Wade, and Fawzia Zawahir. Thanks too to Andi, Markus, and Aden Rindler, Raj Singh and Rekha and Reva Singh-Foo, and Gabriella and Andrew Winters for many happy days. I have to express particular gratitude to Angela Vaughn for being so wonderful to me and my family. Conversations with Sarah Symmons, along with her warm meals and warmer welcomes, have sustained me over many years now. Tania Cleaves and Keren Hammerschlag have read every word of this book in various stages of its development, more than once—it would not have been written without their incisive criticisms, ardent encouragement, and steadfast friendship.

My extended family has always supported me, even though my work has likely seemed arcane to them at times. I would like to thank Katie Boudart; Julito, Oliver, Grace, and Charlotte Ruiz-Gómez; and my in-laws Vram, Aznive, Garen, Sebouh, Vicken, Sébastien, and Inès Yegparian. A special note of thanks to Christina Lehmejian-Karaszewski for always taking an interest in my work, and Mirtha Sadurní for being a model of serenity. I am especially grateful to my brother, Julio Ruiz-Gómez, who has actively helped to make many of my dreams come true.

My late father, Julio O. Ruiz-Gómez, taught me to look everywhere for beauty; he would have been proud that I managed to find beauty even in pathology. My mother, Miriam Ruiz-Gómez, is the most resilient and compassionate person I've ever known. I strive to emulate their quiet courage and their integrity. "Thank you" would never be enough. The lives of my daughters, Sabrina Ruiz Yegparian and Daphne Gómez Yegparian, have spanned this project, and my memory of their childhood is intermingled with the researching and writing of this book. For that, I am both sorry and grateful—they are more wondrous than anything in the histories of art or medicine. My husband and in-house copyeditor, Raffi Yegparian, teases me by asking why I don't study "beautiful" things, not realizing that, thanks to him, I have all the beauty I need. This book is dedicated to them.

INTRODUCTION

Clinicians and Artists

The physician is inseparable from the artist.

—HENRY MEIGE, 1898

In May 1885, art critic and novelist Octave Mirbeau published an article in *L'Événement* in which he characterized the nineteenth century as "the century of nervous diseases." He argued that this was the case because nervous diseases motivated its events and were the focus of its scientific obsession. Thus, Mirbeau writes, "it will perhaps be neither the century of Victor Hugo nor the century of Napoleon, but the century of Charcot." In this largely overlooked article, the author describes in detail one of the celebrated lessons at the Hôpital de la Salpêtrière of Doctor Jean-Martin Charcot (1825–1893), a founder of modern neurology, and the frisson generated by its partially disrobed and hypnotized hysterics. Mirbeau calls for a painting of the famed clinician in his amphitheater as a pendant to Rembrandt's *Anatomy Lesson of Doctor Nicolaes Tulp* (1632, Mauritshuis, The Hague). This would become "the painting of the century" if the artist managed to create a work that was worthy of the model.[1] *Une leçon clinique à la Salpêtrière (A Clinical Lesson at the Salpêtrière)* (1887), exhibited at the Paris Salon exactly two years later, could be viewed as realist painter André Brouillet's (1857–1914) answer to Mirbeau's appeal (fig. 1).

Brouillet's painting—hailed by the *Journal des arts* as "one of the most important works of the Salon of 1887"—celebrates Charcot's renown as the theorizer of hysteria and hypnosis as well as the theatricality of his lectures.[2] His stature rivaled only by Louis Pasteur, Charcot became a celebrity with the help of the contemporary fixation on hysteria and the female patients of the Salpêtrière Hospital in Paris.[3] Charcot was famous in the scientific community not only for his role in spearheading many of the period's most important advancements in the study of neurological illnesses, including multiple sclerosis and Parkinson's disease, but also for his exceptionally effective application of the anatomo-clinical method.[4] Because this method involved correlating signs of disease observed during life with the results of autopsies conducted after death, Charcot benefited immensely from the fact that the Salpêtrière was also a hospice that

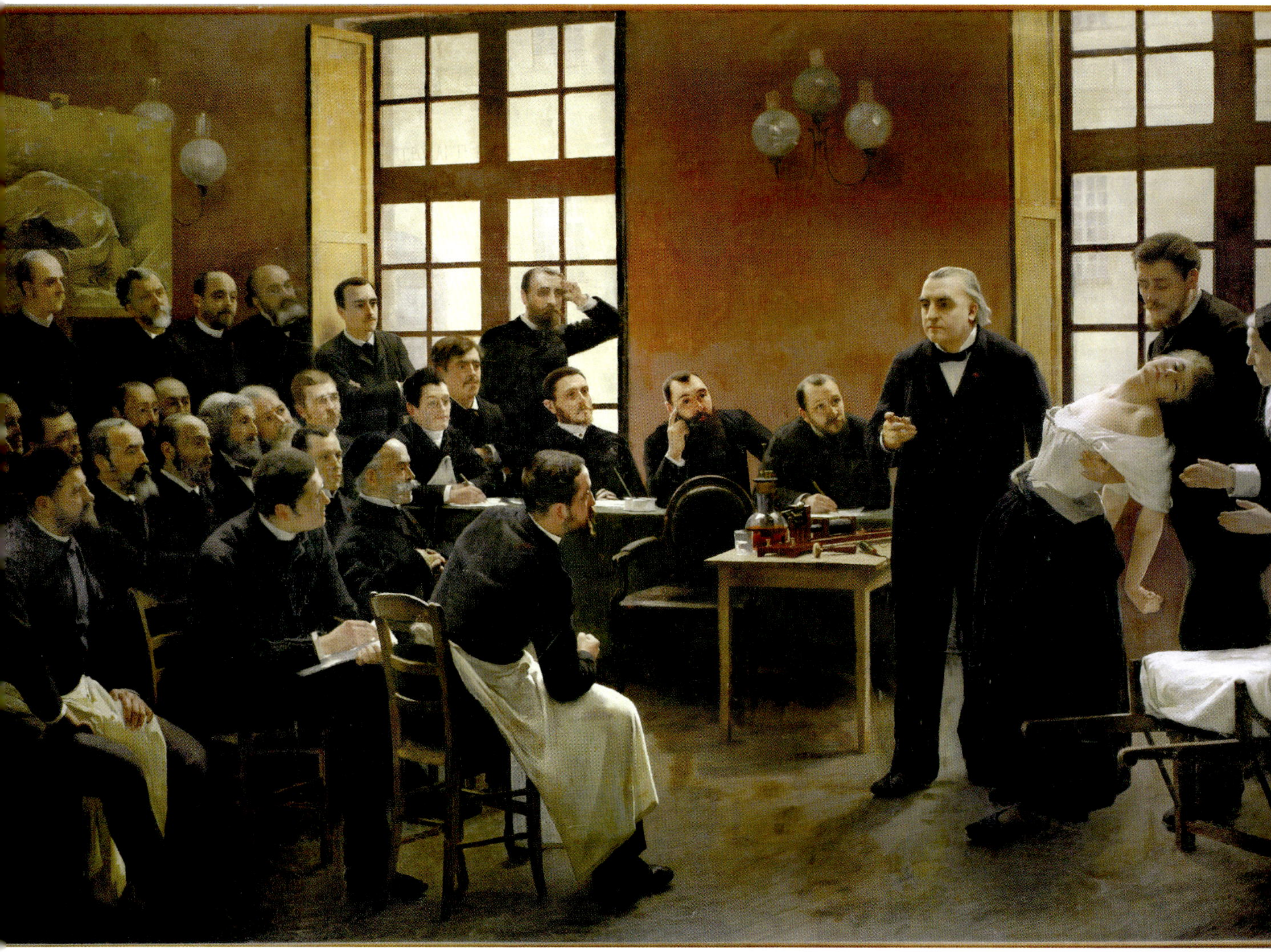

housed and treated individuals for life. In 1882, recognition of the advancements in neurology that had resulted from his studies led the Faculté de médecine to create the first chair in the field, which he accepted. His renown, however, extended well beyond medical circles—he was a celebrity even among the general public. His name appeared several times in the 1880s on the front page of *Le Figaro*, and depictions of the hospital and the pitiable state of its patients were engraved in *Paris illustré* and *Le Monde illustré*.[5] Coinciding with the exhibition of Brouillet's canvas at the Salon, Charcot was portrayed on the cover of the popular *Revue illustrée* standing before a wall of illustrations showing typical hysterical postures, like an artist in front of his own work.[6] The Salpêtrière even appeared in guidebooks at the end of the century, listed alongside the Jardin des Plantes as an attraction on the Left Bank.[7] He was famous outside of France as well; in 1885 the young Viennese doctor Sigmund Freud received a fellowship to study with Charcot and spent almost five months in Paris, dividing his time between the Salpêtrière, the Louvre, and the theater—arguably three interests that were not unrelated.[8]

Fig. 1 (opposite)
Pierre-André Brouillet, *A Clinical Lesson at the Salpêtrière*, 1887. Oil on canvas, 290 × 430 cm. Paris, Musée d'Histoire de la Médecine. Inv. F.N.A.C. 1123. Photo: akg-images / Erich Lessing.

Trained in the studio of Orientalist painter Jean-Léon Gérôme (1824–1904), a personal friend of Charcot's, Brouillet purports to paint a typical lesson in this almost life-size work: Charcot standing dispassionately while discoursing on hysteria and hypnosis before a standing-room-only crowd made up of *le tout Paris*; his protégé, Doctor Paul Richer (1849–1933), sketching or taking notes, just to Charcot's proper right, behind a table where the most modern medical technology is proudly displayed; the young doctor Joseph Babinski (1857–1932) gazing sympathetically at the hypnotized Blanche Wittmann (1859–1913) in his arms (she was known at the time as the "Queen of the Hysterics"); nurse Marguerite Bottard (1822–1906) holding out her hands to ease Wittmann's swoon onto the awaiting stretcher.[9] The lesson's audience is framed by the visual construction of hysteria. Richer's large drawing of a hysteric in the arched back or *arc-de-cercle* pose is tucked subtly but significantly into the top left corner of the painting, both predicting and validating Wittmann's attitude in the right foreground. The female body here is shaped by, and enacts, the representation of illness.

The presence of Richer's drawing and the figure of Wittmann herself attest to Charcot's pioneering use of visual aids in his lectures. He deployed photographs, casts, diagrams, graphs, drawings, lantern slides, and especially patients to help the audience understand his presentations. For example, in Richer's many drawings of Charcot's lessons, one can see bones at the ready on a table or posters displayed on the stage of the Salpêtrière amphitheater. In one of his sketchbooks, Richer drew an attentive technician or junior doctor sitting by a projector in the hospital's amphitheater in front of Tony Robert-Fleury's painting *Pinel délivrant les aliénés de leurs chaînes* (*Pinel Freeing the Insane from Their Chains*) (1876, Paris, Hôpital de la Salpêtrière).[10] This well-known Salon painting represents a scene at the Salpêtrière from the late eighteenth century but uses the vocabulary of the hysterical body codified by Charcot and Richer.[11] Charcot gave primacy to the visual—"the eye that knows and decides, the eye that governs"—and pursued artistic interests throughout his life, incorporating them into his medical career and encouraging them in his students.[12] Indeed, Achille Souques (1860–1944), who did his residency at the Salpêtrière, speculated that Charcot studied nervous diseases specifically because of the unavoidable visibility of their symptomatology: "One may wonder whether the physical deformities, so visible and so common in nervous diseases, had not directed his studies toward this favored branch of pathology."[13] Sigmund Freud thought that Charcot had "the nature of an artist."[14] It is especially appropriate, then, that Charcot would be immortalized in a Salon painting that would become one of the most famous images in the history of medicine.

Clinical Lesson was a realist manifesto: it celebrated contemporary progress while attempting to depict reality "objectively." Realist artworks were therefore often compared to the purportedly objective medium of photography. Charles Ponsonhailhe in *L'Artiste* dismissed *Clinical Lesson* as merely "a large photographic reproduction of a lesson given by a scientist."[15] Critics also noted that observation was central to the realist enterprise, just as it was to science. Louis de Fourcaud insisted that the "modern school" of art had only one method: "honest . . . observation." In the exhibition he was reviewing, which included Brouillet's canvas, he noted that contemporary painting had substituted "mythological scenes" for "humanized gods."[16] In a later essay, he reflected that "the right to portray reality faithfully" is inherent to realism.[17] Peter Brooks argues, "The claim of 'realism' in both painting and literature is in large part that our sense of sight is the most reliable guide to the world."[18]

Charcot's own project echoed that of realist artists: he professed his objectivity while at the same time creating and nurturing an image-making workshop that often prioritized the hand of the artist. The prodigious output in a variety of media from Charcot and the many clinicians who worked under him, who came to be known as the Salpêtrière School, embodies this paradox.[19] Henry Meige (1866–1940), who was a later member of this School and would eventually take on the post of professor of anatomy at the École des beaux-arts, characterized the pathological sculptures produced at the hospital by Paul Richer as "scientific artworks."[20] This term is not an oxymoron: it recognizes Richer's deliberate conflation of scientific objectivity and artistic interpretation and can also be applied to the myriad images and objects illustrating nervous pathology that emerged from the Salpêtrière at the end of the nineteenth century. These "scientific artworks" are the focus of this book.

Scientific Artworks

Pathology and Visual Culture examines an exceptional group of pathological drawings, photographs, casts, and sculptures created by clinicians who knowingly combined scientific knowledge and artistic expression. As head of the medical service at the Hôpital de la Salpêtrière for more than thirty years, Jean-Martin Charcot cultivated the artistic sensibilities of the many doctors who worked under him.[21] The images and objects created by the Salpêtrière School demonstrate not only the selective and interpretive processes inherent to any artistic practice but also an active engagement with contemporary artistic discourses and the history of art, even as these clinicians professed dedication to objectivity. Taking these scientific artworks as my focus, I grapple with the following questions: In what ways can the history of art inform and nuance our understanding of medical imagery? What are the limits of the categories we use to describe medical and artistic imagery? How was the intersection of art and medical science explored and exploited by the Salpêtrière School at the end of the nineteenth century? What new possibilities arose from working within this space, and how did these doctors negotiate its tensions? *Pathology and Visual Culture* argues for the critical importance of art and its histories to an understanding of imagery and objects not traditionally associated with the discipline.

In this book, I analyze works that have languished in storage for decades, including the unpublished and mostly unknown medical albums of the so-called Musée Charcot, the Salpêtrière's museum of pathological anatomy. They have been overlooked in part because they defy clear-cut disciplinary categories and therefore require analysis through new methodological tools if they are to be properly understood. In exploring the artistic output of the Salpêtrière School, I compare it with contemporary paintings and sculptures as well as other objects from the history of art; I put it into dialogue with published memoirs, technical manuals, and art and cultural criticism; and I consider it against medical texts and illustrations by authors both within and outside the Salpêtrière. All of it was created at an intellectual and cultural moment that predated the development of the boundary that now seems to divide medicine and art. This book brings into focus the ways in which the Salpêtrière's images and objects straddle that disciplinary boundary as well as their relevance to the histories of both disciplines. After all, Charcot himself felt equally at home in both medical and artistic circles.

Pathology and Visual Culture moves beyond current medical and art-historical scholarship by questioning and expanding conventional interpretations of medical imagery and objects. Its sustained attention to their production—in a wide variety of media by many clinicians under the aegis of a single figure—enables a uniquely thorough analysis of the ways in which medical science and art were consciously deployed together to create tools for understanding pathology at the end of the nineteenth century. The body of work that constitutes the focus of *Pathology and Visual Culture* attests to these clinicians' negotiation of medical objectivity and artistry. Arlette Farge embraces the complications that arise from the riches discovered in archives, the "details that disabuse, derail, and straightforwardly break any hope of linearity or positivism. This eruption of works and actions shatters established models, broadens the norm, displaces conventional wisdom once and for all, and often adds a certain confusion to things that had been previously considered simple."[22] The mythology of Charcot often starts with the moment when his father forced him to choose a course of study in either art or medicine. The elder Charcot was a carriage builder, "more artist than artisan," and could only afford higher education for one of his sons; since Jean-Martin performed the best in school, he was permitted to choose a profession.[23] Much of the existing scholarship on

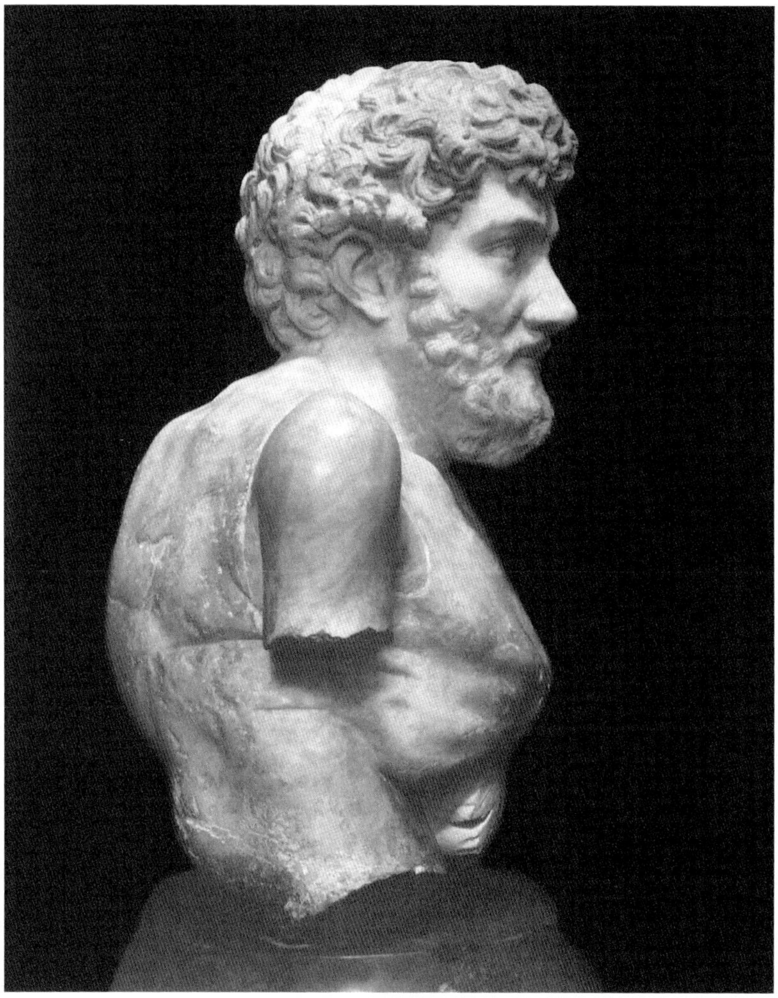

Charcot's engagement with art then jumps to the period of his greatest fame, when he was studying hysteria in the 1880s. These texts overlook the fact that, from the beginning of his career, Charcot envisaged an important role for the clinician in the study of art. *Pathology and Visual Culture* aims to expand the purview of the art historian, just as Charcot wanted to expand the purview of the clinician.

Clinician as Critic and Artist

In the 1850s, as a young physician lacking a hospital post, Charcot did his own version of the Grand Tour, visiting Italy as the private doctor of banker Benoît Fould and starting a personal tradition of filling notebooks with drawings every time he traveled.[24] Already at this early moment in his career, Charcot not only "diagnosed" illness in depicted bodies but also asserted the primacy of the clinician in judging works of art. In 1857, he co-authored an article with the physician Amédée Dechambre (1812–1886) in which they discuss the anatomy of several ancient sculptures, including a bust in the Villa Albani in Rome that was thought to show Aesop (ca. 300 BCE; fig. 2). The authors comment that Lysippus had famously carved Aesop's form by copying a kyphotic model in his studio while taking inspiration from the moral and intellectual character of the fabulist. This, they assert, is the reason for the figure's nudity—not heroic convention but the desire to show a personage almost as well known for the "oddness" (*bizarrerie*) of his body as for the sharpness of his mind.[25]

Fig. 2
Aesop, ca. 300 BCE. Marble. Rome, Villa Albani. Photo: akg-images.

The spinal curvature was modeled "from life," Charcot and Dechambre conclude, but the bearing of the head and even the symmetry of the face do not conform to the same condition.[26] The authors hypothesize that "this anatomical impossibility" shows that the obviously skilled sculptor took certain liberties in order to give the visage a certain noble beauty that was not in line with Aesop's famous kyphosis.[27] While Charcot and Dechambre assert that they would not "describe the bust minutely as we would do for an observation in the hospital," they offer a detailed analysis of the curvature of the spine and its attendant effects on the rest of the torso, abdomen, and neck.[28]

Based on these details, which are "so true, so naturalistic (to use a term from the atelier)," and lacking the evidence of the rest of the body, they ultimately diagnose Pott's disease, a form of spinal tuberculosis that is one cause of this deformity.[29]

Charcot and Dechambre go on to criticize the histories of art, the academies, and the studios of eminent painters and sculptors that incessantly repeat the falsity that the artists of antiquity solely pursued the ideal. Furthermore, they claim, the sculpture of Aesop "introduces to the plastic arts an element of critique whose meaning and scope must be established by doctors."[30] The import of a medical judgment to the artist or art historian is made explicit: the authors declare that medicine plays a role in determining "if this or that imperfection of features, of pose, or of structure belongs to nature or the chisel, and consequently if it shows in the artist great skill or great incompetence."[31] Visible effects of any deformity are not arbitrary, they argue, and that is why only doctors can determine whether the artist was guided by a profound knowledge of nature.[32] Charcot and Dechambre assign to medicine—and, by extension, to doctors—the role of assessing works of art and their fidelity to nature.

Charcot would return again and again to works of art that highlighted the critical role the physician must play in the history of art. He revisited the sculpture of Aesop more than thirty years later in the book he co-authored with Paul Richer, *Les Difformes et les malades dans l'art* (The deformed and the ill in art, 1889).[33] The inspiration for this book and their earlier *Les Démoniaques dans l'art* (The possessed in art, 1887)—which was perhaps not coincidentally published the same year Brouillet's painting appeared at the Salon—came from Charcot's examination of *The Miracles of Saint Ignatius of Loyola* (ca. 1619, Genoa, Church of Jesus and the Saints Ambrogio and Andrea), an altarpiece by seventeenth-century Flemish painter Peter Paul Rubens (1577–1640).[34] Charcot identified the historic belief in demonic possession as a sort of misdiagnosis of hysteria, and he and Richer subsequently acclaimed not only the painter's "scrupulous observation of nature" but also his ability to "copy" it.[35] Since Rubens's works were productive for both science and art, according to the authors, it is unsurprising that his study of a woman possessed by the devil had already been included in a Salpêtrière journal intended for a medical audience.[36] This altarpiece was an especially useful device in battling the popular claim that the Salpêtrière was the center of the hysteria epidemic in France and that the illness itself had been "invented" at the hospital.[37] Charcot and Richer, then, diagnosed illnesses in figures in historical artworks to validate their diagnoses in the present. The Salpêtrière School also called upon a long history of images of the diseased or deformed in order to create powerful and purportedly veridical representations of medical pathology, exemplifying the circular and mutually reinforcing relationship between art and science in the late nineteenth century.

But Charcot was not just a judge of art—he was an artist as well. This is evident in the drawings contained in the notebooks he filled while traveling, the albums of the Salpêtrière's museum of pathological anatomy, and the artworks he designed for his home (see chapter 1). He also curated the spaces of his home and the hospital. Both supporters and detractors of Charcot commented during and after his lifetime on the centrality of art in his neurological practice. In an *éloge* to Charcot, for instance, Pierre Marie (1853–1940) argued that Charcot's (anatomo-clinical) "method" would be better described as his "manner" (*manière*), a term typically used to characterize the work of "the greatest artists." For him, "Charcot was a great artist of medicine!"[38] Moreover, Charcot himself repeatedly equated the artist and the clinician, arguing that "the anatomical pathologist often felt the need to become an artist himself."[39] Five years after Charcot's death, Henry Meige wrote "Charcot artiste," describing the fundamental role that Charcot's artistic sensibilities and practice had played in his personal and professional life. As this chapter's epigraph notes, Meige eulogized the "inseparability" of the physician and artist.[40]

The *Savants-Artistes* of the Salpêtrière

Pathology and Visual Culture furthers Meige's analysis of Charcot's artistic inclinations by expanding it to include the clinicians who came to study with him. I bring to light the work of myriad *savants-artistes* whose contributions have gone mostly unremarked, their work overshadowed by a scholarly focus on the celebrated Charcot himself. The inclusion of the words "Salpêtrière School" in the title of this book is quite intentional. It has become apparent that drawings and ideas are often attributed to Charcot even when they appear in co-authored books and in the Salpêtrière's journals, effectively disregarding the clinicians who worked for and with him. While Charcot's impress would have been manifest in these volumes and these texts would not have been published without his support, his overwhelming public persona has substantially obfuscated the contributions of others and silenced his colleagues' authorial voices.

Many of the pathological images and objects examined in *Pathology and Visual Culture* have received no attention in either medical or art-historical scholarship. For the most part, these are works created by men who saw themselves as clinicians and not artists, though many of them likely gravitated to Charcot because of their artistic interests or inclinations. Even Paul Richer, who was exhibiting realist sculptures and winning prizes at the Salon while working at the Salpêtrière, considered himself first and foremost a doctor (see especially chapter 4). Therefore, these clinicians often did not sign the drawings they created. Many of these works are rather schematic, as they were intended primarily to capture the typical symptom of a particular illness or patient. They were not intended to impress *le grand public* but to improve their own understanding and to inform other physicians of the symptoms and causes of specific pathologies. I consider the information that these images and objects supplied to the medical community that could not be garnered from texts. The fact that the Salpêtrière School created artworks as they conducted research—and not just to publicize their findings—means that art making and the limits of an individual doctor's artistic abilities had an impact on how they conceived of disease. In other words, the way they visualized pathology had an impact on how they understood it.

My contention is that the clinicians who created these works under Charcot's direction engaged with the era's artistic practices and discourses as well as with the history of art. This was inescapable at the Salpêtrière, given Charcot's and Richer's intense focus on art history and the place of their patients *in* that history. Their own position in that history is relevant as well: the anticlerical Charcot takes the place of Saint Ignatius, healing the possessed/hysterics, in Rubens's *The Miracles of Saint Ignatius of Loyola*, the artwork that acted as a self-conscious originary moment for their medicalized history of art.[41] It is inevitable that there would be crossover between fine art and medicine when both Richer and Albert Londe (1858–1917), the Salpêtrière's photographer from the early 1880s, were working between and within disciplines. How could the conventions of the Paris Salon not influence Richer's creations at the Salpêtrière, for example? The critical vocabulary of art history illuminates the works that emerged from the sophisticated laboratories of the Salpêtrière and, at the same time, reveals the inherent limitations of that vocabulary in describing both medical and artistic imagery and objects. Attending more closely to the formal elements of the images and objects produced at the hospital—and couching analysis within a critical art-historical tradition—allows us to better understand the contributions of medical imagery not only to our broader visual culture but also to the history of art itself.

Artistry and Objectivity

The Salpêtrière presents a particularly rich case study of the intersection between the two broad intellectual endeavors of art and medicine, because the clinicians were consciously and actively engaged in both. Consider that Charcot participated in and encouraged art making and art criticism; Richer created artworks for both the hospital and the Salon; and Londe, a professional photographer, directed the hospital's photography studio. Visual images and objects were incorporated into the practice and teaching of medicine at the hospital under Charcot's aegis. They were utilized by Charcot and his many students to capture symptoms, construct archetypes, and understand illness. As I noted earlier, the life-size Salon painting of *Pinel Freeing the Insane* by Robert-Fleury hung in the amphitheater where Charcot gave his famous demonstrations. Art was everywhere at the Salpêtrière. Visual imagery in science and medicine, which, then as now, is used to communicate to both specialists and the general public, has always been socially constructed and inflected by contemporary artistic practices and discourses, and these in turn have been shaped by medicine and science.[42]

In their groundbreaking study, *Objectivity*, Lorraine Daston and Peter Galison use the imagery published in atlases from the eighteenth century through the twentieth to attempt to explain the links between scientific visualization, the "scientific self," and the history of objectivity.[43] They posit that there were three "epistemic virtues" that shaped the role of the scientist across the period: an early "truth-to-nature," which saw sagelike scientists define and depict the "perfect" image, even if it did not exist in nature; "mechanical objectivity," in which scientists attempted to remove themselves from the image because of anxiety about possible influence, leading to the representation of "individual" (as opposed to universal or perfect) examples; and, finally, the later "trained judgment," in which scientists took data and "made sense of it" for viewers, emphasizing the most relevant details and discarding any extraneous information that would only serve to distract. In this account, Charcot's tenure at the Salpêtrière would fall within the period of "mechanical objectivity," epitomized by the photograph as the medical image *par excellence* because of its apparent indexicality and seeming promise of "knowledge unmarked by prejudice or skill."[44] Daston and Galison argue that in this moment, "the scientific self . . . was perceived by contemporaries as diametrically opposed to the artistic self, just as scientific images were routinely contrasted to artistic ones."[45]

Charcot's well-known statement "I am absolutely nothing but the photographer [at the Salpêtrière]; I register [*inscris*] what I see" seems to confirm Daston and Galison's contention that "epistemology and ethos are intertwined: mechanical objectivity, for example, is a way of being as well as a way of knowing."[46] They note, however, that objectivity "is a chapter in this history of intellectual fear of errors anxiously anticipated and precautions taken."[47] This observation, writes D. Graham Burnett in his review of *Objectivity*, "articulates the fundamentally human drama at the heart of the history of science."[48] With this in mind, it is illuminating to reread Charcot's characterization of himself as a "photographer," using the language of "mechanical objectivity" defensively to counter the claim that hysteria was "invented" at the Salpêtrière. The full passage reads:

> It seems that hystero-epilepsy exists only in France and, I could say and it has been sometimes said, only at the Salpêtrière, as if I had created it through the force of my will. That would be a truly marvelous thing, if I could create illnesses in this way, according to my whim and fancy. But, in truth, I am absolutely nothing but the photographer [at the Salpêtrière]; I register [*inscris*] what I see, and it is only too easy for me to prove that it is not only at the Salpêtrière that these things happen. . . . M. Richer, in his book [*Études cliniques sur la grande hystérie ou hystéro-épilepsie*], shows us that in the fifteenth century it was exactly as it is now.[49]

It was as a result of a public attack on his "scientific self" that Charcot fell back on the dominant epistemic virtue—even if the practices of "scientific objectivity" and "artistic subjectivity" at the Salpêtrière were exactly *not* "in reversed-mirror-image relationship to one another," as Daston and Galison claim was typical of this era.[50] Uncoincidentally, Charcot's defense concludes with "evidence" of hysteria found in historical artworks. The second edition of Richer's book *Études cliniques sur la grande hystérie ou hystéro-épilepsie* (Clinical studies on hysteria or hystero-epilepsy), published three years before Charcot's lecture, includes an appendix that maps the presence of "hysteria in art" through representations of the possessed from the fifth century through the seventeenth.[51]

The artistic output of the Salpêtrière School demonstrates the limits of Daston and Galison's elegant theorization. The clinicians' search for the archetype is in some ways analogous to the "perfect example" that Daston and Galison posit as the epistemic virtue of the previous era. The illustrations of "individuals" that captured a particular incidence of disease often stood for the "universal," which Daston and Galison claim epitomized the time of "mechanical objectivity." Yet the Salpêtrière School's belief in the objectivity of new mechanical media is belied by their retouching of photos, a practice whose only apparent purpose is aesthetic (see chapter 2). Their artistic interpretation of pathology in various media, including drawing and sculpture, seems to look ahead to the first half of the twentieth century, when the dominant epistemic virtue was "trained judgment." Of course, Daston and Galison note that these virtues did not arise as a chronological sequence but instead as a "history . . . of innovation and proliferation rather than monarchic succession."[52] Still, the Salpêtrière School, one of the most important producers and distributors of medical imagery in the late nineteenth century, defies the framework in *Objectivity*. *Pathology and Visual Culture* makes a crucial contribution to this debate because of the particular way in which members of the School negotiated the notion of objectivity: by emphasizing their scientific role as clinicians and *at the same time* fostering artistic skill and a detailed study of the history of art. The images and objects considered in this book bear witness to the tangled history of objectivity and the importance of both art history and the critical medical humanities in nuancing and enriching our understanding of that history.

Some scholars have challenged Daston and Galison's central claims about the "scientific self." Joel Snyder, for instance, makes the compelling case that French physiologist Étienne-Jules Marey (1830–1904), well known as one of the inventors of chronophotography, was not attempting to remove his "subjective self" from the mechanical data he produced, chronophotographic and otherwise. Instead, Snyder elaborates, there was "nothing for a mediator to mediate," as the information resulting from his instruments was "outside the scope of human sensibility."[53] Historian of science Theodore Porter disagrees with their contention that a "distrust of self" led the late nineteenth-century scientist to have absolute faith in mechanical objectivity. He argues instead that "objectivity was mainly a positive moral trait" that "did not annihilate judgment but exalted it . . . by conferring a scientific attitude that rose above petty distractions of local circumstance and self-interest."[54] Philosopher Martin Kusch, too, worries that the opposition outlined by Daston and Galison between the epistemic virtue and the scientific self is false: using a visual analogy, he writes, "*Objectivity* comes close to granting this point when the relationship is described as 'yin' and 'yang.' . . . Think of the typical pictorial representation of that relationship: surely, once you have demarcated the yin, you have fully specified the shape of the yang."[55] What if objectivity and subjectivity—"the shadow term that is held to separate art from science"—were not in mutual opposition, since "neither category is stable or sufficient—not for artists and not for scientists"?[56] What if instead we considered them "two faces of the same object," as Charcot and Richer characterized them?[57] In working on this project, it became clear to me that the objective/subjective binary that Daston and Galison posit is too constricting for the scientific artworks produced at the Salpêtrière.[58] Henry Meige understood this, noting that Charcot the physician and Charcot the artist were one and the same, even if for Daston and Galison there was "a scientific self grounded in a will to willessness [*sic*] at one pole, and an artistic self that circulated around a will to willfulness at the other" at that time.[59] The analyses of images and objects in *Pathology and Visual Culture* point to the ways in which the clinicians' mediation, intervention, and "artistry" were productive in their endeavor to accurately diagnose neurological illnesses. The personal and published texts of the Salpêtrière School, including those by Charcot and Richer, frame art and (medical) science—what I am simplifying to "subjectivity" and "objectivity," in Daston and Galison's formulation—as related and requisite in the pursuit of a higher goal, which they call "truth" but that we can characterize as medical knowledge.[60] This is why Meige's term "scientific artwork" encapsulates their project. For Charcot and the clinicians at the Salpêtrière, "subjectivity" was not antithetical to the "scientific self." Quite the contrary: it was essential.

Nervous Diseases

One contention of this book is not only that Charcot and the Salpêtrière School engaged with contemporary artistic practices and discourses but that those practices and discourses came to shape the way they visualized pathology. Medical imagery and objects can inform us about the limitations of vision and knowledge, and they can show us the resulting lacunae differently than texts. Most importantly, they also fashion medical knowledge. Certainly in the case of the Salpêtrière School, images do not belong merely "to science's intelligently crafted apparatus" but are integral to "its cognitive and procedural substance," *pace* Joel Smith.[61] Until now, hysteria has been the primary focus of most relevant scholarship that shares this perspective on the Salpêtrière's voluminous output of visual media. Georges Didi-Huberman's groundbreaking book *Invention of Hysteria: Charcot and the Photographic Iconography of the Salpêtrière* sparked interest in the imagery of hysteria at the Salpêtrière and is important for my understanding of the hospital's artistic production. Didi-Huberman argues that the hysterical body was constructed as an image in the photographs, drawings, and sculptures produced at the Salpêtrière as well as in Charcot's amphitheater. He pays significant attention to the hospital's well-known journal, *Iconographie photographique de la Salpêtrière*, published in the late 1870s, which popularized and disseminated photographs of the hysterical attack. Furthermore, he writes, "I am nearly compelled to consider hysteria, insofar as it was fabricated at the Salpêtrière in the last third of the nineteenth century, as a chapter in the history of art."[62] This statement led me to the profound realization that the Salpêtrière's artistic output could be reconceptualized through art history and its methodologies—that the discipline of art history, of which it forms a part, could facilitate a clearer and deeper understanding of the claims that the Salpêtrière clinicians were making *through* those images and objects.

Though my book casts a wider net than Didi-Huberman's, his work prompted a substantial body of art-historical scholarship that has convincingly demonstrated the influence of hysteria on modern art and culture.[63] Rae Beth Gordon, for example, has written about the immense importance of the "hysterical aesthetic" in Parisian café culture, through which it influenced modern art—including the work of Henri de Toulouse-Lautrec (1864–1901) and Edgar Degas (1834–1917).[64] Other art historians have analyzed the connection between the images of hysteria and art—for instance, Anthea Callen also sees Charcot's influence on Degas, and I have written elsewhere of the way sculptor Auguste Rodin (1840–1917) interpreted and manipulated the postures of the hysterical attack to create a distinctly modern portrayal of the human condition.[65] With the exception of chapter 2, which delves into the Salpêtrière's retouched photographs of hysterical patients, *Pathology and Visual Culture* moves away from hysteria. My aim is to widen the scope of art-historical analysis to take in other neurological conditions treated at the hospital and to broaden the discussion of Charcot's work and that of his protégés. Nor does this book discuss hypnosis, a practice used by Charcot in his study of hysteria that was also sensationalized at the time, becoming a subject of public fascination and scientific debate in its own right.[66] Rather, *Pathology and Visual Culture* is about "nervous diseases" at a moment when they were being identified and attempts were being made to understand them. From today's perspective, Charcot's neurological discoveries are much more significant than any of his claims about hysteria; he made important advances in the study of epilepsy, stroke, multiple sclerosis, neuropathic arthropathy ("Charcot joint"), and neurodegenerative syndromes such as amyotrophic lateral sclerosis (still known in France as "Charcot's disease") and Parkinson's disease, among many other neurological disorders.[67] Visual images were a vehicle for those discoveries.

Contrary to what one may assume from the existing scholarship, I argue that artistry at the Salpêtrière was not limited to a single field, such as hysteria. Nor was it exclusive to a select group of notables like Charcot, Richer, and Londe. Rather, it was an integral aspect of the ethos and protocol of the hospital's medical service, practiced by figures including Paul Regnard, Loreau, and other lesser-known or (currently) unknown individuals. These clinicians saw patients daily, discussed their case histories with Charcot, and utilized artistic practices not only to capture their patients' pathologies but also to determine what those pathologies were. This book attempts to recuperate both this "lost" history of medical imagery at the Salpêtrière and the story of some of the patients who were observed, drawn, sculpted, photographed, and dissected so as to uncover as much detail as possible about the personal histories of the individuals whose likenesses were rendered in various visual media at the hospital.[68] Unfortunately, as there is very little information about most of these patients, it is difficult to gain much insight beyond what can be gleaned from the medical "specimen" on display. While these patients are mostly silent witnesses to the artistic practices of the Salpêtrière School, they also constituted the source material and subject matter for its artistic creations and, as such, were absolutely essential to the hospital's larger artistic and medical project.

Though after death they were completely passive recipients of the medical gaze, in life, the hospital's patients participated in the creation of artistic images by actively engaging with the clinicians who re-presented them. They had some kind of power in those relationships, though it was clearly unbalanced. In many images, patients look directly into the camera or at the clinician portraying them. "Staring ... is an intense visual exchange that makes meaning," Rosemarie Garland-Thomson has written, "recast[ing] starees as subjects not objects."[69] Some patients exercised a measure of control. For instance, novelist Alphonse Daudet (1840–1897) recounts the disruption of one of Charcot's lessons by a hysteric named Balmann who refused to "perform," as she was jealous that another patient, named Daret, had been allowed to appear first. Revealing the slippage between art and medicine typical of the Salpêtrière and those who knew of its practices, Daudet compares Daret to "the dummy in the [artist's] studio, even more docile and more flexible," because she allowed her "sad body" to be moved and manipulated in any way the clinicians wished.[70] As Arlette Farge acknowledges, even though "the archive collects characters," their "names, when revealed, in no way lift their anonymity."[71] I am aware of the sensitive nature and ethical dangers of illustrating—or re-illustrating, since many were published at the time—the images of patients who did not give consent in ways that would be acceptable today.[72] By including them here, I follow historian of medicine Jennifer Wallis, who writes of her own engagement with photographs of patients that "in analyzing and re-purposing images we enter into (and alter) the present and future readings of those images."[73] I have attempted to recover as much of the patients' biographies as possible to call attention to the ways in which the images might demonstrate their agency and to critically contextualize the use of their (re-)presentations, which are central to the argument of this book. While I recognize that these actions do not and cannot return to these individuals the dignity they deserve, I do hope that they will at least help bring to the fore the fundamental role these patients played in the founding of modern neurology.

Entwined Practices

Pathology and Visual Culture explores the various media found in the albums of the Salpêtrière's museum of pathological anatomy, wax casts made in its casting studio, and the sculptures produced in the artist's atelier on its grounds in addition to the well-known photographs of hysterics captured both inside the hospital's wards and outside in its courtyards. The examination of mostly unknown and unpublished material allows for a thorough mapping of the hospital's sophisticated artistic production, but it also necessitates an attentiveness to the differences among various media and their own individual histories within the larger history of art. These material histories structure the book, as the focus largely shifts in each chapter to a different medium (drawings, photographs, casts, sculpture) and producer (Charcot, Regnard, Loreau, Richer). The importance of attending closely to material history was introduced to me in Ludmilla Jordanova's pioneering *Sexual Visions: Images of Gender in Science and Medicine Between the Eighteenth and Twentieth Centuries* (1989). Her discussion of wax anatomical models, the most influential chapter of her book for my own project, showed "the gendered character of natural knowledge."[74] Anthea Callen's scholarship, also attentive to material histories, has similarly shown me the inseparability of art and (medical) science. Her book *The Spectacular Body: Science, Method and Meaning in the Work of Degas,* which inspired my own journey into the intersection of art and medicine, was a radical intervention in the art-historical canon when it was published in 1995. Her work over the last twenty-five years on Paul Richer and on the École des beaux-arts has been key to my understanding of Richer's transition to that Parisian institution.[75] It remains an essential part of the exponential increase in scholarship in the visual medical humanities in recent years.

Pathology and Visual Culture also contributes to the burgeoning field of the visual medical humanities that sees the visual itself as a "mode of intervention and critique."[76] The recent scholarship of art historians such as Suzannah Biernoff, Gemma Blackshaw, Keren Hammerschlag, Allison Morehead, Kathleen Pierce, Susan Sidlauskas, and others demonstrates that medical imagery cannot be properly understood or interrogated without recourse to art-historical methods and that thinking about art and visual culture through the prism of the history of medicine yields unexpected interpretive riches. Moreover, I see myself participating in a critical medical humanities that is "not only sensitive to imbalances of power, implicit and explicit, but include[s] activist, sceptical, urgent and capacious modes of making and re-making medicine."[77] The analyses in this book provide new insights into how Charcot and the Salpêtrière School conceived and established the field of modern neurology through imagery and objects that could be articulate or mute, effective or unhelpful, but always loaded with meaning. As Jennifer Tucker argues, "There is nothing self-evident about the concepts of science, history of science, or scientific illustration. Far from belonging to the order of things, scientific representations have been exposed as visual artifacts that are bound to the times and places of their creations."[78] The visual has been a key element in the conceptualization and understanding of the body, especially in Western medical history.

Pathology and Visual Culture follows Des Fitzgerald and Felicity Callard's theorization of an "entangled" medical humanities: "What holds together much of the research employing 'entanglement' is an intuition that some set of things, commonly held to be separate from one another (indeed, that define themselves precisely with reference to their separability) . . . not only might have something in common, but also, in fact, may be quite *inseparable* from one other."[79] This notion of "entanglement" underlies the analyses in *Pathology and Visual Culture*, especially because of Charcot's and the Salpêtrière School's knowledge of and comfort with both art and medicine. The

School's illustrations of illness in two and three dimensions are impoverished and, in some cases, incomprehensible without an understanding of art and its history. For these clinicians, art and medicine were entangled practices—or perhaps it would be more accurate to use the more positive term "entwined."[80]

In the last ten years, a number of studies have engaged in innovative ways with Charcot's artistry. My book builds on Mary Hunter's *The Face of Medicine: Visualising Medical Masculinities in Late Nineteenth-Century Paris* (2016), in which Brouillet's canvas is used as a springboard into a discussion of how "realist modes and media dealt with the challenge of representing hysteria."[81] Whereas Hunter focuses her insightful analysis on the ways in which realisms "went mad" at the Salpêtrière by examining its clinicians' use of various media to visualize hysteria, I instead look at the Salpêtrière School's wider neurological practice and how it navigated the intersection of art and medical science. In *Performing Neurology: The Dramaturgy of Dr Jean-Martin Charcot* (2016), Jonathan Marshall, a scholar of performance, discusses the theatrical strategies that Charcot used in his lessons, from a Wagnerian aesthetic to a "Brechtian" mode *avant la lettre*.[82] Elements of Marshall's analysis have been useful for my study, such as his discussion of the way that Charcot's lecture style facilitated the fragmentation of the patient's body in the amphitheater. In *Charcot in Morocco* (2012), historian Toby Gelfand examines the journal that Charcot kept while traveling in North Africa in 1887, which reveals the "priority of the visual over the written record."[83] During this trip, Charcot clearly had in mind Eugène Delacroix's illustrated travel notebooks, and we know that Charcot kept some of Delacroix's original drawings of Morocco handy in his office drawer.[84] In comparing the two, Gelfand reveals the same entwinement of (medical) objectivity and (artistic) subjectivity that is my focus here. Charcot "explicitly invokes the painter's eye by using the word 'painting' ['*tableau*'] . . . and again by his desire to see a scene which Delacroix painted [a Jewish wedding]." But, Gelfand continues, "Significantly, the verb 'to see' ['*voir*'] is employed nearly forty times in the absence of a first person voice (*on voit, se voit, il faut voir, laisse voir*, etc.) as compared with only five times in the active form (*je vois*) thus underscoring the putative objectivity of the observer who transmits what is seen or to be seen." He concludes, "The Moroccan journal as a whole conveys a passion to see."[85]

Gelfand was a co-author, with Christopher Goetz and Michel Bonduelle, of the indispensable biography of Charcot, which follows the midcentury panegyric published by Georges Guillain and the novelistic *Monsieur Charcot de la Salpêtrière* (1993) by psychiatrist and writer Jean Thuillier.[86] Charcot's biographers have all recognized his artistic sensibility as a key to understanding his medical and popular success. His artistic production, and that of the Salpêtrière School, has also been the focus of scholarship by medical doctors themselves, such as Goetz, a practicing neurologist, and Olivier Walusinski.[87] The most important recent intervention was *Charcot, une vie avec l'image* (2013) by Catherine Bouchara, a psychiatrist at the Salpêtrière who specialized in hypnosis. Her copiously illustrated book serves as a visual biography of the neurologist and helpfully includes previously unknown and mostly personal drawings and photographs from the archives of the Vallin-Charcot Family. However, Bouchara seems unable to distinguish Charcot's hand and therefore misattributes several images: drawings created by more skilled clinicians—principally by Paul Richer—are attributed to Charcot. She assumes that the unsigned drawings in the Musée Charcot albums or those found in his papers are all by Charcot.[88]

The publication of Bouchara's book prompted an exhibition in the seventeenth-century church on the grounds of the Salpêtrière in 2014. It gathered drawings, photographs, sculptures, casts, films, and objects from the collections of the Musée de l'Assistance Publique–Hôpitaux de Paris, the École nationale supérieure des beaux-arts, and private collections, among others, as well as installations by contemporary artists that created "a bridge . . . between Charcot's visual thinking and contemporary thought, between art and mental health."[89] Given Bouchara's own specialization and the fact that she was the principal curator, the exhibition approached its subject more from the perspective of psychiatry (especially in relation to hysteria) than of neurology; it also included the same misattributions as the book. The exhibition nonetheless attempted to dissolve the boundaries between art and medicine, both in Charcot's practice and historically, to stunning effect. It is worth noting that a projection of Brouillet's canvas hung over the crossing of the church–cum–exhibition space, above Charcot's autopsy apron and his robes from the Institut de France (he was inducted into the Académie des sciences in 1883), in a hagiographic scene that was reminiscent of an altarpiece.

The Case Studies

After its exhibition in 1887, Brouillet's *Clinical Lesson* took on a life of its own: it was reproduced in French and international newspapers and journals, reimagined as caricature, reexhibited at the Universal Exposition of 1889, and translated into a wax sculpture and a popular print.[90] It acquired personal significance for figures as noteworthy as Sigmund Freud as well as for the anonymous individual who used a small copy of it to make a collage that was tipped into a volume of the *Iconographie photographique de la Salpêtrière*. Details of the painting illustrated books and articles, as did a photograph of a solitary Charcot that served as evidence of Brouillet's use of photography. Each chapter of *Pathology and Visual Culture* is introduced with an iteration of *Clinical Lesson*, serving the dual purpose of providing "intelligent commentary" on the original and setting the stage for the individual case studies that begin in chapter 1, "Curating Pathology at the Musée Charcot."[91] Charcot opened a museum of pathological anatomy in 1878 that came to be known as the Musée Charcot. It did not resemble other nineteenth-century medical museums, with their clinical look and vitrines full of specimens or casts: instead, it was "very elegantly decorated," as Charcot himself noted, with furniture of dark wood, sculptural ornamentation commissioned from a contemporary artist, and an idiosyncratic group of medical objects. These included a sculpted pathological portrait made by Richer, the latest medical equipment, a vitrine of skeletons, a full-body wax cast referred to as the *Ataxic Venus*, and a series of albums maintained by the clinicians at the hospital. Pasted into these extraordinary albums are drawings, photographs, charts, graphs, fragments of case notes, and scholarly citations that refer to the patients and illnesses treated in the hospital.

The goal of this chapter is twofold: first, to bring to light the Musée Charcot's contents and décor and their relationship to Charcot's own home and its curated spaces, and second, to consider what the images in the museum's albums reveal about the Salpêtrière School's working practices and their use of art making to better understand the pathologies they encountered in the hospital. I see the albums as microcosms of the (no longer extant) museum, a space made up of disparate elements created by a variety of hands that only cohere when understood as a kind of portrait of Charcot himself. In essence, the museum resembles a *Wunderkammer* more than a modern medical museum.

Each of the remaining chapters focuses on a particular medium. Chapter 2, "The Art of Retouching at the Salpêtrière," examines in detail a forgotten album of photographs made in preparation for the first volume of the *Iconographie photographique de la Salpêtrière*, published by Charcot's protégés Désiré-Magloire Bourneville and Paul Regnard. In this album, many of the photographs show evidence of retouching, a practice that has gone almost unremarked in the scholarship on the famous photographs of hysterics at the Salpêtrière. This album was a working document whose pages clearly show the complexities in deciding which images to include and how to manipulate them to maximum effect. Several of the pages of this album include specific instructions to the retoucher on their versos.

I analyze closely the images of hysterics from this album, comparing them to the original, unretouched versions and considering the possible reasons for the often extensive changes made to these purportedly objective documents. Much of the retouching is poorly executed, suggesting that the clinician and amateur photographer Paul Regnard also tried his hand at "correcting" the images. While some of the modifications serve to highlight a hysterical contracture or emphasize an expression, in most cases they do not serve any clear "scientific" purpose but rather appear to be principally aesthetic. In fact, as a result of dubious aesthetic and practical choices or clumsy implementation, the retouching often proves completely counterproductive, unintentionally obfuscating a photograph's subject or its details.

Returning to the Musée Charcot, chapter 3, "The *Ataxic Venus*: Between Portrait and Specimen," considers the so-called *Ataxic Venus*, the most famous object in the museum. This polychrome full-body wax cast was created by Loreau, the head of the Salpêtrière's casting studio (about whom little is known), and shows a patient named Berthelot, who had locomotor ataxia caused by tertiary syphilis. Charcot exploited Berthelot's illness—using, among other props, this uncannily life-like cast, photographs of her, and even her actual skeleton, which was extracted after her death and preserved for display—to establish his international reputation. Like photography, another indexical medium, wax casting creates the illusion of objectivity even as it displays the results of myriad artistic decisions. The *Ataxic Venus* is a spectacular medical object whose production required exceptional artistic and technical skill, but it is also an arresting portrait of a patient and of her illness. Its affective power comes not only from the deformities that mark this body but also from the way it refers to art-historical precedents. It was, furthermore, in dialogue with contemporary polychrome sculpture exhibited in the Salon and elsewhere.

Because Berthelot seems to have left no verbal trace whatsoever in the many texts on her illness written by Charcot and the Salpêtrière School, I use the words of the novelist Alphonse Daudet, who also had locomotor ataxia and was one of Charcot's private patients. His posthumously published *La Doulou* (*In the Land of Pain*, 1930) recounts its excruciating symptoms. I use the autobiographical text as a sort of surrogate for Berthelot, to attempt to approximate and articulate her (unknowable) experience and to assist me in understanding and explaining the emotional power of the *Ataxic Venus*. This striking wax cast is, I argue, not only a portrait of Berthelot and locomotor ataxia but of pain itself.

The final chapter, "Paul Richer, Sculpting Pathology," treats a series of four sculptures made at the Salpêtrière by Richer in the 1890s, while he was also exhibiting realist sculpture at the Salon. Like the wax cast of Berthelot, they depict patients at the hospital. However, Richer's sculptures more obviously betray the artistic choices made as he crafted these patient portraits, despite the fact that they were compared to photographs.[92] Sculpting allowed Richer to convey likeness, pathology, and pathos.

This chapter considers Richer's pathological portraits, produced in an atelier at the hospital, in relation to his "fine art" practice and to the broader contemporaneous discourse on realist sculpture. I argue that Richer played with artistic conventions and with art-historical precedents in crafting these portraits that depict clearly identifiable individuals while representing "types" (of illness). He was an autodidact with strong connections in the art world and a prodigious knowledge of art history who wrote extensively about both artistic anatomy and the intersection of art and medicine. All of this would stand Richer in good stead when it was time to embark on the second half of his long and fruitful career.

Pathology and Visual Culture ends with a coda, "The Salpêtrière at the École des Beaux-Arts," that sees Richer leave the Salpêtrière after a quarter-century to teach anatomy at the École des beaux-arts, where he would train art students for the next twenty years. He focused there on creating athletic male bodies instead of the sickly, and predominantly female, body that had served previously as his standard subject. Richer insisted, however, that his work at the École did not signal a break from his earlier focus on pathology. For him, there was no distinction between the "scientific self" and the "artistic self."

CURATING PATHOLOGY AT THE MUSÉE CHARCOT

I

I urge you to continue sketching: it is a good way to occupy one's spare time; science and art are allies, two of Apollo's children.

—JEAN-MARTIN CHARCOT, UNDATED

In the autumn of 1885, a twenty-nine-year-old Sigmund Freud arrived in Paris for the first time, having been awarded a travel grant from the Faculty of Medicine of the University of Vienna to spend five months working at the Salpêtrière with the internationally renowned Jean-Martin Charcot.[1] The time he spent with Charcot would dramatically change the direction of his research and alter the course of twentieth-century thought. Freud's letters to his then fiancée, Martha Bernays, recount his joys, fears, frustrations, and pleasures, his experiences in museums and at the Salpêtrière, and his encounters with Charcot. After their first meeting, he gave a detailed description of the celebrated clinician: "At 10 o'clock M. Charcot arrived, a tall man of 58, wearing a top hat, with dark, strangely soft eyes (or rather one is, the other is expressionless and has an inward cast), long wisps of hair stuck behind his ears, clean shaven, very expressive features with full protruding lips—in short, like a worldly priest from whom one expects a ready wit and an appreciation of good living."[2]

Freud intended to focus on the microscopic study of children's brains in the pathological laboratory of the Salpêtrière, but he soon found that the laboratory was not only unsuitable for an "extra" worker but also lacked organization.[3] This marked a turning point in Freud's career—it was then that he shifted his attention to hysteria and hypnosis. He was so excited by the presentations he had witnessed in Charcot's amphitheater that he attempted to use hypnosis as a treatment in his own practice upon his return to Vienna. Less than ten years later, Freud and Josef Breuer would publish *Studies on Hysteria* (1895), which included the case history of the hysterical patient "Anna O," who inadvertently led to the development of the "talking cure."[4]

An additional cause for Freud's shift to hysteria and hypnosis could have been his fascination with Charcot's personality and compelling neurological discoveries. Freud wrote to Bernays in November 1885: "Charcot, who is one of the greatest physicians and a man whose common sense borders on genius, is simply wrecking all my aims

Fig. 3 (opposite)
Sigmund Freud's London study, with a print of Brouillet's *A Clinical Lesson at the Salpêtrière*. Photo: Freud Museum London.

and opinions. I sometimes come out of his lectures as from out of Notre-Dame, with an entirely new idea about perfection."[5] It is widely known that Charcot had an incalculable impact on the founder of psychoanalysis—Freud considered himself Charcot's pupil his entire life and even named his firstborn son Jean-Martin in honor of his mentor.[6] Freud was also clearly taken with the idiosyncratic décor of Charcot's home when he attended the famous receptions the family hosted every Tuesday evening from October through May. He likely would have agreed with Henry Meige's sentiment that "no frame could have been better harmonized with Charcot's personality."[7] Charcot fashioned the Salpêtrière's museum of pathological anatomy in the same style. Both spaces seem to have left an indelible impression on Freud, whose own study would eventually be crowded with sculptures on all its surfaces and images on all its walls.[8] Freud, too, created a perfect "frame" in which to study—and be studied. Prominently displayed in his consulting room from his years in Vienna until his death was a reproduction of Brouillet's *A Clinical Lesson at the Salpêtrière*.[9] In his London home, Charcot hovered both literally over the famous couch where Freud codified the move from looking to listening and figuratively over the creation and evolution of psychoanalysis (fig. 3).[10]

As Ludmilla Jordanova has argued, prolonged looking at an individual is rarely sanctioned in society, but exceptions include the acts of examining portraits and examining patients.[11] In the image by Brouillet, the collective gaze of the men in their funereal bourgeois costumes on the left is fixed on the group of figures on the right—fixed on what could be described as the active construction of medical knowledge—thematizing the late nineteenth century's obsession with medical voyeurism, a phenomenon that pervades the anatomical museums of the period.[12] Significantly and not coincidentally, in 1875 Charcot proposed to the Assistance Publique the creation of a museum that would complement the "living pathological museum" of the Salpêtrière.[13] He reasoned that "the clinical and anatomo-pathological riches that [the Salpêtrière] holds . . . are not utilized as widely as they deserve to be."[14] By 1879, he could thank the administration for the hospital's new photography studio and electrotherapy room as well as "an anatomo-pathological museum, perfectly arranged, [and] very elegantly decorated."[15]

Like the Brouillet painting, which reveals little about hysteria or hypnosis except a visible (and, some argue, invented[16]) bodily attitude that signified the disorder, the Musée Charcot offered a partial and idiosyncratic vision of nervous disease. While illumination had been the presumed goal of anatomical museums since the Enlightenment, the exhibits here did not clearly signal pathology. In the mostly unknown and unpublished albums from the Musée Charcot's collection—albums that replicate the museum's methodology in miniature—drawings and photographs appear alongside more "objective" graphs and diagrams to represent the pathologies seen at the Salpêtrière.[17] While most of the images included in these albums clearly show patients with various disorders, in many of the most accomplished drawings, illness is harder to recognize. Many of the drawings are more likely to recall precedents from the history of art than illustrations seen in contemporary medical journals. These images may equivocally

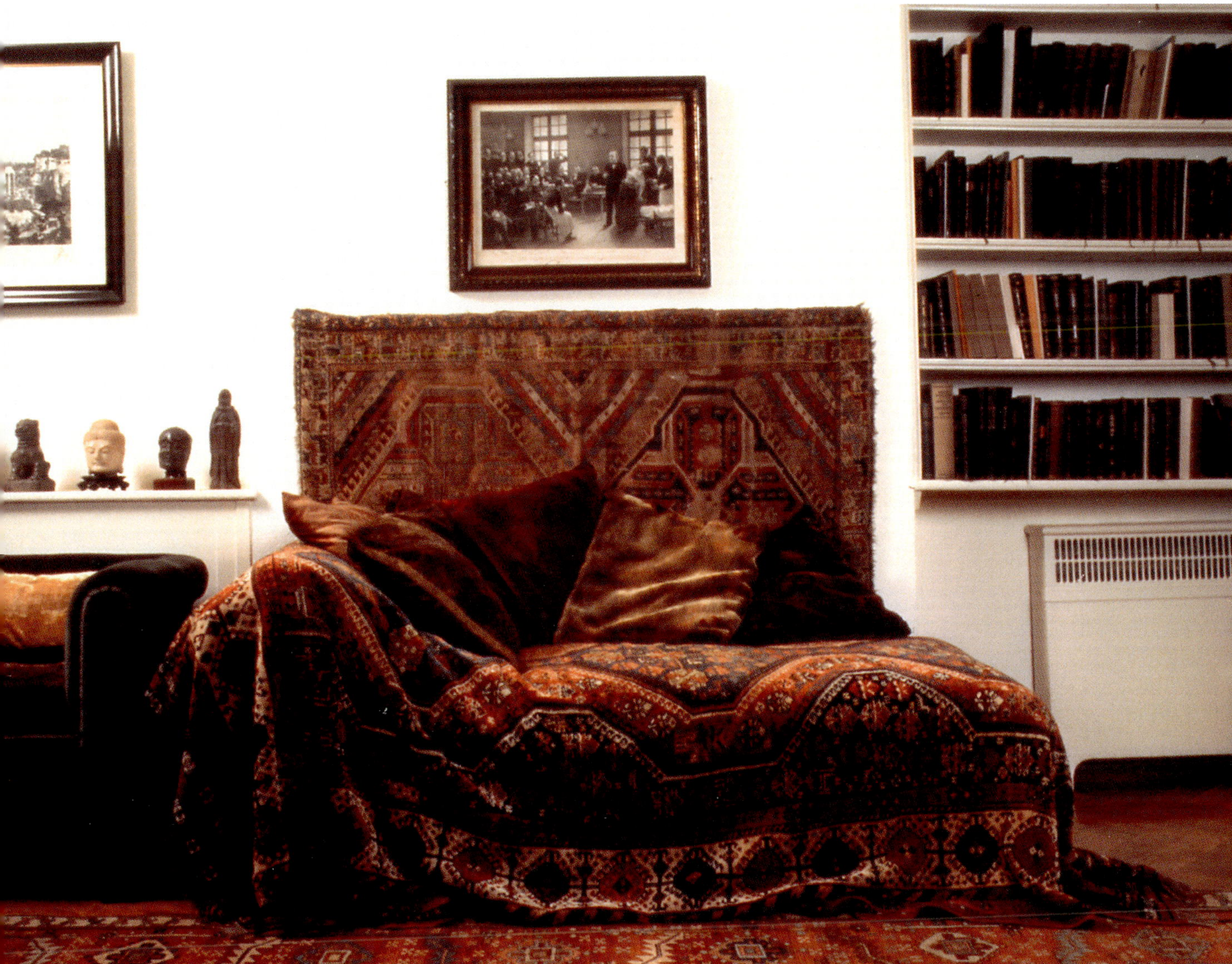

Fig. 4
Photograph of the Musée Charcot, ca. 1894. From F[ernand] Levillain, "Charcot et l'École de la Salpêtrière," *Revue encyclopédique* 10 (March 1, 1894): 112. Photo © The British Library Board (P.P.4283.k.).

illustrate illness, but they unequivocally show their makers' artistry. In this chapter, I argue that, like the anatomical specimens, sculptures, wax casts, medical equipment, and reproductions of artworks in the Musée Charcot—or the objects in an early modern *Wunderkammer*—the albums' contents cohere only when recognized as the collection of a single individual: the museum's formidable founder, Jean-Martin Charcot.

The Musée Charcot

Charcot advocated the creation of a pathological anatomy museum at the Salpêtrière, arguing that it would be a place "where, at little cost, the most interesting [pathological] pieces would be gathered, more varied and more numerous than anywhere else."[18] The fullest description of the completed Musée Charcot, which is no longer extant, comes from Belgian philosopher and psychologist Joseph Delboeuf. He recounts a visit to the Salpêtrière alongside the historian Hippolyte Taine in the mid-1880s to witness firsthand the hypnosis of Blanche Wittmann:

> [The session] took place in a large room, a kind of museum, whose walls, even the ceiling, are decorated with a considerable number of drawings, paintings, engravings, photographs sometimes showing scenes with various individuals, sometimes a single patient naked or clothed, standing, sitting or reclining, sometimes one or two legs, a hand, a torso, or another part of the body altogether. All around, cupboards with skulls, spines, tibias, humeri showing this or that anatomical feature; all over the place, on tables, in vitrines, a pell-mell of jars, instruments, devices; the image in wax, not yet completed, of an old woman, nude and lying on a kind of bed; busts, including that of [Franz] Gall, painted green.[19]

While the Musée Charcot has been mentioned by Mary Hunter, Andreas Mayer, Gérard Tilles, and others, there has been no extended discussion of its contents in either art-historical or medical scholarship.[20] Much can be discerned from the only known photograph of the space, probably taken in the early 1890s, which shows a curious group of objects and images that coalesce under the umbrella of medical evidence (fig. 4).[21]

Starting with the back wall, we can see a portrait in profile, perhaps of a notable medical figure, placed high up in a thick, imposing frame. Next to this painting hangs what seems to be a reproduction of an artwork, likely one in which Charcot and Richer retrospectively "diagnosed" an illness visible at the Salpêtrière—a practice that the pair continued in the two books they wrote together. In 1885, a writer for the *New York Medical Record* noted that, in addition to photographs of patients, on the walls hung engravings of "famous paintings from different European museums" that showed the possessed being healed, demonstrating "perfectly the fact that hysterical and epileptic

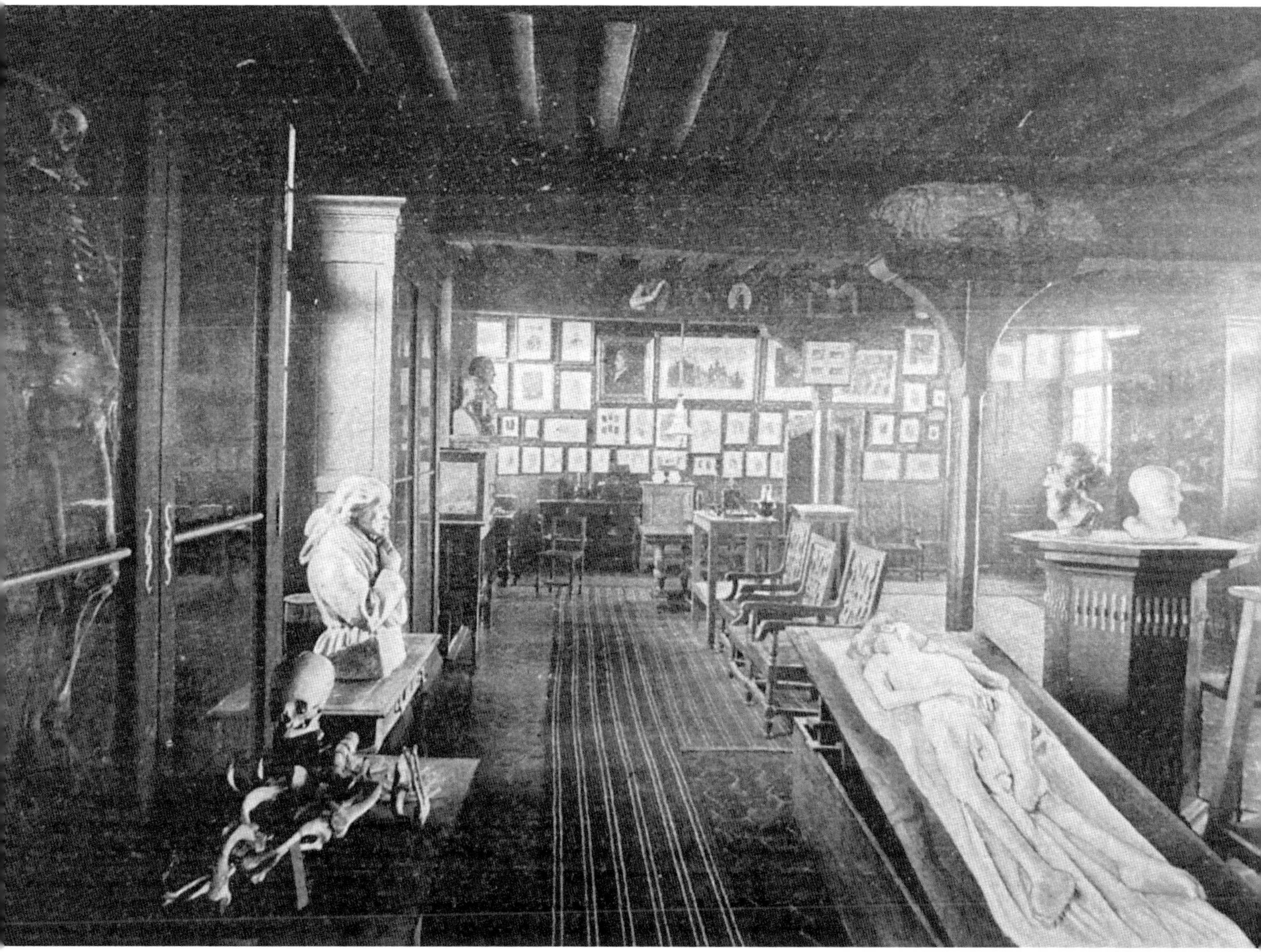

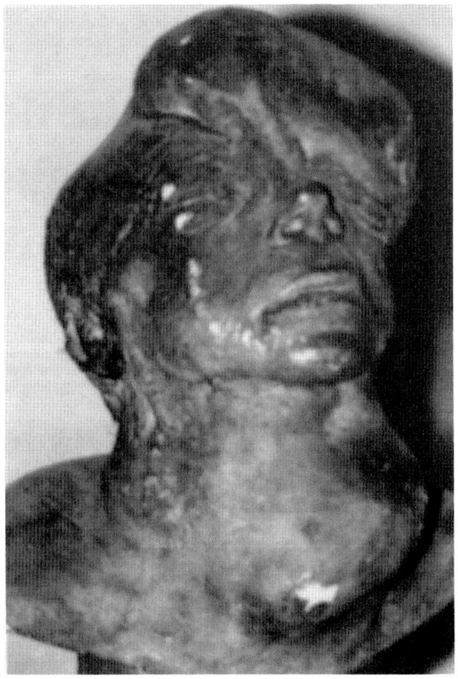

Fig. 5
Photograph of a plaster cast of a patient with neurofibromatosis from the Musée Charcot. From Philippe Ricou, Véronique Leroux-Hugon, and Jacques Poirier, *La Bibliothèque Charcot à la Salpêtrière* (Paris: Éditions Pradel, 1993), 31, fig. 25. Photo courtesy of Véronique Leroux-Hugon.

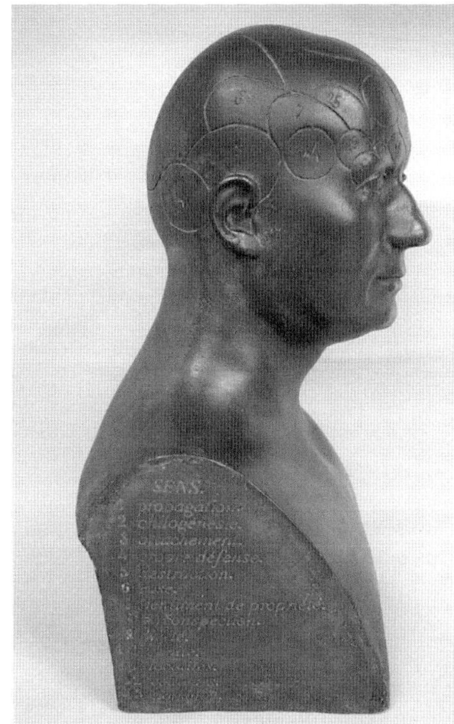

Fig. 6
F. Deniau, *Tête de Gall* (*Head of Gall*), nineteenth century. Painted plaster, 52 × 30 × 30 cm. Paris, Musée de l'Assistance Publique–Hôpitaux de Paris. Inv. AP 2003.7.9.2. Photo: AP-HP/musée–F. Marin.

attacks were well studied by artists in past centuries and were accurately reproduced in painting."[22] There are also other (unidentifiable) portraits of notable figures, likely influential medical men. This wall calls to mind Charcot's office and consulting room at the hospital, described by Alphonse Daudet as exhibiting "photographs, primitive Italian and Spanish paintings representing saints in prayer, ecstatics, convulsives, demoniacs, the great religious nervous disease, as they say at the asylum."[23] Meige corroborates this account, writing that the walls, painted black, displayed "reproductions of all the artistic findings relating to hysteria," while Georges Guillain notes that it included a "large portrait with a dedication from the English neurologist John Hughlings Jackson."[24]

The still life from Brouillet's *Clinical Lesson* is replicated on a small table located next to the ornate wooden chairs in the center of the room.[25] Above it, relief sculptures are just visible on the beams supporting the ceiling, where one can see the bust of a figure in profile, who seems to be reaching up. We know that Charcot commissioned wax reliefs for the room by a contemporary sculptor, Henry Cros, whose work he also purchased for his home (see chapter 3).[26] A visitor to the museum derided this element of the eccentric decor: "Let us note . . . the garish ornamentation that has been smeared on the beams protruding from the ceiling."[27] On a high plinth to the right of the photograph sits a sculpture, no longer extant,[28] of a person with neurofibromatosis, along with what may be a phrenological bust (fig. 5). Below them, the vertical lines on the plinth seem to indicate storage for images that could be pulled out and viewed by the visitor, as typically found in art galleries and museums; perhaps they needed to be kept in the dark for conservation reasons.

There are two busts on a cabinet visible to the left of the photograph. Here, the dark green bust of Franz Joseph Gall (1758–1828), the German founder of phrenology, takes center stage (fig. 6). Created by an F. Deniau, the sculpture is both a portrait and a phrenological head, with notations on the pate and keys on the side of the bust referring to Gall's system of identifying behaviors and traits on the skull.[29] Blanche Wittmann, while under the hypnosis that Delboeuf witnessed in the museum, was asked to kiss this bust of Gall at the suggestion of the physician Charles Féré and did so "amorously" on both cheeks.[30] Delboeuf notes that this bust was surrounded by "a collection of heads with bumps on their skulls catalogued according to [Gall's] system." Moreover, he mentions that "in glass vitrines all around the room are arranged and labeled bones, the head of [Paul] Lebiez, the skulls of other criminals, [and] the brains of forgers and thieves."[31] Like other medical museums of the time, such as the Musée Dupuytren, Charcot's museum included wax casts and the skulls of criminals that could serve as examples for medical study.[32] Lebiez and his accomplice Aimé Barré were guilty of an infamous murder and guillotined on September 7, 1878. A long article in *Le Figaro* the next day detailed the execution and cited Lebiez's last words to his father: he did not want his head cast because he wanted to disappear forever.[33] However, his "head" may have ended up at the Salpêtrière because Charcot played a role in the execution. The École de médecine claimed Barré's corpse, which was unwanted by the murderer's family, and Charcot presided over the dissection and various medical experiments performed on the head and body that very afternoon.[34]

In the left foreground of the photograph, the pathological portrait by Paul Richer of a woman with labio-glosso-laryngeal paralysis (see fig. 75), discussed at length in chapter 4, sits next to a partial, bony body and a vitrine of skeletons. This includes the skeleton of the patient whose postmortem cast lies on a table in the center of the museum, a sculpture called the *Ataxic Venus* that is the focus of chapter 3 (see fig. 51). The cast is retouched in the photograph to make its contours distinct in the room's low light. Even in this documentary photograph of the museum space, artistic intervention was deemed necessary.

Other objects not visible in the photograph could be included in this eclectic mix. Journalist and art critic Maurice Guillemot mentions that high up on the walls of the museum are some of the "large drawings by Paul Richet [*sic*], charcoal highlighted with white, that show all the different poses of the patient during a [hysterical] attack."[35] These must have recalled for visitors Brouillet's Salon painting, in which Richer's large drawing of a hysteric in the *arc-de-cercle* pose matching Guillemot's description is conspicuously displayed. The museum also likely exhibited fragments of bodies cast from patients, illustrating various illnesses seen in the hospital. Extant plaster hands from the Musée Charcot show, for instance, hysterical contractures or symptoms of Parkinson's disease (fig. 7). They are rendered hyperrealistically and serve their didactic purpose as simulacra of and proxies for the absent patients. The cracks or chips in the casts point to their handling and use as teaching aids in the museum or in the amphitheater. These cast fragments also recall the artist's atelier and the art gallery. Samuel

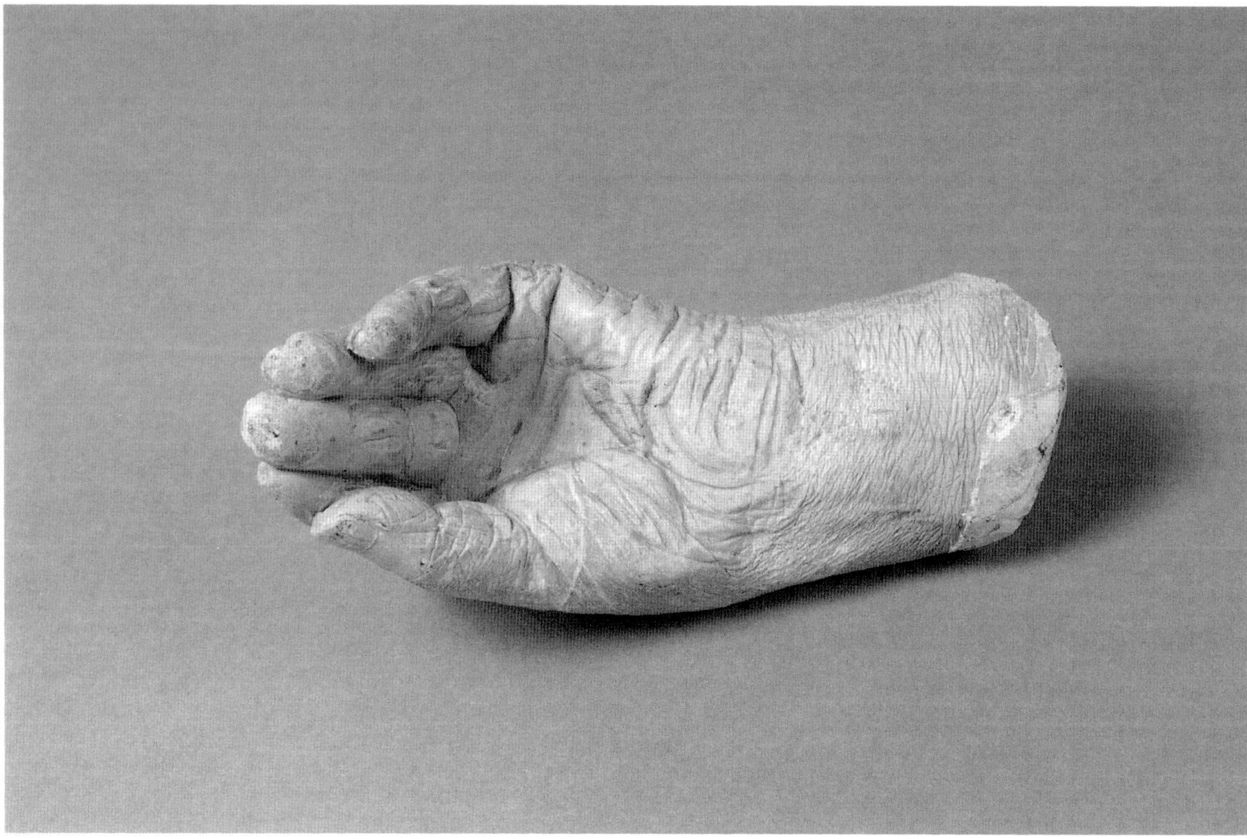

Fig. 7
Anonymous, *Main parkinsonienne* (*Hand of a Patient with Parkinson's Disease*), end of the nineteenth century. Plaster cast, 19 × 8 × 8 cm. Paris, Musée de l'Assistance Publique–Hôpitaux de Paris. Inv. AP 2003.7.9.1. Photo: AP-HP/musée–F. Marin.

Alberti writes that "human remains in anatomy museums mirrored architectural and statuary remains elsewhere.... Dismembered body parts had classical equivalents in the fragments of statuary and classical ruins that flooded Northern European galleries from Italy and Greece."[36] They could also link the atelier, the museum, and the album. The contracted cast hand of a patient named Bourdy, for example, has a metal ring at the amputated end so that it could be hung and studied, like the cast heads and body parts in Adolph Menzel's *The Studio Wall* (1872, Hamburg, Kunsthalle) or some of the hands in Auguste Rodin's atelier.[37] Bourdy's hand and lower arm also appear in an album, in a fine pen-and-ink study by Richer dated November 21, 1882.[38] An annotated but less detailed copy of this drawing is also in the collection of the École des beaux-arts, where Richer would spend the second half of his life as professor of anatomy.[39]

In the Musée Charcot, then, the human body was simultaneously absent and ubiquitous, except when the patients themselves were "displayed."[40] For instance, Delboeuf described Wittmann as "a real living laboratory specimen" as she wandered hypnotized through the museum, echoing Charcot's own characterization of the entire hospital as a "living pathological museum." On her quest to kiss the bust of Gall, she inspired Delboeuf to suggest that "with her, one can explore the human body as meticulously and more demonstratively than with a cadaver."[41] The scientific riches offered by the live patient complemented the museum's deathly remains, wax casts, and artworks.

Charcot on the Boulevard Saint-Germain

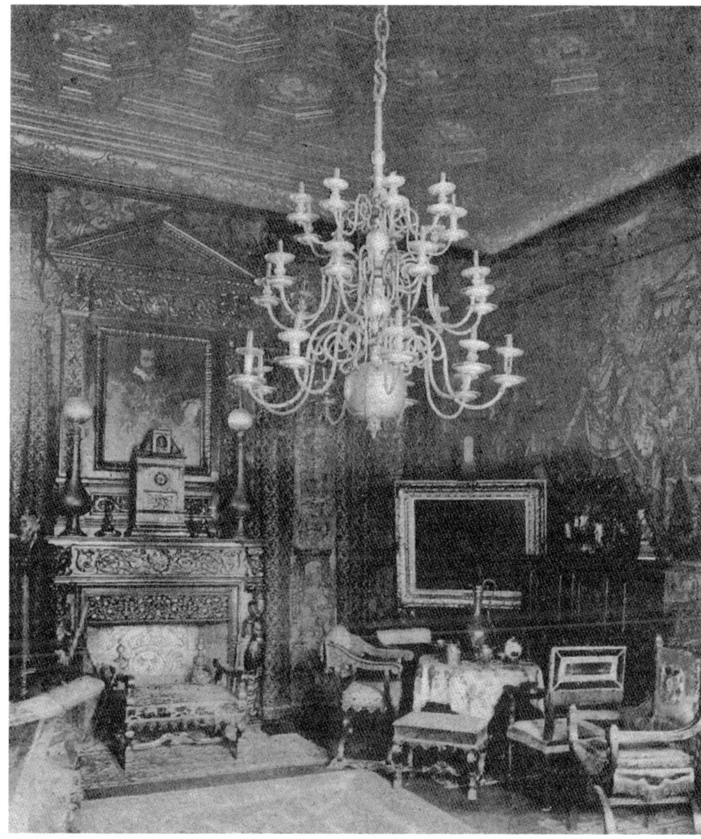

Fig. 8
Le Salon. Le Plafond à caissons a été peint, et le lustre émaillé, par Mme Charcot (The Living Room: The Coffered Ceiling Was Painted and the Chandelier Enamelled by Mme. Charcot). From Gustave Goetschy, "Les Femmes du monde artistes. Madame Charcot," *Revue des arts décoratifs* 20, no. 1 (1900): 44. Photo © The British Library Board (PP.1803.LAG).

According to medical historian Michael Sappol, during the nineteenth century "membership in the [medical] profession was consolidated by a common culture of collectorship." He specifies that "in formal medical discourse the specimen was accounted as an educational aid.... Informally, there was the pleasure of acquisition and possession and a connoisseur's appreciation of the artistry of the preparation."[42] This connoisseurial spirit is made manifest in the wooden armchairs, striped rug, and dark-paneled walls of the lavishly appointed museum at the Salpêtrière. Reproductions of artworks hung on the walls, and, as was noted above, the polychrome wax sculptures of Henry Cros covered some of the room's wooden supports. This museum, therefore, resembled less a clinical space than the physician's study or indeed Charcot's own home, the "magic castle in which [Charcot] lives," as a dazzled Freud described it after his first visit.[43]

Most accounts of Charcot's grand home on the Left Bank were adulatory and praised, in particular, the creations of Charcot and his wife, Augustine (née Victoire Augustine Laurent), who together ran an atelier where the family engaged in the design and decoration of furniture, among other artisanal pursuits.[44] In fact, after their purchase of the Hôtel de Varangeville on the fashionable Boulevard Saint-Germain, the Charcots added two wings: one contained Charcot's expansive two-story library, and the other, his wife's studio.[45] Their art collection included paintings by Francisco Goya, Hubert Robert, Jean-Honoré Fragonard, and Camille Corot, while cabinets displayed Asian *objets d'art*. Walls were decorated with Renaissance tapestries, and windows were adorned with stained glass depicting religious figures from the fourteenth century through the sixteenth. Charcot collected sculptures in wood, marble, and bronze and heavy antique furniture from Italy, Holland, and France in the style of Louis XIV and Louis XVI.[46] Writer, politician, and former Charcot student Léon Daudet described the family home as being in "the style of the Middle Ages"; he wrote that it was "a questionable and romantic style, but luxurious" (fig. 8).[47] Charcot's home office included bookcases of his own design that were based on those in the Medici Library in the Convent of San Lorenzo in Florence. Stained-glass windows lent this room "a rather mystic appearance, with lighting effects resembling those of a church."[48] The style of the family home was aggressively maintained; Charcot removed and sold the sumptuous Rococo

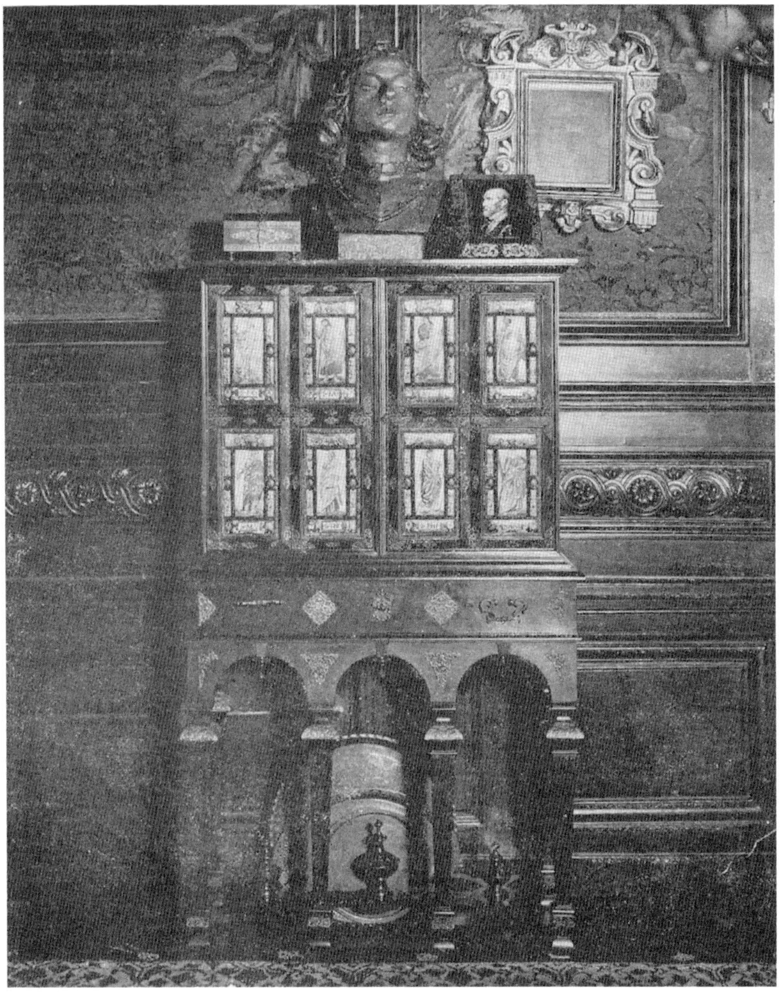

Fig. 9
Salon. –Cabinet orné de plaques en émaux de Limoges, dessinées par le Dr Charcot. Les cuivres ajourés sont de Mme Charcot (Living Room: Cabinet Decorated with Limoges Enamel Plaques Designed by Dr. Charcot; The Openwork Brass Is by Mme. Charcot). From Gustave Goetschy, "Les Femmes du monde artistes. Madame Charcot," *Revue des arts décoratifs* 20, no. 1 (1900): 45. Photo © The British Library Board (PP.1803.LAG).

boiserie from his *hôtel particulier* because it was not to his taste.[49] Meige's observation about Charcot's home was astute: "This frame was also his masterpiece."[50]

This was a "frame" that Charcot played a significant role in crafting. He was much more than a collector of the objects displayed in this "curious family museum"—he was also a co-creator.[51] The Goncourt brothers acerbically commented on the "archaic bric-a-brac of modern manufacture" that filled the home, likely alluding to the fact that Charcot and his family designed and created much of its decoration.[52] Unsurprisingly, gender defined the family members' roles: Charcot designed while his wife and daughters crafted. Augustine Charcot was the daughter of a wealthy clothier and art collector, Charles Vincent Claude Laurent (known as Laurent-Richard), and the widow of Edmé Victor Durvis. According to Gustave Goetschy, she "had inherited from her father an artistic sense *très juste* and her love of beautiful things [*oeuvres*]."[53] She knew how to work metal, leather, glass, and wood and make pottery and ceramics; she even had a specially designed oven installed in her home so that she could bake her pieces at the requisite high temperatures.[54]

Goetschy devoted an article in the *Revue des arts décoratifs* posthumously to Augustine Charcot. In it he illustrates, for instance, a cabinet from the family's salon, with ceramic panels designed by Charcot representing the "Apostles of [Leonard] Limousin," and the fireplace in their dining room with faience designed by Charcot after a sixteenth-century original, executed by his wife (fig. 9). Goetschy tellingly notes that Charcot excelled at the "art of appropriating" works by "better" artists, such as Albrecht Dürer, whose work the neurologist would have encountered on his holidays around Europe.[55] Dürer seems to have been a favorite, as Charcot decorated the internal façade of his *maison particulier* with copies of his illustrations for *Das Narrenschiff* (*Ship of Fools*) by Sébastien Brant, published at the end of the fifteenth century.[56] It seems that Charcot focused his artistic energies on the copy, whether in the decorations of his home or the illustrations of his patients' bodies in the museum and its albums.

Charcot decorated his home office in the same style. In the designs for the stained-glass windows and the painted *boiseries* of the ceiling, he copied the kingly decorations visible in the Louvre and the princely ornament in the medieval Château de Tarascon.[57] These sources were perhaps indicative of his pretensions. Léon Daudet paints a colorful picture of the private patients waiting for a consultation in Charcot's home: "People with atrophied muscles spread their emaciated limbs on griffins, wurms, or gargoyles."[58] In a revealing comment, Charcot's student Fernand Levillain wrote that the house on the Boulevard Saint-Germain revealed its owner to be "not in effect a systematic collector, but a very eclectic artist."[59] The house served not merely as a "frame" for its owner but as a kind of canvas for an evolving self-portrait.

The idiosyncratic personal style visible in the Charcot family home—"a singular taste for the aesthetic," as Meige describes it—extended to the museum at the Salpêtrière and led to confusion as to whether it functioned as Charcot's personal study at the hospital.[60] When describing the Musée Charcot, Guillemot characterized it as "the office of Doctor Charcot, which one should perhaps call a museum."[61] Others thought that it was the antechamber of his office.[62] This uncertainty is a reflection of the fact that, like his home and the artworks he bought and designed, the museum and its contents referred unmistakably back to Charcot himself. Indeed, the Musée Charcot resembled an aristocratic cabinet of curiosities more than a "modern" medical museum, like the ones founded in 1867 at the Hôpital Saint-Louis for dermatological diseases or in 1880 at Bicêtre, Paris's hospice for men, by neurologist and politician Désiré-Magloire Bourneville (1840–1909).

After working with Charcot, during which time he published the *Iconographie photographique de la Salpêtrière*, Bourneville left for Bicêtre and founded a museum that focused on children with physical and mental disabilities.[63] It had simple straight-backed chairs, a wall of floor-to-ceiling vitrines with a dangling skeleton and neatly displayed plaster casts on its shelves, a back wall with an orderly arrangement of framed images, and another wall of windows with tidy table-height glass cases and a sculpture of a child standing guard over the room. The space, flooded with bright light, did not have any "extraneous" or distracting elements, and it appears—at least on the surface—to be rationally organized.[64] In contrast, the Musée Charcot, with its decorative relief sculptures, striped runner, and hodgepodge of objects, frames, and furniture, is far more idiosyncratic. Its contents reflected the categories found in the cabinet of curiosities, which has been called the precursor to the nineteenth-century anatomical museum: *naturalia* (objects taken from nature, including "monsters"); *scientifica* (scientific instruments); and *artificialia* (man-made objects, such as medals or artworks).[65]

Sappol asserts that collecting "was a quasi-erotic quest. . . . The collector prided himself on his erudition and acumen, cultivated a love of the grotesque, beautiful, and obscure, and took sensuous delight in the fine craftsmanship, creative presentation, and quality of anatomical objects, whether taken from real bodies or molded in wax or other media."[66] The act of voyeurism is implicit in the Salpêtrière's curated space of nude bodies, revealed organs, and concretized pathology. Like the cabinet of curiosities, the medical museum was essentially concerned with seeing, knowing, touching, classifying—and, we might add, possessing.[67] The same could be said of the albums collated by Charcot and his students (now mostly owned by the Musée de l'Assistance Publique–Hôpitaux de Paris, hereafter Musée de l'AP-HP).[68] They can be seen as microcosms of the Musée Charcot. Their contents detail the minutiae of patient's bodies during life and after death and bear witness to the ways in which illnesses were seen and understood by the clinicians at the Salpêtrière.

Charcot's "Paper Museum"

The Musée Charcot albums comprise a diversity of drawings, photographs, charts, and graphs pasted onto their faded, stained, and sometimes damaged blue pages with very little explanatory text. Only some of the images have captions indicating diagnoses, patient names, or references to medical articles that reveal more details about particular cases. A wide variety of styles and hands is evident, but unfortunately, most of the drawings are anonymous. Among those that do bear signatures, some are by doctors who are or were well known, like the pathologist Édouard Brissaud (1852–1909). Others are by practitioners who are forgotten or more obscure, such as a P. Savard, who contributed a watercolor from 1874 of a left breast stricken with cancer; an article in the *Bulletin de la Société anatomique de Paris* several years later singles out Savard's drawings for being "very accurate."[69] Early drawings by Charcot are pasted alongside images by others from decades later, indicating that these albums were "living" documents that could be amended or updated as necessary. Each of the albums "bears the marks of its own history as an object": on some of the pages, images have been roughly cut out (for teaching purposes? for sale? as a keepsake?), leaving captions with names and diagnoses beneath gaping holes through which photographs from subsequent pages stubbornly persist despite the turning of pages, assuming one identity after another from the orphaned captions.[70]

Martha Langford has written eloquently of the ways in which family photographic albums act as repositories of memory. She posits that "the rule of randomness and its resistance to reading" applies in the album, in part because of missing "titles, dates, and other signposts."[71] The reading of the album brings forth a kind of performance, which likely took place among Charcot and his protégés even though there is no record of who exactly looked at the Musée Charcot albums or whether they ever left the museum.[72] The albums, like the museum, acted as sites where a global medical world was convened, through the inclusion of letters and images sent by other clinicians, references to articles or sources in international journals, and so on. In this, too, the albums reflect the well-traveled and internationally known Charcot. More importantly, Langford argues that "the album as collection (the paper museum) groups objects, or images of objects, that somehow relate. How so is not always very clear. Experience suggests that at some point in the process, either reason or passion was in control." Langford's theorization of the "paper museum," which combines "reason or passion" and a performative reading, is a productive lens through which to view the albums of the Salpêtrière clinicians. Their peculiar system of representation has resulted in albums full of visual documentation aimed at gaining insight into their patients' various neuropathologies, which incongruously, at least to the eyes of a layperson, are not necessarily self-evident. As a result, the albums and many of their contents are remarkably ambiguous, often suggesting a pleasure in the very acts of depicting the body specifically and art-making generally. The "album-collection," Langford notes, "looks like its subject category, until it suddenly mutates into another form of acquisitive desire."[73]

The Salpêtrière's clinicians made equivalences between different modes of observation in the albums and different kinds of objects in the museum. As Anthea Callen has observed, "For Charcot and the Salpêtrière School, the scientist's sight constitutes 'truth.'"[74] In other words, these different kinds of "evidence" were on equal footing, through an emphasis on the visual and through the vehicle of the clinician. And while I am keen to bring to light the contributions of many clinicians inside and outside the Salpêtrière, the albums, like the museum itself, highlight the illnesses that Charcot chose to study at the hospital. Despite the plurality of hands that composed them and the opacity of the selective criteria for their contents, the albums point to Charcot himself. They are a portrait of the man and his interests.

Just as the museum's collection appeals almost exclusively to the visual sense—Charcot was called a "visuel" by his student Sigmund Freud—the albums similarly contain a wide variety of visual "evidence" for the nervous diseases studied at the Salpêtrière.[75] "To see was to understand," as Meige wrote of Charcot's use of drawing during his lessons.[76] For instance, the test results recorded in the graphs in Album AP 2003.7.2.3 (Paris, Musée de l'AP-HP) date from between 1882 and 1885 and were captured by Gilbert Ballet (1853–1916), who appears in Brouillet's canvas and would go on to become an important figure in French psychiatry. The name of the patient, along with the corresponding volume and page number of the case notes, illness, and sometimes age and the date of the test, is noted on each page. Some even specify the ward at the Salpêtrière where the patient could be found. These large black graphs with white lines indicate the intensity of an epileptic seizure or the contractions of the masseter muscle in the jaw. Now faceless patients such as Roudier, Barbant, and Rivière can only be recuperated through these rudimentary analyses of their symptoms.

Album AP 2003.7.2.2 (Paris, Musée de l'AP-HP) contains illustrations of tissue, organs, and sections of the body. Some were skillfully drawn while others were hastily colored onto templates or quickly sketched freehand. The volume is entitled "anatomie pathologique," although it begins with "normal" anatomy. Colored pencils recreate the detailed topography of parts of the body of adults, children, fetuses, and even a guinea pig, many labeled in pen and helpfully accompanied by a key. A number of the drawings picture diseased lungs and date from 1877 to 1878, though there are some by Charcot from as early as thirty years before, such as a watercolor titled

Fig. 10
Paul Richer, *Grosjean*, June 18, 1878. Drawing in pencil. Located in Album AP 2003.7.2.2 of the Musée Charcot anatomie pathologique. Paris, Musée de l'Assistance Publique–Hôpitaux de Paris. Inv. AP 2003.7.2.2. Photo: AP-HP/musée–author.

Fig. 11 (opposite)
Anonymous, *Portrait d'un homme* (*Portrait of a Man*) (factual title), end of the nineteenth century. Photograph pasted on cardboard. Located in Album AP 2003.7.1.5 of the Musée Charcot anatomie pathologique. Paris, Musée de l'Assistance Publique–Hôpitaux de Paris. Inv. AP 2003.7.1.5. Photo: AP-HP/musée–author.

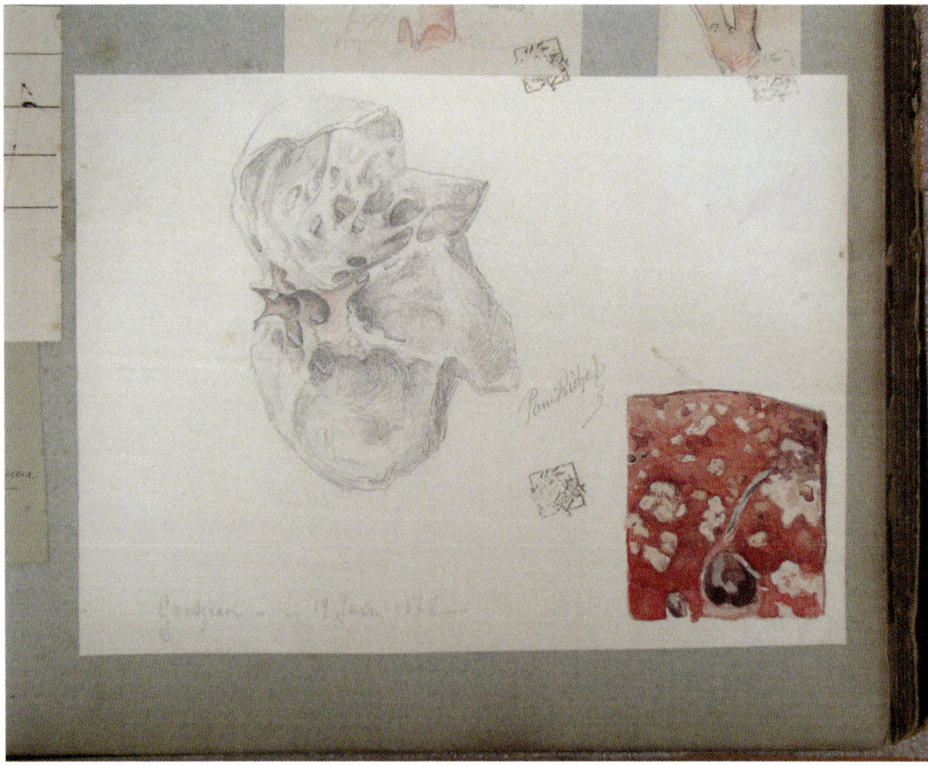

simply "Cholera 1849." While the patient is often unnamed, pride of place is granted to the physician who donated the specimen, such as Alfred Hardy (1811–1893), Louis Landouzy (1845–1917), and Ernest Mesnet (1825–1898); some patients were cared for at the Hôtel Dieu or the Hôpital de la Charité. There are colored drawings cut out and pasted onto other, darker sheets, which are, in turn, pasted onto the album's pages. These detailed body parts are macabre *papiers collés avant la lettre*. Some are hyperrealistically detailed, while others are schematically figured. Drawings by Richer in this album distinguish different parts of the body in shades of gray with hints of other colors, which is interesting given that he was color blind (fig. 10).[77]

Several albums mostly comprise photographs, many of which are uncaptioned; text could have, in Roland Barthes's formulation, "permitt[ed] me to focus not simply my gaze but also my understanding."[78] In many cases, the absence of accompanying clinical information means that the purpose of the photographs is difficult to ascertain, but the individual agency of the patient models comes through clearly in their unconventional postures and expressions. A young man, suited and seated, presents his wrinkled brow and direct gaze to the camera, the contour of his pointed pate outlined against the dark background (fig. 11). His striking face seems to betray consternation even as he acquiesces to having his photograph taken, suggesting "both resistance and complicity."[79] Yet even this photograph hints at "the usually invisible lines of social power in the world of medicine," to use Sander Gilman's words.[80] An inadvertent fingerprint on the photographic print serves as a poignant reminder of the clinician's power, holding the man's fate, so to speak, in his hands.

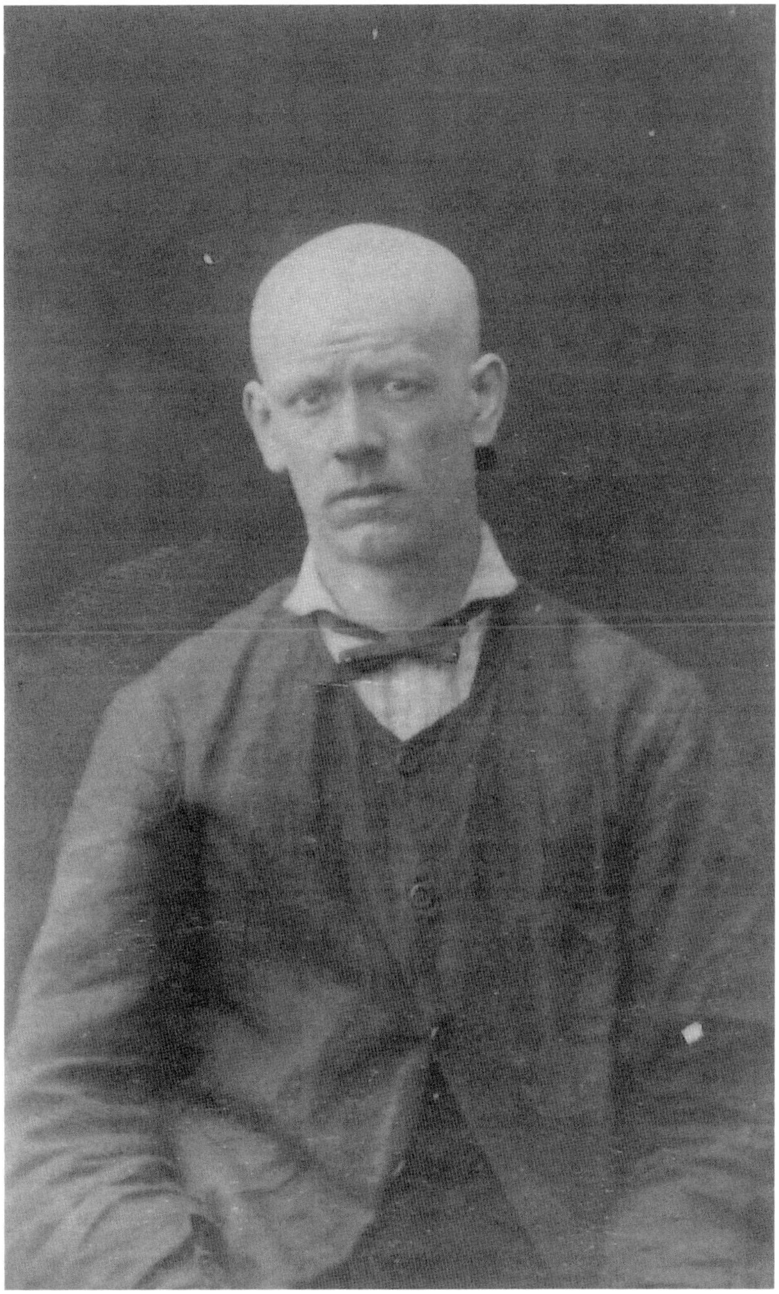

The powerful and voyeuristic gaze of the clinician dominates many of the images in the Musée Charcot albums, which often show scenes of discomfort and vulnerability. In Album AP 2003.7.1.4 (Paris, Musée de l'AP-HP), there are hands and feet uncontrollably clenched or flexed, atrophied limbs, pained or vacant faces, disfigurements impassively captured from different angles. In a revealing example from another album, a patient with an enlarged hand tries to hide from the gaze of the camera, which serves, in this instance, as a coercive instrument of the medical profession's power (fig. 12).[81] This juxtaposition of healthy and morbid was typical of Albert Londe's practice under Charcot. As in this case, abnormal appendages were usually photographed next to "normal" ones.[82] Moreover, Londe developed the stand on which a patient could pose his or her hands; in *La Photographie médicale* (1893), he includes an illustration of it and notes that the camera must be placed at the same angle as the stand to avoid distortions.[83]

There is an especially unexpected album in which the images of famous individuals—scientists, intellectuals, artists—have been neatly affixed, one above the other (Album AP 2003.7.2.4, Paris, Musée de l'AP-HP). A few prints reproduce instead details of Renaissance and Baroque paintings. The celebrities include writers, politicians, composers, philosophers, princes, and kings as well as painters; on one of its pages, portraits of Raphael, Michelangelo, and Dürer share the viewer's attention. The captions are mostly written in German, while at least one lists its maker on the back: A. Girard at 9, quai Voltaire.[84] A number of the album's images include the same border, indicating that they were printed (and bought) in a series. It is tantalizing to consider the role that this album may have played in the Salpêtrière's museum of pathological anatomy. There could have

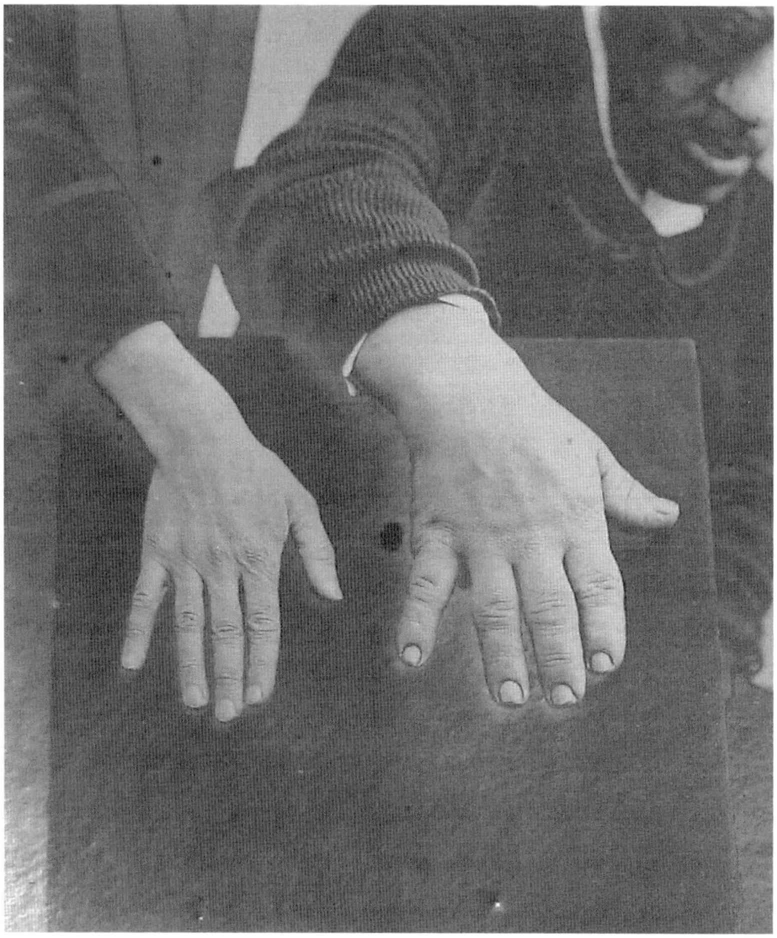

Fig. 12
Anonymous, *Mains* (*Hands*) (factual title), end of the nineteenth century. Photograph pasted on cardboard. Located in Album AP 2003.7.1.2 of the Musée Charcot anatomie pathologique. Paris, Musée de l'Assistance Publique–Hôpitaux de Paris. Inv. AP 2003.7.1.2. Photo: AP-HP/musée–author.

been a vestigial interest at the Salpêtrière School in the already discredited pseudoscience of physiognomy, which purported to identify the relationship between the features of the face and the character of these great men; certainly, physical features continued to play a role in the understanding of "genius" at this time.[85] The so-called bust of Gall in the museum is evidence of their interest in phrenology. Or perhaps Charcot and the doctors who worked under him hoped to see their own images one day in a similar album.

Instances of exchange in these albums signal the importance and extent of international communication in the field of medicine in the late nineteenth century. In Album AP 2003.7.1.5 (Paris, Musée de l'AP-HP), there are a few images of a sectioned brain, annotated "G. Burckhardt-de Waldau-près Berne," presumably from either Gottlieb Burckhardt (1836–1907) himself, director of the Waldau Psychiatric Clinic from 1875 to 1882, or from one of his publications. In the 1880s, Burckhardt, the first modern psychosurgeon, wrote about traumatic hysteria.[86] A letter addressed to Charcot by American neurologist Royal Wells Amidon (1854–1938) is pasted alongside a photograph and its brief caption in Album AP.2005.0.27.1 (fig. 13). Sent in 1884, the letter includes regards to Mme. Charcot and "John" (presumably Jean-Baptiste Charcot) as well as a nostalgic reference to an earlier time in Paris, suggesting that Amidon had spent time at the Salpêtrière and in the Charcot family home. The enclosed cabinet card captures, in his words, "the result, the fruit, you may say, of one of the few 'cases' we sometimes meet in the course of our dreary existence over here in New York." The caption to the photograph describes the patient's condition as "'word deafness' or 'word blindness' with no paralysis, or true aphasia."[87] An autopsied brain, in profile, rests on a frayed cloth laid on top of another textile, the rough texture of which fills the rest of the image. This specimen of an abnormal organ is framed tightly at the center of this vertical photograph, a format more typical of, and better suited to, a portrait. But, of course, this *is* a portrait of a patient, with the name of the photographer printed along its bottom edge: "Thomas, 717 6th Avenue." The photographic studio of S. A. Thomas was only a few blocks away from

Amidon's home on 41 West Twentieth Street in Manhattan. An obituary printed in the *Photographic Times and American Photographer* in 1894 states that Thomas "made a specialty of the portraits of children."[88] In this case, presumably an anomaly in his oeuvre, Thomas took a "portrait" of Amidon's dead patient, whose illness—and, seemingly, essence—was captured, self-evidently for Amidon and presumably for Charcot, in this photograph.

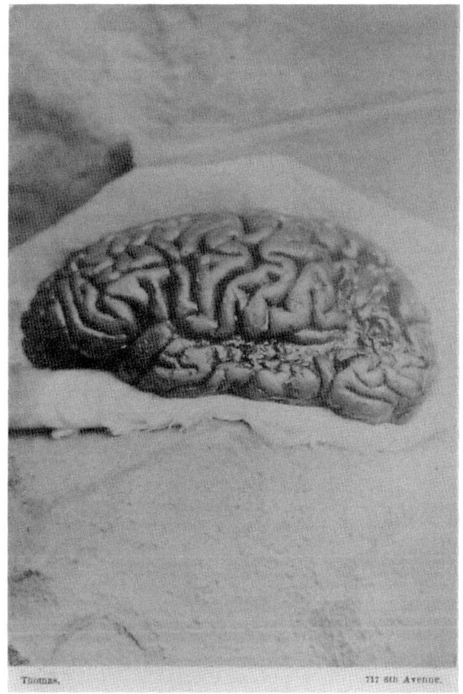

Fig. 13
S. A. Thomas, *Cerveau* (*Brain*) (factual title). Salted paper photograph pasted on cardboard. Located in Album AP 2005.0.27.1 of the Musée Charcot anatomie pathologique. Paris, Musée de l'Assistance Publique–Hôpitaux de Paris. Inv. AP 2005.0.27.1. Photo: AP-HP/musée–author.

Thomas made a habit of stamping promotional messages onto the back of his cabinet cards. One reads "photographic artist"; another is in the shape of a painter's palette on which is written the photographer's name and address, along with the words "Rembrandt effects."[89] Thomas must have prided himself on the artistry of his photographs, and this sepia-toned cabinet card is no exception. The stamp brings to the fore the impossibility of removing individual interpretation from the results of the supposedly "objective" medium, even in a photograph of an internal organ. This cabinet card is especially intriguing, as it was presumably taken in order to share medical knowledge between specialists in nervous diseases. This was also the function of the medical museum, where rare or "signature" illnesses were put on display to edify and excite the (medical) visitor. Thomas's cabinet card stands as a mise en abyme of the tangled relationship between art and medicine concretized in the albums, exhibited in the museum, and cultivated by Charcot.

The diversity of the images in the albums and the Musée Charcot itself challenge anthropologist Elizabeth Hallam's notion of the "anatomical intermediality" in play in the anatomy museum. Its objects, images, and texts "become echo chambers of repeated yet modified fragments. These references and entanglements are significant in practice, as students learning anatomy are expected to visualise the internal dimensions of an integrated living body built up from the visual and manual exploration of dissected bodies and inanimate models. Thus anatomical intermediality aids the imagining of an integrated rather than a dismembered anatomy."[90] A pathological museum highlights aberrance rather than normality. Regardless, they both share the exhibition of real or represented bodies, either whole or in fragments. It is difficult to imagine a body coming together—or "integrating," to use Hallam's word—through the disparate images in the Musée Charcot or its albums.

Curating Pathology

According to Eilean Hooper-Greenhill, following Michel Foucault, a "curatorial" gaze came into being in postrevolutionary France that "paralleled" the medical gaze.[91] Both are exemplified by Album AP 2003.7.2.1 (Paris, Musée de l'AP-HP), which includes a variety of images by different hands mostly showing the surfaces of the body. Like the museum, this album contains many types of evidence, including a page of illustrations of ears, each rendered in pen, graphite, colored pencils, and red chalk; a sketch in the style of a chronophotograph, capturing the movement of a hysteric during an attack; dissections depicted with colored pencils or in pen; a graphic rendering of a "scintillating scotoma" visualized during a migraine by a doctor named Millioti and recorded "from life [*dal vero*]," as we are told in the Italian text below;[92] a drawing by Charcot of a melancholic woman; photographs of excised bones next to prints of bodies deformed by locomotor ataxia;[93] and drawings of a man with Parkinson's disease wearing a fez, among others. The mixture of living and lifeless, indexical and artistic, was typical of the eclectic clinical practice at the hospital. The album's drawings by Paul Richer especially demonstrate the artistic aspirations that are apparent in much of its medical imagery.

This album's first page has an accomplished drawing of a young woman's visage alongside three drawings of Élisabeth Porreau, whose case was key to Charcot's identification of amyotrophic lateral sclerosis (ALS) or motor neuron disease, still known in France as Charcot's disease (fig. 14).[94] One of Charcot's most ferocious detractors, Félix Platel, who went by the *nom de plume* of Ignotus, wrote on the front page of *Le Figaro* about one of the neurologist's famous lessons in the amphitheater in which he "exhibited" a patient with ALS. Platel described the woman as "a statue of Despair" and, after she was unveiled like a sculpture "on inauguration day," he compared her to Auguste Clésinger's infamous *Femme piquée par un serpent* (*Woman Bitten by a Snake*, 1847, Paris, Musée d'Orsay).[95] The public was fully aware of Charcot's penchant for art, and his lectures and patients were often discussed in those terms.

In the larger sketch of Porreau on her deathbed, her body is shown to the knees. The figure's atrophied legs emerge from a sketchily drawn blanket, and her arms show contractures at both wrists so that her hands sit uncomfortably on her prone body, while her shoulders and head rest almost vertically against a large pillow. This drawing bears the signs of Charcot's inexpert draughtsmanship: ink over faint pencil lines, roughly capturing the shape of the body but having difficulty with foreshortening, and the strangeness of the visage (several more drawings of her face by the same hand appear on the next page). Crude lines compose the body and the face as well as the drapery around the figure and the drool that "constantly" escaped the patient's mouth. The two drawings below of Porreau's face are more carefully crafted, and only their juxtaposition with the image of the prone patient above confirm that they show the same person. They ignore the atrophied torso and the contorted hands to capture instead the fact that all the muscles of her face were "in a permanent state of contracture." The focus is on her staring eyes and her mouth, which was "always wide open."[96]

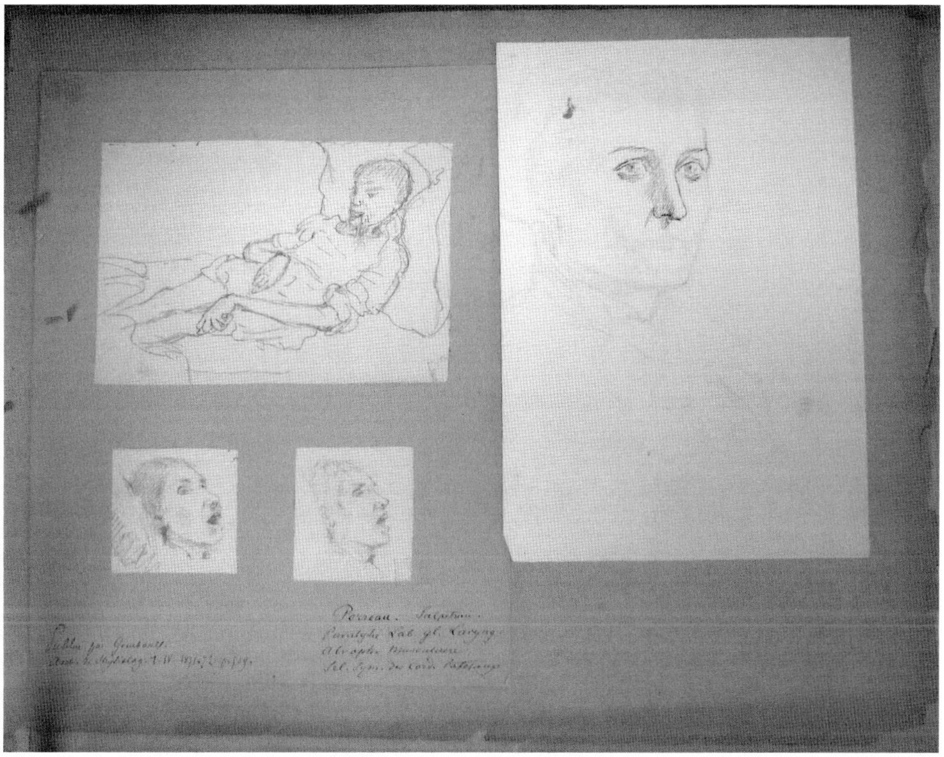

Fig. 14
Poireau, Paralysie glosso-labio-laryngée atrophie musculaire (*Poireau* [Porreau], *Labio-Glosso-Laryngeal Paralysis Muscular Atrophy*), ca. 1871. Drawing in pencil, 31.2 × 23.7 cm. Located in Album 7 of the Musée Charcot anatomie pathologique. Paris, Musée de l'Assistance Publique–Hôpitaux de Paris. Inv. AP 2003.7.2.1. Photo: AP-HP/musée–author.

The group of drawings in the album must have been done between July 11, 1871, when the fifty-eight-year-old Élisabeth Porreau entered the Salpêtrière, and her death three months later, on October 25.[97] These details are provided in a reference written underneath the drawings: Charcot's student and collaborator Albert Gombault (1844–1904) published an article on this patient in the *Archives de physiologie normale et pathologique*. It described in detail her symptoms during life and the revelations of her autopsy, which led Gombault to posthumously diagnose primary lateral sclerosis (*sclérose primitive des cordons latéraux*). He concluded that the paralysis of her facial muscles was merely a secondary symptom.[98] The drawings of Porreau, which focus primarily on her face and the symptoms of labio-glosso-laryngeal paralysis, are ultimately misleading, even if they capture an important part of her case history. It is probable that the caption that notes her illness was written after Gombault's article was published, as it includes his final diagnosis. Or, perhaps, the drawings and her name were included in the album only after her case history was published, as they are pasted onto a separate piece of blue paper, which was apparently glued later into the album.

Opposite these is a portrait of a woman's face on a larger white sheet, likely done by Paul Richer. She stares sternly off the side of the page, her strong cheekbones and chin lightly sketched by a clinician, her hair neatly tied behind her head and her collar decorated with a bow. The contours of her visage are drawn in pencil, but her nose, eyes, and eyebrows, along with the shading that gives them volume, have been rendered in pen.

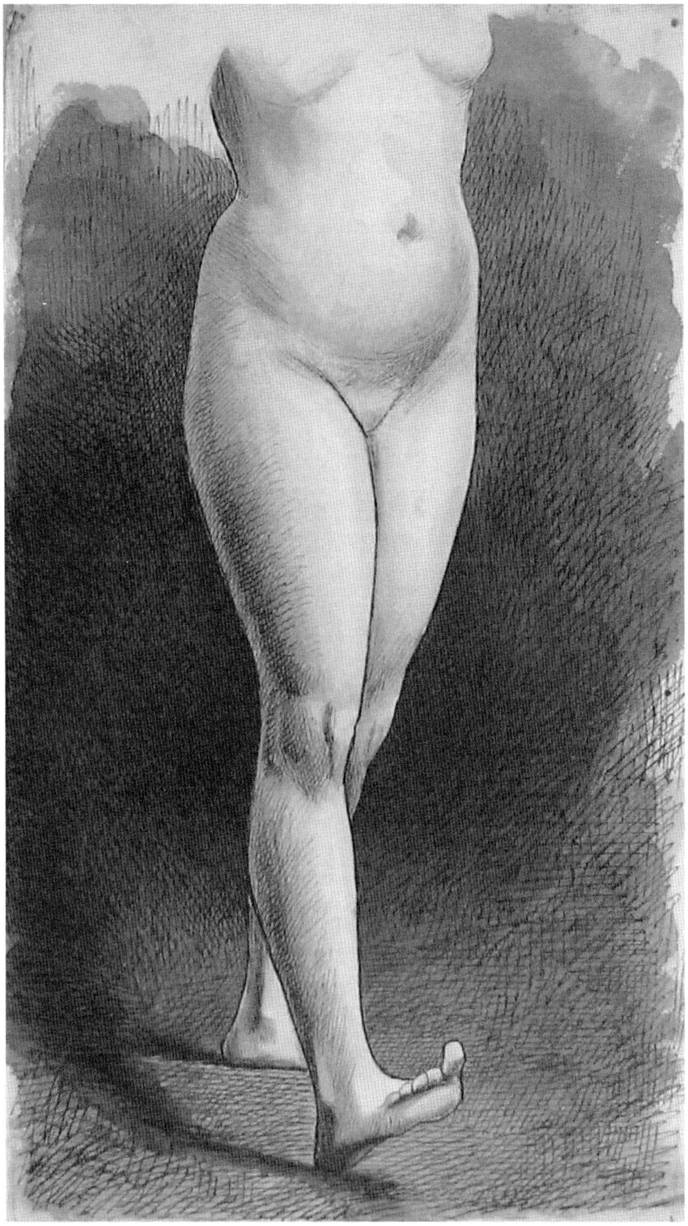

The unsigned drawing is mute—without a caption, a name, or a diagnosis, the reason for this drawing's inclusion in the album remains a mystery. The woman pictured does not, on the surface, appear to be ill. If she is not a patient, then why was her portrait included in this album? If she is a patient, then what does this skillful rendering reveal? At the very least, it inadvertently highlights the clumsiness of the portraits of Porreau on the same page.

Another drawing that appears later in the album, made with pen and black ink and gray wash, resembles an *académie,* the drawing of a live model that was considered an indispensable part of a student's training at the École des beaux-arts (fig. 15).[99] The woman's body is rendered from the chest down, and her gait seems to be the focus. Her strong legs and thick waist are sharply contoured in black, while her torso and breasts are suggested in shades of gray. Regular hatch marks give the legs volume and provide varying depths to the background. The figure's right leg is shown taking a step, heel down and toes in the air. The position of the back foot, of which only the heel is visible, would suggest that the patient is not, in fact, shown walking but simply putting her foot forward. The toes of that right foot are almost caricatured—the big toe in particular is raised up, while the others are differentiated only by the thin lines separating them. The body and the background gradually dissolve as they reach the top of the page; the wash of the background ends in puffs of gray and black. The *savant-artiste* has sensitively drawn the roundness of the stomach, the dot of the navel, and the shading of the breasts. And while the *mons veneris* is central to the image—it forms a V that points directly down to the right foot—it is hairless, following academic conventions. Of course, pubic hair would not have given the viewer any more information about the disorder we are meant to recognize here—whether to include it or not was ultimately an aesthetic decision, just as it was to include the breasts, as they add nothing to the factual data the drawing is meant to impart.[100]

Clearly a gifted artist, knowledgeable in artistic conventions, created this *acéphale*. A simple line drawing could have conveyed the basic information about these legs and this body—and, in fact, only a schematic version of the drawing was ultimately published, the angle of the upper body shifted back slightly to render the pose more precarious.[101] The published illustration is signed by Paul Richer and depicts the hysterical contracture of the entire right leg, which was so severe that the patient could not sit down. The case history was taken in 1882 and published seven years later in the second volume of the *Nouvelle Iconographie de la Salpêtrière*, the hospital's journal of medico-artistic case studies and articles on neurological disorders, published annually between 1888 and 1918. This patient was exceptional, Richer tells us, because the contracture was very unusual, especially resistant to treatment, and therefore persisted for years before spontaneously resolving. Richer calls this a "forme cérébrale" of hysteria, as opposed to the more common "forme spinale"; because it disappeared during sleep, the contracture had to be the result of unconscious forces.[102] The drawing in the album is as exceptional as the case because of the care and pleasure evident in its creation: in the subtle gradations of shadow in the background and the figure's own cast shadow, in the wash that lends volume to the woman's belly and hints at her breasts. W. J. T. Mitchell has written of the double meaning of "drawing": "an act of tracing or inscribing lines, on the one hand, and an act of pulling, dragging, or attracting, on the other, as when we talk of a horse-drawn buggy, drawing water from a well, drawing back a bowstring to release the arrows of desire, or 'drawing and quartering' a human body in that most grotesque form of capital punishment. . . . Drawing draws us on. Desire just *is*, quite literally, drawing, or *a* drawing—a pulling or attracting force, and the trace of this force in a picture."[103] Richer's drawing reveals a delight in art-making in addition to—or, perhaps, rather than—an unusual hysterical symptom. As an obituary noted, he handled the burin as delicately as the scalpel.[104]

Fig. 15 (opposite)
Anonymous, *Corps féminin* (*Female Body*) (factual title), end of the nineteenth century. Drawing in pencil with watercolor on paper. Located in Album 7 of the Musée Charcot anatomie pathologique. Paris, Musée de l'Assistance Publique–Hôpitaux de Paris. Inv. AP 2003.7.2.1. Photo: AP-HP/musée–author.

Richer's *Hands*

Richer is likely the anonymous artist responsible for a number of drawings of hands, two of which are sketched in red chalk (*sanguine*), a medium associated more with fine art than with medical illustration. Since Richer joined the Salpêtrière in January 1878, and the albums of the Musée Charcot hold a spate of unsigned but skilled drawings dated from that year, it is my contention that Richer began filling page after page with drawings upon his arrival.[105] His facility in drawing had brought him to Charcot's attention in the first place. As a medical student in Paris in the 1870s, he began frequenting Charcot's celebrated lessons at the École de médecine. There Richer once heard Charcot declare the need for a medical study of the hand, which required, "besides medical knowledge, a bit of artistic talent."[106] Richer then sought out his friend Henri Meillet and offered to do the illustrations for his medical thesis on *Des déformations permanentes de la main* (Permanent deformities of the hand).[107] In the second plate of the thesis, one sees hands transformed by rheumatism, gout, and Parkinson's disease, some copied from a patient at the Salpêtrière and others from plaster casts from "the collection of M. Charcot" in the Musée Dupuytren.[108] Some are delineated with fine hatch marks that convey the deformity of bone under wrinkled skin, while others are much more quickly rendered. The young Richer was "discovered" at the defense of Meillet's thesis, where Charcot, the principal examiner, exclaimed: "You could make a diagnosis from these drawings!"[109] He further asserted that Richer could revive a medico-artistic practice in the tradition of Adriaan van den Spiegel, Thomas Bartholin, and Andreas Vesalius, "whose magnificent plates remain famous."[110] Charcot immediately offered Richer an internship at the Salpêtrière during his fourth year of studies (in 1878). As one of an elite coterie of *internes*, Richer would be not just a student of the famed neurologist but also a collaborator.[111] By nurturing a modern-day descendant of these eminent sixteenth- and seventeenth-century anatomists, Charcot endeavored to establish his hospital as an internationally renowned producer of medical imagery. He also found a kindred spirit in the younger doctor, who shared his interest in the intersection of art and medicine; of course, they would later co-author two popular books in which they diagnosed illnesses in people represented in artworks of the past.

Richer's only formal artistic training seems to have occurred in school in his hometown of Chartres, where he started drawing classes at the age of eight. He regularly won drawing competitions in his youth.[112] As he was color-blind, he channeled his artistic talents into drawing and, later, sculpture (see chapter 4). He began sculpting around the age of forty and submitted his first sculpture to the Salon in 1890, regularly exhibiting there in subsequent years. Critics immediately recognized that Richer's artistic practice, like Brouillet's, was invested in realism, a movement committed to depicting contemporary life.[113] (Let's remember that Brouillet gave him a place of prominence in *Clinical Lesson*.) Gustave Larroumet, for example, in response to five sculptures that Richer submitted to the Salon of 1892, noted his "realist spirit."[114] Richer's fine art, in other words, attempted to capture the world around him as "objectively" as possible, and he saw his naturalistic sculptures of laborers—sower, harvester, blacksmith, and the like—on a continuum with his medical practice.

Perhaps Charcot was especially impressed by Richer's illustrations because, decades before, Charcot's medical thesis had included his own drawings of hands; one of these, showing the effects of rheumatoid arthritis, is also included in this album.[115] Another page shows the palm and the back of the same hand in two drawings in red chalk likely done by Richer (fig. 16).[116] All the fingers except the thumb exhibit a lateral bend in the direction of the little finger, a common deformity resulting from rheumatoid arthritis. Whether looking at the back of the hand or the palm, the deformed joints force the bent fingers to spiral out in a shape that can be likened to a shell or a star. The triangular form of the hand in the drawings, along with the hint of lower arm, makes them resemble arrows pointing downward. The artist has used a light touch with the red chalk to create the contours of the dramatically distorted hand as well as the hatch marks that lend it volume. The beauty of these sketches belies the painful deformity

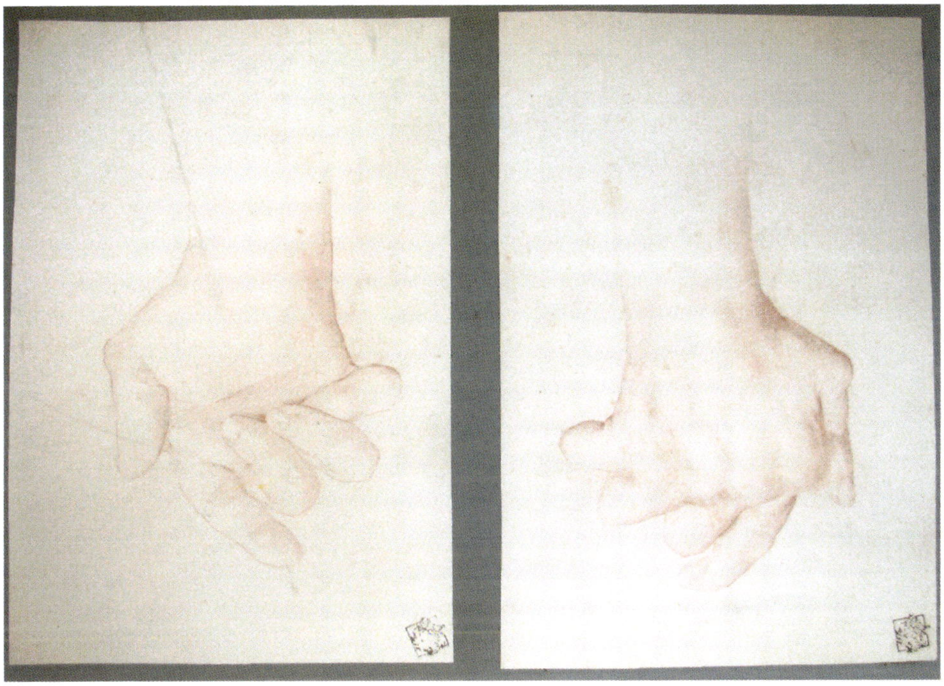

Fig. 16
Anonymous, *Poignée* (*Fist*) (factual title), end of the nineteenth century. Drawing in pencil on paper. Located in Album 7 of the Musée Charcot anatomie pathologique. Paris, Musée de l'Assistance Publique–Hôpitaux de Paris. Inv. AP 2003.7.2.1. Photo: AP-HP/musée–author.

they depict. It is poignant to think of the skill and dexterity of the artist's hands in rendering images of a hand that was likely rendered almost useless by arthritis. In a text entitled "Dialogues sur l'art et la science" (Dialogues on art and science) from 1897, Richer discusses the process of creating a drawing from life: "While copying nature very sincerely, the artist who creates a drawing, that is, a reduced reproduction of the model, is led to suppress a great number of useless details while accentuating other features, and, in doing so, he imparts his personal stamp on the work that reveals the originality of his temperament."[117] These fine drawings capture the salient characteristics of the diseased limb, but what stands out most is the artist's re-presentation of them. The "real" hand is faithfully "copied," but the artist's signature style is also vividly apparent.

The use of *sanguine*, too, shows Richer's artistic ambitions. The medium, utilized typically for preparatory studies, was rarely employed in the second half of the nineteenth century.[118] It harks back instead to the Old Masters of seventeenth- and eighteenth-century France. Richer's drawings do not appear to be preparatory studies—instead, they delight in the beautiful tonal effects facilitated by red chalk. The hands are centered on the sheet and parallel to the picture plane, rendered in a style that was used commonly in medical photography but also in early portraiture. These are portraits not only of the symptoms of the illness that deformed them but also of individual hands, rendered with care. Perhaps they show the progress of rheumatoid arthritis in the hands of the same Salpêtrière patient Richer depicted for Meillet's thesis.[119]

Hands are the focus of other pages in this album as well, presented in various states of dissection, among them three skillful pen-and-ink drawings (fig. 17). In the

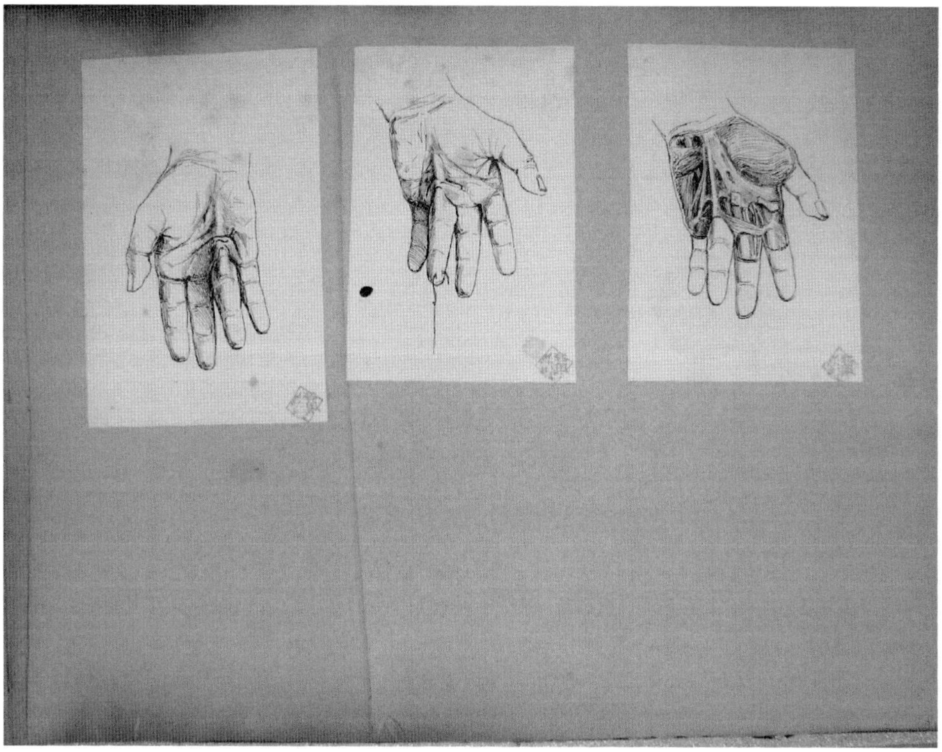

Fig. 17
Anonymous, *Mains* (*Hands*) (factual title), end of the nineteenth century. Drawing, 37 × 46.5 cm. Located in Album 7 of the Musée Charcot anatomie pathologique. Paris, Musée de l'Assistance Publique–Hôpitaux de Paris. Inv. AP 2003.7.2.1. Photo: AP-HP/musée–author.

second image, the left hand is suspended from a hook that pierces the tip of the ring finger. The sketch focuses our attention on the tendon bulging through the skin of the palm, wrenched by the hook from which it would have been suspended (the drawing has been pasted into the album upside down). The third drawing shows what is presumably the same hand after the skin has been removed from the palm, revealing the internal anatomy. On the next page of the album are glued four sheets with six sketches of these same hands, done quickly but deliberately in pencil. These include views of the hand from the side and another stage in the dissection of the left hand. It seems that these pencil drawings were originals from which the three on the previous page were selected and copied in black ink, perhaps in preparation for publication. It is worth noting that the original pencil sketch of the dissected left hand does not include the (undissected) thumb; this has been added to the ink drawing, where it looks malformed, as if the artist were unsure of himself. Having no model, or even a sketch from which to copy the thumb, it is evident under close inspection that this part of the work is more tentative. For these clinicians, having a "real" model to copy from was critically important. Their artistry stems not from their powers of invention but from their meticulous study of the model, just as Charcot needed to copy the Old Masters for the decorative additions to his home.

Two other drawings in this album, dated 1878, were likely done by Richer. One shows us *Gireudot la vieille (The Elderly Gireudot)*, a woman with large, bright eyes and a partially opened mouth, in the three-quarter view that Richer seemed to prefer

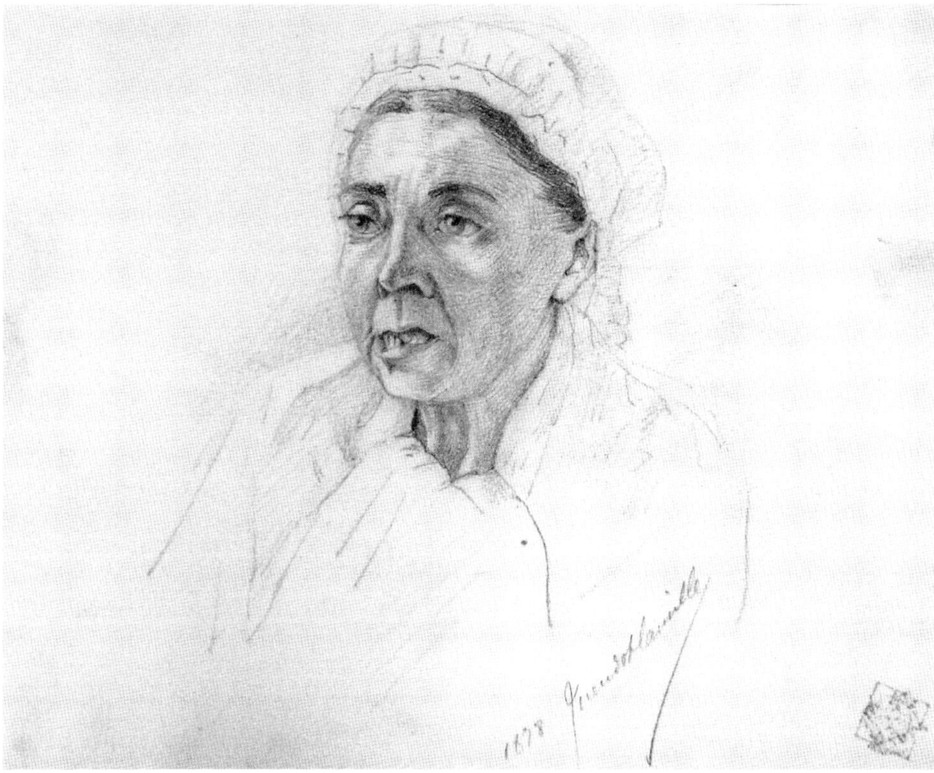

Fig. 18
Anonymous, *Gireudot la vieille (The Elderly Gireudot)*, 1878. Drawing in pencil, 17 x 21 cm. Located in Album 7 of the Musée Charcot anatomie pathologique. Paris, Musée de l'Assistance Publique–Hôpitaux de Paris. Inv. AP 2003.7.2.1. Photo: AP-HP/musée–author.

and would have been a natural choice from his position on the side of a hospital bed (fig. 18).[120] The confident hatch marks render the contours of her face; the light shining from her proper right highlights her forehead, nose, and slack lower lip that reveals a row of uneven teeth. Equal attention has been paid to her tensed neck, unlike her clothes and bonnet. The artist has, however, made sure to include the cloth tucked into her dress like a bib, most likely to catch drool. The elegant drawing quietly suggests this symptom of her infirmity, unlike the rough sketch of Porreau at the start of this album, though perhaps the two women had the same illness. Gireudot's eyes command as much attention as her mouth and give us a sense of this patient's identity, despite their apparent expression of fear or shock. It is as much a portrait of an individual as a study of a symptom, in stark contrast to drawings that share the album page—the tongue and uvula of a patient named "Lambert" from February 20 (1878?), where body parts stand in for the patient.

Juxtapositions

The tongue that veers to one side was the focus of Charcot's and Richer's later study of a grotesque mask from the church of Santa Maria Formosa in Venice, in which they determined that the seventeenth-century artist who made it must have witnessed firsthand a person with a hysterical glossolabial hemispasm.[121] Citing John Ruskin's

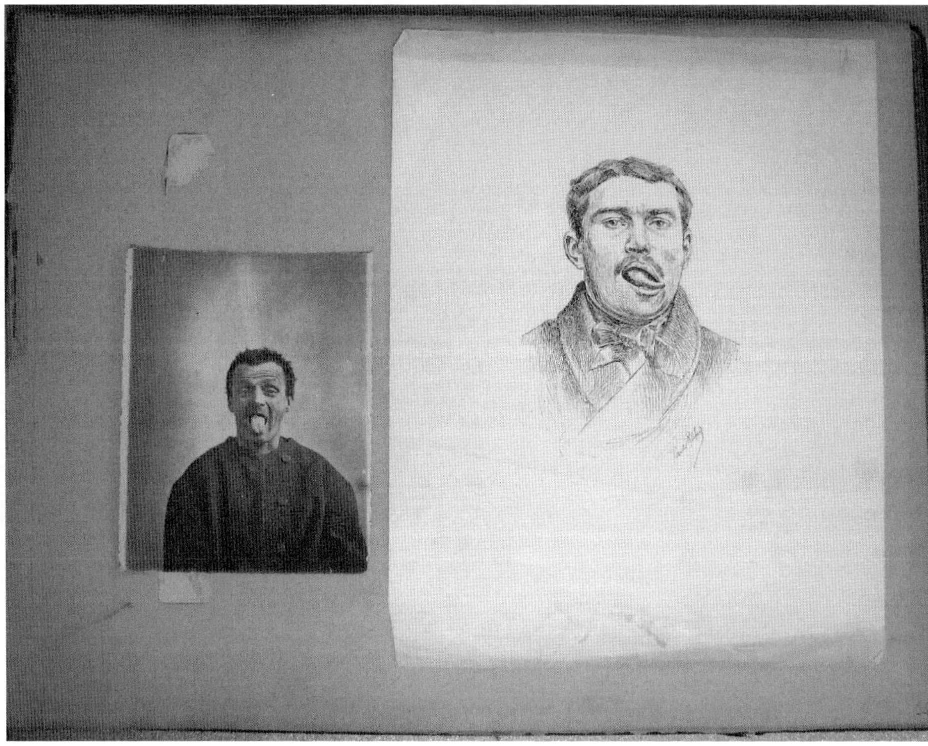

Fig. 19
Anonymous, *Homme qui tire la langue (Man Sticking Out His Tongue)* (factual title), end of the nineteenth century, photograph pasted on cardboard, 16 × 13 cm, and Paul Richer, drawing on paper. Album 7 of the Musée Charcot anatomie pathologique, plate 24. Paris, Musée de l'Assistance Publique–Hôpitaux de Paris. Inv. AP 2003.7.2.1. Photo: AP-HP/musée–author.

description of the mask in *The Stones of Venice* (1851), Charcot and Richer hypothesize that, instead of creating an "artistic fantasy," the sculptor must have "met on his way, seen with his eyes, seized in passing and reproduced with accuracy" a person with an illness that, in Charcot's day, was to be found in the wards of the Salpêtrière.[122] The doctors philosophize that nature "in its variety of forms is a source of inexhaustible richness wherein are mingled beauty and ugliness, the harmonious and the deformed and all degrees in between."[123] Using the language of the day, they write that the mask is a masterpiece of "naturalist" art.[124] A pen and black ink drawing by Richer that was included in the article graces another page of this album, alongside a photograph of a man showing us his tongue with only one tooth visible (fig. 19). In his "Dialogues," Richer wrote about the disadvantages of the photograph in comparison to the artist's sketch: "Despite his best efforts, the photographer will always be inferior to the illustrator. The objective is merciless. While reducing, it ignores nothing. . . . In the photograph, nature appears, so to speak, diminished, shrunk, while in a drawing of the same size, it retains or even expands the character of grandeur of which it is truly invested."[125] Richer's sitter is certainly more "presentable" than the patient in the photograph; his cravat and jacket, as well as his neatly combed hair and moustache, look relatively fashionable. In contrast, the messy hair and overly large jacket with big buttons of the photographed patient make him look like a modern-day Pierrot. While the open mouth gives us a glimpse of a single front tooth, his deeply furrowed brow makes it seem that sticking his tongue out requires exertion. The drawing may have allowed

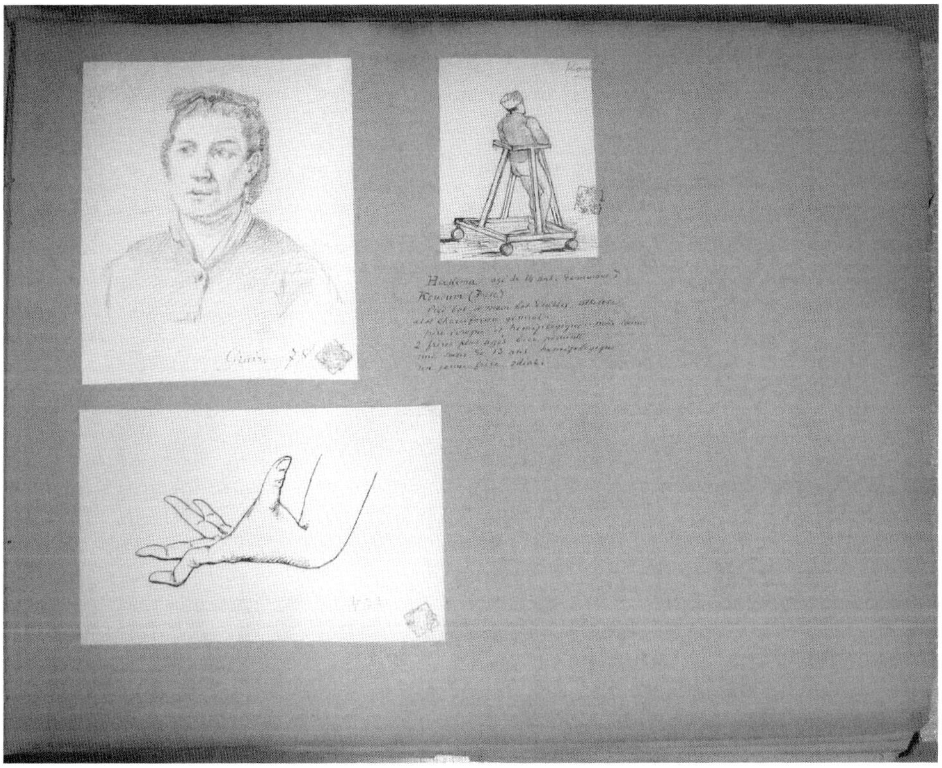

Fig. 20
Anonymous, *Dessins* (*Drawings*), ca. 1878. 37 × 46.5 cm. Located in Album 7 of the Musée Charcot anatomie pathologique. Paris, Musée de l'Assistance Publique–Hôpitaux de Paris. Inv. AP 2003.7.2.1. Photo: AP-HP/musée–author.

Richer to normalize the symptom by granting him artistic license to craft a patient from a different class and with a different psychological profile.

Sharing a page with a drawing of a young boy held upright in a wheeled wooden frame and a drawing of a dramatically contorted hand is a bust-length portrait of a patient named Grain, another pencil sketch likely done by Richer and dated 1878 (fig. 20). Grain's expression appears slightly confused or uncertain. Her left eyebrow is raised quizzically as she looks off to the side. A flouncy bow sits incongruously on her neatly pinned-up hair, and there is no immediately visible symptom—like the unfinished portrait at the start of this album, this drawing does not clearly display a malady. Her mouth is slightly open, as though caught mid-speech, and so it appears to refer back to the *portraits parlants* of a previous century. I wonder if the image "spoke" to the clinicians, communicating knowledge of its illness that is inscrutable to us now. Immediately below is simple but accomplished pen drawing of a hand. The wrist is painfully bent, as in a hysterical contracture, but the strained fingers stretch out with the palm open. This sketch has been placed upside down, as the numbers written on the sheet make clear, so that the hand seems to be opening to catch the image of Grain above.[126]

To the right of these two drawings is a pen-and-ink sketch, possibly by Charcot, of a boy standing upright in a device that acts as a sort of scaffolding, with four wheels at its corners. This is an exceptional image in the context of this album, in that the text below gives a brief case history of a fourteen-year-old boy named Hoekema, who lived

Fig. 21 (opposite)
Anonymous, *Femme avec problème vasculaire et schéma* (*Woman with Vascular Problem and Diagram*) (factual title), end of the nineteenth century. Drawing in pencil on paper. Located in Album 7 of the Musée Charcot anatomie pathologique. Paris, Musée de l'Assistance Publique–Hôpitaux de Paris. Inv. AP 2003.7.2.1. Photo: AP-HP/musée–author.

in the small town of Koudum in the Netherlands. Charcot could have seen him on one of his holidays, when he typically traveled around Europe, visiting museums and seeing patients. According to the text, Hoekema had a clubfoot and two clubhands, and both his father and one of his siblings were hemiplegic, exhibiting a lack of control or weakness on one side of the body. Only part of the word "Koudum" appears at the top right, indicating that the sketch was cut out, perhaps from a notebook. The boy is shown nude from the waist down, but his hands are not visible, and only a small bit of a foot can be seen. The import of the sketch, then, appears to be the mobility aid designed to help the child: the uppermost edges of the frame support his elbows while the base keeps him balanced and upright, despite the tilt of his body. If there is a connection between the portrait, the hand, and the device in these drawings, a reason for them to be pasted onto the same page, it is now lost to us.

Drawings of a patient named Marguerite Moutarde include various details of her body, a full portrait of her alive, and a postmortem sketch of the culprit in her death—her own heart (fig. 21). She had osteomalacia, a softening of the bones comparable to rickets in children, now easily treated with vitamin D and calcium supplements.[127] During Charcot's time, however, as the cause was unknown, osteomalacia was untreatable and generally fatal.[128] Moutarde's case is exceptionally illuminated in the album, as there are four pages dedicated to it, including a page that provides notes from her autopsy. Drawings of her whole body and details of its interior and exterior cover three pages. Moutarde entered the Salpêtrière in August 1851, by which point she could no longer walk. Her bones were so fragile that a nurse broke one in changing her sheets.[129] Her case history, outlined in a medical thesis on osteomalacia by Paul Bouley, notes that her physical ailments began after moving to Paris from her home in the Ardennes in 1841 to work at the Grand-Condé, a Left Bank department store. She was "malnourished," Bouley notes, and lived in a room without sunlight. Within a couple of years, her clothes felt loose and friends commented that she appeared to be shrinking. She visited a doctor who was only able to examine her superficially, because she did not want to undress; by the time the clinicians at the Salpêtrière drew her naked body over and over again, her modesty must have suffered too. Little by little over the course of her illness, she lost most of her teeth, her thighs bowed, and she felt terrible pain. Various bones in her body fractured; coughing led to broken ribs. She was bedridden for ten years at the Salpêtrière.

In the drawing, Moutarde's nude body seemingly floats without support. Her only clothing is a bonnet covering the back of her head, its border ringing her face like a halo. Two other pages show sketches of her hands and feet, the rolls of fat in her inner thighs, the soft flesh of her stomach and breasts silhouetted against her arms. Her body is cut up in these small sketches, pasted grid-like onto the album's blue pages, fetishized by the clinician. These changes of focus—from one part of the body to another—appear to be an attempt to capture evidence of Moutarde's malady on the surface of her body, over which the clinician's gaze ranges obsessively, almost cinematically. "The intercostal spaces had largely disappeared" and her spine had become concave, leading to

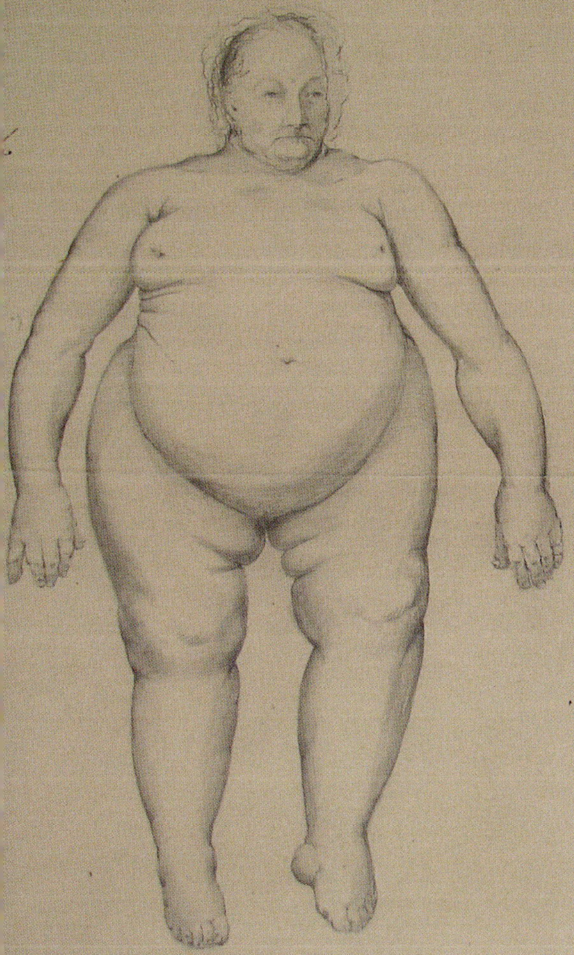

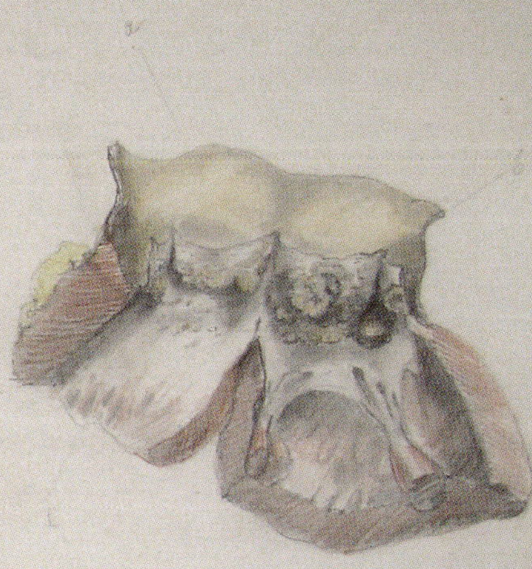

Charcot delin. ad naturam

Anévrisme valvulaire :
Valv. Sygmoïde,

Moutarde
ostéomalacie,

an "extremely short" torso—this was presumably the reason for the attention paid to her chest.[130] Bouley notes that the fingers of her hands seem to come back on themselves with "flattened" tips (*en raquette*); this is especially noticeable in her right hand, rendered as a fragmented whole and in detail in the album. Moutarde attributed this to the fact that she used her fingers to help prop herself up in bed. Her pelvis tilted in the wrong direction, so in the drawing it seems tucked under her large abdomen. The medical thesis also comments on the "deep folds" of her inner thighs and Moutarde's pointed feet, which form a straight line with her legs. It is possible to read the text as "explaining" the images and the way in which the clinician's gaze has zoomed in to capture areas of her body.

But the sketched details offer little information beyond what is already imparted in the rendering of her entire body. Moreover, the strangeness of this drawing belies the "truthfulness" implicit in the close study of the patient. The artist's point of view appears to hover over the bed to which Moutarde was confined at the time the drawings were made. This is an impossible position, and the lack of anecdotal detail, such as the bed or the sheet on which she must be resting—usually included in drawings of patients—further obfuscates the clinical setting. Like the *gisante* in Pablo Picasso's *Demoiselles d'Avignon* (1907, New York, Museum of Modern Art), she appears at first glance to be standing on limp feet that could not support her. It is only upon closer inspection that it becomes clear that she has sprung up onto the yellowed sheet of paper from a prone position.

Moutarde died "in 1863 or 1864" not of the illness purportedly chronicled in these drawings but of ulcerative endocarditis.[131] Bouley notes bluntly that the autopsy did not include an examination of her bones. Charcot's own sketch of her dissected heart is glued next to the one of Moutarde's body, the juxtaposition exemplifying Foucault's claim that the interior organs have become the site where "bodies and eyes meet."[132] Like an artist, Charcot annotated it in Latin: "*Charcot delin. ad. naturam.*" Her cut-open heart spreads out like wings, and its contours and spaces are rendered in red, yellow, brown, and gray. It is faintly labeled "a," "b," and "c," but the key is nowhere to be found. This colored drawing overpowers the image of Moutarde while alive: it is more vivid than her living body, which is also much smaller in scale. This drawing illustrates Charcot's comment that "pathological anatomy, as it penetrates further into the intimacy of the tissues, simultaneously becomes more animated, more alive."[133] In the album, the cause of Moutarde's death brutally overshadows the illness that affected her daily in life.

A final example from this album shows a photograph of the Farnese Hercules (ca. 216 AD, Naples, Museo Archeologico Nazionale) paired with two photographs of a boy taken from the back and the side (fig. 22). This is certainly not an accidental pairing, as the three images are all framed within a single black-and-white border. At first glance, it would appear that the classical sculpture is providing an ideal to which the boy's oddly muscular body can be compared, though the patient's body is not posed frontally like the sculpture. The child appears to be supported by an individual whose white-cuffed arm is visible on the far right. The reason for the comparison with the sculpture is discussed in an extensive five-part article in the *Archives générales de médecine* from 1868 by Charcot's friend and mentor, the physiologist Guillaume Duchenne de Boulogne (1806–1875). In it, Duchenne recounts the comment of another physician when looking at a boy with pseudohypertrophic paralysis: "It is the child of the Farnese Hercules."[134] Children with this disorder—now understood to be caused by a gene mutation and known as Duchenne muscular dystrophy—develop an exaggerated musculature that paradoxically coincides with a progressive weakness in the body, one that eventually leads to paralysis and death. Duchenne argues, "The Farnese Hercules is the ideal of physical strength in antique statuary. . . . Its musculature is admirable in its proportion and above all its naturalness. . . . To compare it with the monstrous musculature of the hypertrophic paralytic would be to mistake its aesthetic beauty."[135]

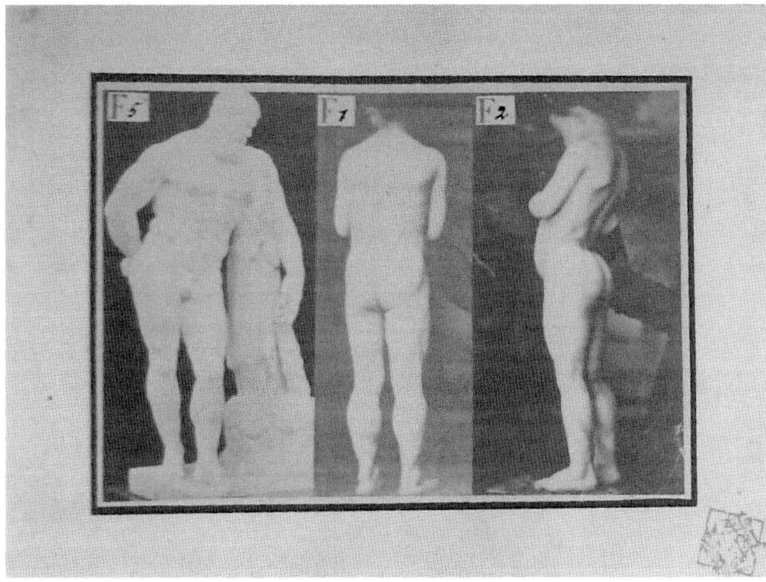

Fig. 22
Anonymous, *Postures d'hommes* (*Male Postures*) (factual title). Salted paper photographs pasted on cardboard. Located in Album 7 of the Musée Charcot anatomie pathologique. Paris, Musée de l'Assistance Publique–Hôpitaux de Paris. Inv. AP 2003.7.2.1. Photo: AP-HP/musée–author.

The two photographs paired with the Farnese Hercules are reproduced as drawings in Duchenne's article. We learn that they show a seven-year-old boy brought to him in 1858, whom he immediately photographed because of the striking contrast between the muscles of his lower and upper body.[136] Incongruously, this child had "the muscles of an athlete" yet could not stand without support and spent most of his time sitting or lying down.[137] For Duchenne, this boy was the perfect "example and typical case" of this illness.[138] As many historians have noted, his reliance on photography influenced Charcot, who called Duchenne his "master of neurology" and gave the elder physiologist access not only to the research facilities at the Salpêtrière but also to its patients.[139] In return, Duchenne taught Charcot "the fine points of medical photography," in Gilman's words, and may have encouraged Charcot's early interest in the diseases of the nervous system.[140] It is no wonder, then, to find Duchenne's theories represented in the albums of the Musée Charcot. One could argue that his use of classical sculpture was fundamentally different from that of his colleague Charcot, who used comparisons of sick bodies and artworks to demonstrate the important role of clinicians in the study of art while affirming the existence of contemporary disorders (like hysteria) and validating his own diagnoses. In this comparison by Duchenne, we are shown instead a sort of *faux ami*: the bodies look similar to the uninitiated but are, in fact, very different. However, Duchenne himself contradicts this theory when he states, "This false Hercules-child recalls only the School of Michelangelo [and not the Farnese Hercules], which, driven by the power of [Michelangelo's] conceptions, had the ambition to represent physical strength better than nature by exaggerating the musculature, an exaggeration that could be forgiven only because of his genius."[141] Perhaps this juxtaposition from the 1860s gave Charcot the idea to compare pathologies to artworks in the first place.

Many of the images in this album seem at first to have nothing in common. But, in fact, they do: the clinicians' unabashed belief in the importance of visual description, the weight given to representation (over, say, text), and the apparent delight in those depictions. Charcot encouraged sketching in a letter to his son, who was following in his footsteps and studying medicine, by asserting that "science and art are allies, two of Apollo's children."[142] He clearly saw his and the Salpêtrière School's endeavor as both scientific *and* artistic.

The Laughing Cavalier

While many of the images in the albums of the Musée Charcot are enigmatic, striking, and even troubling, the most curious is perhaps the final one in Album AP 2003.7.1.5: a creased reproduction of *The Laughing Cavalier* (1624, London, Wallace Collection) by Frans Hals (ca. 1582–1666). The reproduction is pasted horizontally to make it fit on the page (fig. 23). The poor-quality black-and-white print of Hals's painting of a twenty-six-year-old model, who looks directly at the viewer with a jauntily cocked head and sly smile, contrasts with the medical imagery shown in the albums. Remember that Souques claimed that the visible symptoms of nervous disease likely led Charcot to privilege this "branch of pathology" in the first place, yet the signs of disease on many of the bodies in these albums are remarkably inarticulate.[143] Many of the faces, however, like that of the *Laughing Cavalier,* convey a strong sense of inner life (see fig. 11).[144] Joshua Reynolds, first president of the Royal Academy of Arts, complimented exactly that quality in Hals's portraits.[145] Wielding a paintbrush instead of a camera, Hals seems to penetrate the body's surface, but with the intention of expressing character rather than pathology.

Seymour Slive has described Hals's sitter as "one of the most familiar characters in the history of Western painting."[146] Charcot may have first encountered the painting as a reproduction in the *Gazette des beaux-arts* in 1865, in an article that discussed the Pourtalès sale in Paris in which it was being auctioned; the astronomical price paid for it by Lord Hertford in a bidding war with Baron James de Rothschild likely stoked the public's interest in the work.[147] The *Laughing Cavalier* may display a pathological symptom relevant to the clinicians at the Salpêtrière—after all, they published many "medico-artistic" case studies in the *Nouvelle Iconographie de la Salpêtrière* in which they diagnosed figures in past artworks. However, neither the *Laughing Cavalier* nor any other of Hals's works is analyzed in the journal.[148] Hals is also missing from Charcot and Richer's two popular books on the possessed, deformed, and ill in art in which they chart the "invasion of pathology into art."[149]

Richer claimed that science and art were simply "two different manifestations of the same principle: Truth," echoing the sentiment that Charcot shared in the letter to his son.[150] In their view, both science and art were united in a concern with knowledge and, specifically, with nature. This attention to nature was also a well-known characteristic of seventeenth-century Dutch painters like Hals, whose "realism" was touted by historians and artists in France during Charcot's time.[151] Charcot's personal art collection included paintings by Hals's contemporaries: Gabriël Metsu, Ludolf Bakhuizen, and Jan Steen. He owned significant works by Steen, including the *Marriage at Cana* (1676, Pasadena, Norton Simon Museum), and his paintings were used more than once to illustrate articles in the *Nouvelle Iconographie de la Salpêtrière*.[152] The style of Hals's painting would certainly have been to Charcot's taste, and he may have felt a kinship with the Dutch master who was also a keen observer.

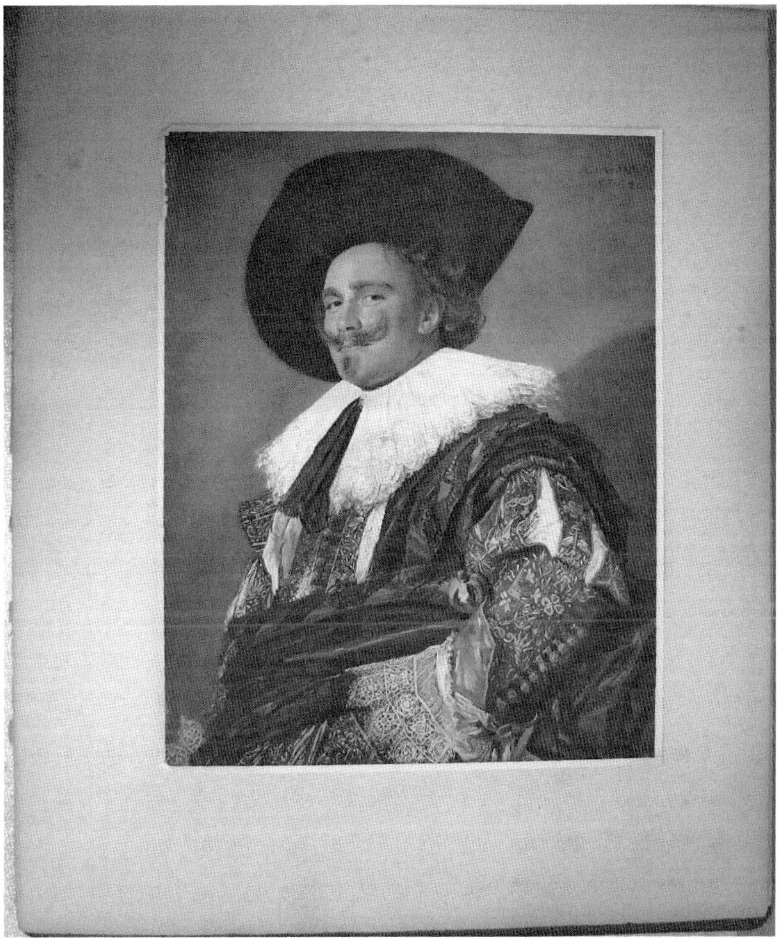

Fig. 23
Frans Hals (after), *Cavalier* (factual title), twentieth-century reproduction. Copy on paper. Located in Album 7 of the Musée Charcot anatomie pathologique. Paris, Musée de l'Assistance Publique–Hôpitaux de Paris. Inv. AP 2003.7.1.5. Photo: AP-HP/musée–author.

Charcot's focused attention while examining a patient's body was similar to the close looking required by the artist sketching a model or by the connoisseur studying a work of art. The neurologist believed that one of the keys to an accurate diagnosis was to view the (nude) body, which he often did in silence while patients were paraded before him.[153] According to Meige, Charcot exhorted clinicians to "look, to look again and to look always, it is only thus that one comes to *see*"—not unlike a teacher of the fine arts.[154] Let us recall the epiphany that Charcot had in front of Rubens's *Miracles of Saint Ignatius of Loyola*, as well as Charcot's and Richer's later lionization of that artist's "scrupulous observation of nature."[155]

The reproduction of the *Laughing Cavalier*, along with other examples from these albums, evinces an engagement with both the history and practices of art that seems incongruous in a clinical setting at the end of the nineteenth century. They also point to an equivalence between the albums and the museum itself, which also exhibited reproductions of artworks alongside clinical specimens. Many of the albums' images and the museum's objects are more successful at eliciting pathos than depicting pathology.[156] The shared origin of "pathos" and "pathology" in the emotions points to the Salpêtrière School's delight, or thrill, in the compulsive representation of ailing bodies that is also at odds with our conventional understanding of "objectivity" at the end of the nineteenth century. Hunter affirms this point: "Although medical men and artists emphasized the objectivity and reason of their realistic objects, whether in paint, wax, photography, or print, pleasure and subjectivity were a vital component of creating and collecting bodies."[157] Sappol, too, writes that the cabinet of curiosities and the anatomical museum "responded to and fostered a pleasure principle."[158] The albums in the Musée Charcot, as well as the museum itself, showcase the evident pleasure in collecting, categorizing, observing, rendering, and illustrating illness.

Anthropologist Nélia Dias comments that medical collections can be read "as the history of constant, regular and endless attempts to find adequate and accurate means to translate the real."[159] For Charcot and the members of the Salpêtrière School, one way to "translate the real" was with the help of the aesthetic or artistic. As we have seen, there are images in these albums that reveal very little about pathology, yet the *savants-artistes* clearly delighted in crafting them. Beautiful drawings in red chalk, comparisons to ancient sculpture, and delicately rendered portraits of patients actually tell us almost nothing about illness, but they do betray the clinician's interest in the aesthetic. The images in Charcot's "paper museum" are critically confounding—they point to the challenges or even impossibility of "fixing" illness in the visual but also to the revelatory potential of those same images. In their very resistance to being read, they tell us about Charcot's and the Salpêtrière clinicians' interests, desires, and pleasures. The albums they curated call for an intimate reading of the images, either by one observer or by a very few, sharing the experience as pages are turned. This is not the ordered logic of a medical case history but the seemingly haphazard assembly of a scrapbook. The volumes of the *Nouvelle Iconographie de la Salpêtrière* respond to the albums' disjointed coverage of neurological conditions. In fact, in the first line of volume 1, editors Paul Richer, Georges Gilles de la Tourette, and Albert Londe state that their intention in founding the journal was "to take advantage of the many illustrations that are added each day to the albums of the Salpêtrière."[160] The *Nouvelle Iconographie* served as an organizing framework to help them penetrate the albums' chaotic mass of images and tease out the clues and diagnoses that these clinicians suspected lay within. Freud reports a discussion with Charcot in which the elder clinician stated that, while theory is useful, "it doesn't prevent things from existing" (*ça n'empêche pas d'exister*).[161] What exists—what is representable—is not always evident or clear-cut.

Like the Musée Charcot itself, the albums ultimately tell us as much, if not more, about Charcot's research and artistic interests during his long career at the Salpêtrière as about the state of medicine at the end of the nineteenth century. These albums are not just a collection of pathologies but a dossier of particular interests. Like the cabinet of curiosities, their underlying conceit points to one individual. These albums were not compiled solely by Charcot, of course. And while I am attempting to recuperate the other contributors to these albums, the fact that these albums had Charcot's name on their covers only highlights the self-referential nature of the whole enterprise. These albums serve as a kind of portrait of Charcot himself.[162]

In a letter from 1879 sent to his wife from Italy, Charcot expressed privately a fear that his love of art was in tension with his talent for medicine. "For sure," he wrote, "if I had doctors in my family, I also had some painters. My heart is torn between the two."[163] And while one could argue that the images in the Musée Charcot albums similarly show a tension between artistry and objectivity, it might be more accurate to say that they testify to the fact that Charcot and his collaborators could not—and ultimately did not—have to choose between them. As Jordanova argues, "Anything in the cabinet-of-curiosities tradition has a particular epistemological status, because its purpose is to induce wonder, not to convey systematic scientific information."[164] The images in these albums also testify to the misery and pain experienced by many of the nameless or silent patients at the Salpêtrière. Perhaps the most profound characterization of the museum comes from Guillemot, who described the museum as the "sad archives of a suffering humanity."[165]

With the controversial clinician's unexpected death in 1893, the Musée Charcot's inherent and intimate association with its eponymous founder resulted in its decline, and its scientific artworks gradually disappeared from view.[166] While Charcot's brilliant neurological discoveries and experimental diagnostic tools would earn him worldwide renown during his life, many of his theories posthumously fell into disfavor.[167] Almost thirty years after his death, Léon Daudet would claim that Charcot's artistic legacy had overshadowed his clinical reputation, writing that "the great artist is favored over the great scientist."[168]

THE ART OF RETOUCHING AT THE SALPÊTRIÈRE

2

Retouching . . . can always alter truth.

—ALBERT LONDE, 1883

Critics described Brouillet's *A Clinical Lesson at the Salpêtrière* as realist, in part because of its photographic quality (see fig. 1). The purportedly objective medium of photography was frequently invoked as a basis for comparison with realist artworks, in which artists attempted to capture "snapshots" of modern life. Linda Nochlin argues that "it is part of Realist mythology" that the artist, like a camera, "produces his picture merely by looking at and recording what he sees."[1] At the time of the 1887 Salon, Gustave Ollendorf commented that it was as if Brouillet had left Charcot's lesson with "a precious instantaneous photograph" of the scene, while the critic for *L'Artiste* sneered that *Clinical Lesson* was nothing more than "a large painted photograph."[2]

In 1894, the year after Charcot's death, Fernand Levillain illustrated in *La Revue encyclopédique* a full-length photograph of Charcot by Albert Londe, head of the Salpêtrière's photographic service, and claimed that Brouillet had "copied [it] without modifications" (fig. 24).[3] The similarities between the photograph and the painting are striking: the angle of the head, the wave in the hair, the tensed hand, and the position of the body are all the same. Even the curve of his trousers along his left calf match in the two images, although Charcot's left leg is almost completely hidden behind the swooning figure of Blanche Wittmann; here the passages of paint are especially awkward and suggest that the artist struggled to create a convincing figure. One critic in 1887 noticed this and remarked that Charcot looked as if he was "drowning in his trousers and frock coat."[4] The shadow in the photograph that falls across the left side of Charcot's face and the highlights on his right hand also closely match those in Brouillet's painting. The criticism posed by critic Charles Ponsonhailhe—that in Brouillet's painting "all the actors are frozen"—does not seem far off the mark.[5] The use of a photographic portrait attests to Charcot's (or, at least, Londe's) collaboration in the making of this image and Charcot's desire to be the subject of a grand history painting; Richer's drawing of Brouillet in the act of painting this canvas demonstrates, too, that the members

Fig. 24
Photographie de Charcot ayant servi à Brouillet pour l'exécution de son tableau (Photograph of Charcot that Brouillet Used in the Making of His Painting). From F[ernand] Levillain, "Charcot et l'École de la Salpêtrière," *Revue encyclopédique* 4, no. 78 (March 1, 1894): 113. Photo © The British Library Board (P.P.4283.k.).

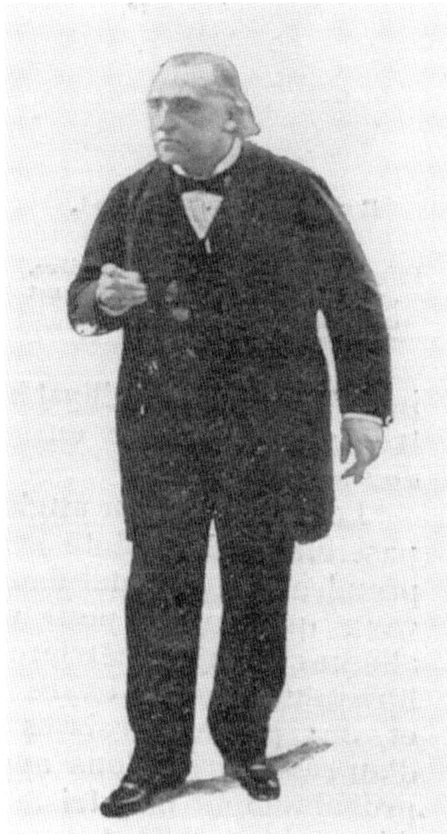

of the Salpêtrière School were involved in its creation.[6]

That Charcot would allow a photograph of himself to be used by Brouillet should not come as a surprise. As noted in the introduction, Charcot famously allied his own practice to the medium, stating, "I am absolutely nothing but the photographer [at the Salpêtrière]; I register [*inscris*] what I see"—even if he might have done so defensively.[7] The Salpêtrière was among the first hospitals to have its own photography studio; the Assistance Publique granted funds for its creation in 1878.[8] It seemed logical to annex a new casting studio to it, linking the two indexical media, and a M. Loreau headed both.[9] In 1882, Charcot hired the young "chemist" Albert Londe, who became director of the photography studio upon Loreau's departure from the hospital two years later, making him the first photographer in France to be paid an official salary for work as a researcher.[10] Londe would become an important theoretician and practitioner of photography as well as an inventor of cameras.[11] He collaborated with Étienne-Jules Marey around 1883 to create a new camera that used a clockwork mechanism to successively uncover its nine lenses arranged in a circle.[12] He also wrote extensively about the use of photography in medicine and predicted in *La Photographie médicale, application aux sciences médicales et physiologiques* (Medical photography: Application to medical and physiological sciences) (1893) that photography studios would soon be obligatory in all medical facilities.[13] In addition to other innovations in medical photography, he developed an electric camera that could capture a succession of images of a patient while allowing the doctor to remain by her side.[14] He followed Charcot by writing a manuscript on hysteria in art, which would have been illustrated with his photographs of paintings and prints.[15] In a lecture given to the Conservatoire national des Arts et Métiers in 1888, Londe cited the words of one of his contemporaries, the astronomer Pierre Janssen, that the photographic plate was the "retina of the scientist, but a retina quite superior to the human eye; because, on the one hand, it keeps the trace of the phenomenon that it has perceived and, on the other, in certain cases, it sees even more."[16] This philosophy led Londe to maintain two sophisticated studios inside the hospital and on the grounds.[17] There, the entirety of a hysterical attack could be conveniently snapped in a series of chronophotographs, or, through the use of tools and props such as gongs, hypnotized patients could be frozen into poses for easy photographing.[18] Judging a series of Londe's chronophotographs that captured the acrobatics of a nude male hysteric, Charcot used aesthetic criteria: "This whole part of the attack is, in the case of G . . . , perfectly beautiful, if I may put it that way. . . . You see that from the point of view of art, the images [of G . . .] leave nothing to be desired, but in addition they are for us very instructive."[19] For Charcot, then, the photos of hysterics had both clinical utility and artistic merit.

The history of the hysteria "epidemic" and Charcot's role in it are well rehearsed, and the many uses of photography at the Salpêtrière—both before and after Londe's arrival—have been explored in depth in the art-historical scholarship. In fact, the photographs produced by the hospital and published in the *Iconographie photographique de la Salpêtrière* (*IPS*) are the focus of most of the scholarship in the humanities on Charcot and his students. And while these photographs are sometimes erroneously attributed to Charcot himself or to Londe[20]—even though the latter arrived at the hospital *after* this journal ceased publication—it is well known that, under Charcot's direction, Désiré-Magloire Bourneville and Paul Regnard (1850–1927) were responsible for the *IPS*. As its title suggests, the *Iconographie photographique de la Salpêtrière* provided a photographic record of the disturbing, discomfiting, and sometimes provocative postures largely of hysterics, but also of epileptics, during an attack. Published in three volumes between approximately 1876 and 1880, it was one of the most important sources for images of hysteria in the late nineteenth century, inspiring novelists with its displays of erotic irrationality and supplying artists with a vast new visual lexicon with which to modernize their work.[21] The images of the *IPS* are so striking, often even spectacular, that they have largely monopolized scholars' attention, eclipsing the other significant and fascinating medical imagery and objects produced at the hospital that are discussed elsewhere in this book.

The attention paid to the hysterics Charcot studied—and to his influence on Freud—has led to a misidentification in much current scholarship of Charcot as a psychiatrist, or alienist, in the language of the day.[22] Significantly, Charcot thought hysteria was a neurological disorder, and it became one of his foci when the administration of the Salpêtrière decided to separate the hospital's population of hysterics and epileptics from those who were insane; the former were assigned to Charcot's medical service.[23] Charcot and Pierre Marie wrote about hysteria that "we do not know anything about its nature, nor about any lesions producing it; we know it only through its manifestations, and are therefore only able to characterize it by its symptoms, for the more hysteria is subjective, the more it is necessary to make it objective, in order to recognize it."[24] Charcot spent the last decades of his career focused on the visible signs of hysteria, while searching, without success, for a lesion in the nervous system that could explain it.

Louis Aragon and André Breton celebrated the photographs of Augustine—a "delicious" hysteric from the Salpêtrière whose image appeared in the second and third volumes of the *IPS*—in "Le Cinquantenaire de l'hystérie," published in *La Révolution*

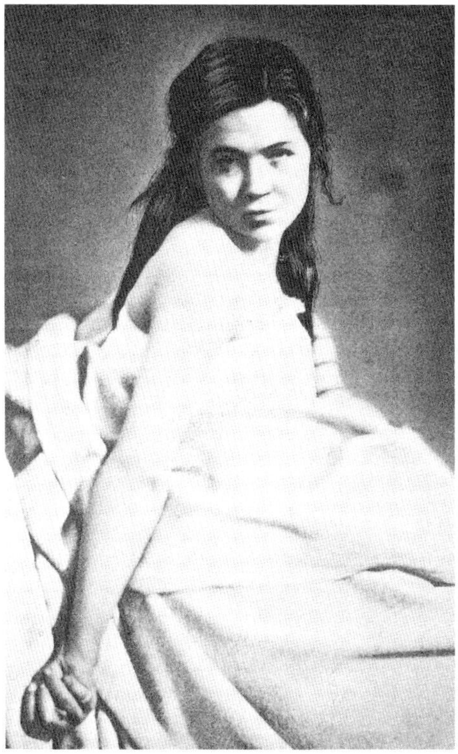

Fig. 25
Hystéro-épilepsie. Contracture (Hystero-Epilepsy: Contracture). From [Désiré-Magloire] Bourneville and P[aul] Regnard, *Iconographie photographique de la Salpêtrière*, vol. 2 (Paris: Bureau du Progrès médical / Adrien Delahaye, 1878), plate 30. Courtesy of the Wellcome Collection.

surréaliste in 1928. And while the Surrealists claimed that hysteria was "the greatest poetic discovery of the late nineteenth century,"[25] Georges Didi-Huberman instead asserted, in the book that ignited scholarly interest in the photographs taken at the Salpêtrière, that Charcot invented hysteria. In *Invention of Hysteria: Charcot and the Photographic Iconography of the Salpêtrière*, Didi-Huberman claims that the visual output of the hospital's laboratories and teaching spaces constructed the hysterical body as an image.[26] To put it another way, the hysteric was already an image—both at the Salpêtrière and in the public imagination—before her photograph was even taken.

Moreover, for Didi-Huberman, "photography was ideally positioned to crystallize the link between the fantasy of hysteria and the fantasy of knowledge."[27] By the 1870s, photography was an important tool in the positivist arsenal, but it had also facilitated the creation of a medical aesthetics, visible in the illustrations of, for instance, the *Revue photographique des hôpitaux de Paris*, of which Bourneville had been a co-founder and editor before working on the *IPS*. As an illness that relied on visual symptomatology for its diagnosis, hysteria lent itself to the photograph's ability for "foresight," in Didi-Huberman's words: photography seemed to both anticipate and then capture the postures of the hysterical attack.[28] Yet the theatrical poses that were caught on the photographic plate were often blurry, difficult to read, and enigmatic. They required both Bourneville's text in the *IPS* and later the synoptic table drawn and assembled by Paul Richer—in which many of the hysterics' poses in Regnard's photographs were copied and subsequently codified—to give them meaning (see fig. 28). According to Didi-Huberman, the practice of photography was both "factitious" and "in fact (irrefutable, even if contingent)"; at the Salpêtrière, photography too was "hysterical."[29] For him, the photographs are symptomatic of the machinations and manipulations at the heart of Charcot's enterprise and the spectacle of hysteria, which are the central concern of his book. He does not attend to the material qualities of the photographs themselves, which explains his lack of interest in the widespread use of retouching in the *Iconographie*. He only notes that some of the photographs of Augustine are retouched, such as one that, he claims, needed corrections because of "a ruined proof" and another in which the exposure time created a blurry image.[30]

One of the few scholars to discuss the retouching of these photographs is psychoanalyst Daphne de Marneffe, who compares the importance of the visual for Charcot and the verbal for Freud in how they understood and catalogued the (female) experience of hysteria. In "Looking and Listening: The Construction of Clinical Knowledge in Charcot and Freud," de Marneffe focuses on the photographs of Augustine from the second volume of the *IPS* and analyzes the ways in which they reify the usually chaotic physical signs of the hysterical attack (fig. 25).[31] It is worth quoting her insightful comments about the retouching at length:

> The use of painterly techniques to retouch his [Charcot's] photographs probably seemed a necessary enhancement rather than a selective distortion. The alignment of Augustine's photographs with representational traditions in art is effected through both the application of paint and the use of pose. A striking feature of the series taken as a whole is the liberal use of white paint or gouache on the surfaces of the drapery, and in some cases on Augustine's hair. Paint may have been applied in some cases to compensate for variable depth of field or badly focused shots; however, its application constitutes an aesthetic choice. . . . These images, ostensibly taken at the precise moment of a hysterical attack, look timeless. They are made weighty and solid, and Augustine, surrounded by her heavy drapery, is imbued with static permanence. The addition of paint creates a contrast in dimensions and surfaces that renders Augustine's skin comparatively soft and luminous. Her vitality becomes tender and seductive in juxtaposition with the painted fabric. The photographs belie the prevalent notion of hysteria as an illness almost defined by the changeability of its manifestations.[32]

De Marneffe rightly identifies the overarching role aesthetic criteria play in the retouching of Augustine's photographs, though in referring to them as "Charcot's" photographs she, like most other scholars who discuss these images, denies agency to Regnard. The corrections to the photographs do not generally serve to clarify a symptom, though they can sometimes be used to emphasize one: in plate 16, which shows Augustine in a "tetanic" state, the lines of white gouache on the pillow, sheets, and hospital gown draw the viewer's attention to the contractures of her face and hands. In the case of plate 28, the extensive retouching fashions a more three-dimensional body; however, the foreshortened right forearm clearly posed a challenge that was beyond the retoucher's skill (fig. 26). The clumsily redrawn hand creates a point of tension within the image, a sort of lacuna in the intended illusion where the photograph's inscription and the retoucher's (lack of) artistry clash.

In most cases the retouches add nothing to the medical meaning of the image but reinforce its art-historical derivation and aspiration. In plate 20 of the second volume of the *Iconographie*, for instance, Augustine looks up to heaven (fig. 27), the retouched whites of her eyes echoing the tearful gaze of Titian's *Penitent Magdalene* (1560s,

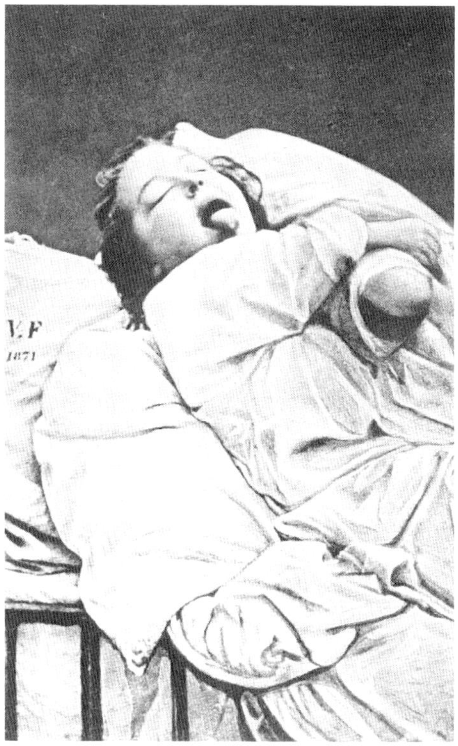

Fig. 26
Début d'une attaque. Cri (Beginning of an Attack: Scream). From [Désiré-Magloire] Bourneville and P[aul] Regnard, *Iconographie photographique de la Salpêtrière,* vol. 2 (Paris: Bureau du Progrès médical / Adrien Delahaye, 1878), plate 28. Courtesy of the Wellcome Collection.

Saint Petersburg, The State Hermitage Museum). White highlights flow down her long, unkempt hair and her hospital gown, giving a sculptural volume to her body while, like the Magdalene, emphasizing the garment that seems to be tantalizingly slipping off her shoulder. The retouched sheets gather around her waist like the Magdalene's shawl or a voluminous skirt, but instead of an ointment jar and a skull, Augustine's attribute is the asylum bed whose headboard is outlined behind her.

By the second volume of the *IPS*, in which Augustine's photographs first appear, both the photographs and the retouching exhibit a sophistication that is lacking in the comparatively amateurish first volume. This might in part explain the appeal of the photographs of Augustine, which also constitute one of the most complete sets of images presented of a given patient in the *Iconographie*. In the preface to this second volume from 1878, Bourneville and Regnard thank the director of the Assistance Publique for funding a photography studio at the Salpêtrière. They also comment on the introduction of photolithography in the current volume. "This process," they note, "thus gives all the guarantees of veracity inherent in the photograph, along with the advantages of impressions in greasy ink."[33] No doubt owing at least in part to the new dedicated studio at his disposal, Regnard's technique improved dramatically: in the second volume the lighting is more even, the patients more in focus, the background less distracting, and the retouching generally more polished.

This chapter will focus on the earlier photographs of volume 1 of the *Iconographie photographique de la Salpêtrière*, when Regnard was only beginning to learn his craft and when the aesthetic criteria applied to the images are far more visible. I look closely at photographs tipped into that first volume as well as a little-known volume of the *IPS* that appeared *earlier*, of which, as far as I know, there is only one extant copy.[34] Furthermore, I will examine an unpublished album of photographs taken by Regnard that has languished in the archives of the Assistance Publique—a working document between these two "first" volumes of the *IPS*.[35] The retouchings evident on the unpublished album's photographs and confirmed in writing on their versos raise profound questions about the "truthfulness" of the clinical photograph. They also cast in high relief the issues surrounding the purported objectivity of the photograph and, significantly, of the clinician (or clinicians) who commissioned the retouching. This unique document illuminates some of the decisions made by Regnard (and possibly also Bourneville and Charcot) in choosing the photographs for the widely disseminated first volume of the *IPS*—as well as why and how he manipulated them. The changes wrought on the photographs of hysterics and epileptics reveal outright indifference to the notion of "mechanical objectivity" at the Salpêtrière.

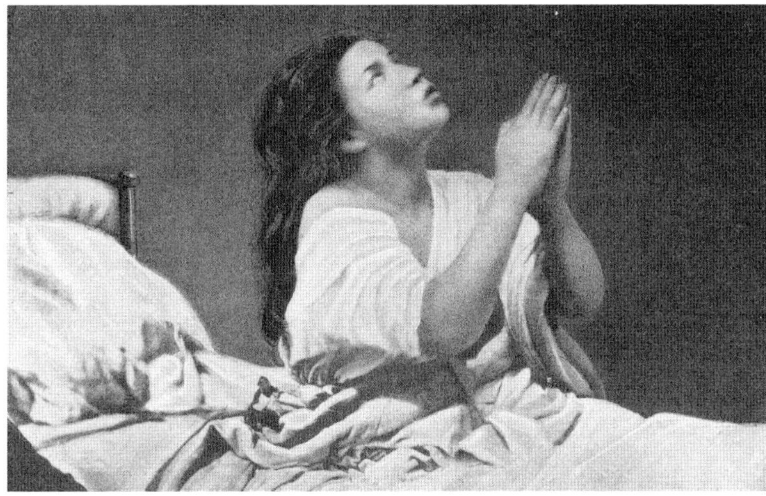

Fig. 27
Attitudes passionnelles. Supplication amoureuse (Passionate Attitudes: Amorous Supplication). From [Désiré-Magloire] Bourneville and P[aul] Regnard, *Iconographie photographique de la Salpêtrière*, vol. 2 (Paris: Bureau du Progrès médical / Adrien Delahaye, 1878), plate 20. Courtesy of the Wellcome Collection.

The Prehistory of the *Iconographie photographique de la Salpêtrière*

The medical profession understood the potential value of photography from its beginnings. In 1840 the invention of photomicrography by Alfred Donné of the Charité hospital in Paris brought the "industrial process" to the service of medicine, allowing the scientist to capture and preserve images otherwise invisible to the naked eye.[36] About ten years later, photography was used for the first time for comparative medical records in France and Germany.[37] Most famously, in the middle of the nineteenth century, Hugh Welch Diamond began to photograph the women under his care in the Surrey County Asylum, establishing what would become a long tradition of portraiture of the insane.[38] Not coincidentally, Diamond was the resident superintendent of the asylum and founding member of the Royal Photographic Society of London, a fact that attests to the close links between medicine and photography at the time. The well-known comments Diamond made in 1856 to the Royal Society of Medicine are instructive, because many of the values that he attributed to photography were still current twenty years later, when the camera entered the Salpêtrière. Diamond's address was about the "peculiar application of Photography" at the asylum, which allowed the doctor "to listen, with the picture before him, to the silent but telling language of nature."[39] He emphasized the particular efficacy of the photograph to "confirm and extend" any written or verbal description.[40] More importantly, he underlined the "unerring accuracy" of the photograph, which provided a "perfect and faithful record" of mental illness.[41] By the time the Salpêtrière volumes were published, then, there was an established tradition of medical portrait photography.

The photograph's indexicality purportedly assured that what was captured was "an unmediated transcription of the real."[42] By indexicality, I mean of course that it is a direct transcription, made "naturally," without human intervention. The simplest example of an indexical trace is a footprint in the sand. The photographic process—light bouncing off an object, captured by chemicals on a negative—was thought to be equally indexical. The impartiality of the camera was lauded by a Reverend H. J. Morton in an article from 1864 entitled "Photography as an Authority": "The camera's eye of microscopic minuteness and exactness of vision, has behind it a crystal plate that has no partiality, and the fingers of the sun that paint the pictures which that crystal surface bears, are vibrations from a great burning heart that throbs with no human passions."[43] In fact, as Peter Hamilton explains, in the nineteenth century "the term 'photography' itself was widely used as a synonym of objective knowledge."[44] And while the camera as scientific tool gave the illusion of total objectivity, what was captured on the photographic plate could similarly be considered objective "evidence." In the words of Elizabeth Edwards, "The role of photography was to create 'virtual witnesses' of scientific observation, and of the creation of scientific fact."[45] Duchenne de Boulogne, Charcot's mentor and friend, confirms its role as witness when he writes in relation to his experiments that photography "will permit readers to attend, so to speak, my electro-physiological experiments, and to judge the worth of the conclusions that I draw from them."[46] Photography was generally touted as an exact, modern, and objective transmitter of knowledge, with medical photography in particular exhibiting demonstrable, repeatable truths, useful in diagnosing symptoms.

However, the prevailing discourse was often undermined by photographic innovators, scientists, and even members of the general public. As scholars like Marta Braun, Tania Cleaves, Josh Ellenbogen, Robin Kelsey, Katherine Rawling, and others have shown, the reality of photographic practice problematized any sense of its being unmediated or objective. The physiologist Étienne-Jules Marey, for instance, created chronophotographs of human and animal movement that produced images impossible to see with the naked eye; Marey himself called chronophotography "an artifice."[47] Kelley Wilder has similarly written about physicist Henri Becquerel's photographs, in which he attempted to make radioactivity "perceptible."[48] In her important article "Camera Medica," Erin O'Connor asserts that the camera—a "mindless eye"—is indiscriminate and that medical photography, therefore, "centres its truth claims in its technical insipidity" rather than in objectivity.[49] André Gunthert has reiterated in several texts that photography is not a "'natural image' but an image in which nature has been constructed."[50] Photography's publics also play a central role in our understanding of the nineteenth-century context. Tanya Sheehan and Jennifer Tucker have both demonstrated that photography's role as "witness" was not taken as a given in the nineteenth century; instead, not only did its authority need to be constructed through a belief in the skills of its makers but it could easily be lost as the image moved between different domains and publics.[51]

While photographs are the best-known images from the Salpêtrière, some scholars have rightly suggested that Charcot was not a keen advocate of photography; as the discussion of the Musée Charcot albums in chapter 1 demonstrates, he saw it as one useful tool among many.[52] Perhaps because of the especially enigmatic nature of hysteria, he and his protégés chose photography, that most "objective" medium, to illustrate published case studies of epileptics and hysterics. Hysteria's irregular symptomatology, which included paralysis, convulsions, and fainting, had puzzled doctors since the

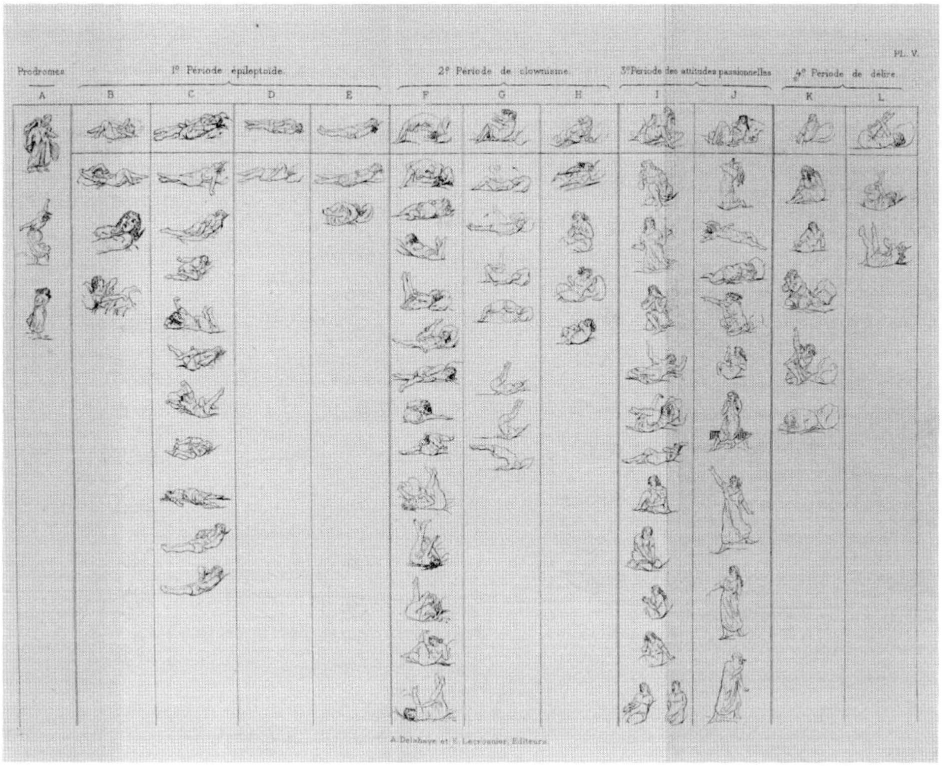

Fig. 28
Paul Richer, *Un tableau synoptique de la grand attaque hystérique . . .* (*A Synoptic Table of the Hysterical Attack . . .*). From Paul Richer, *Études cliniques sur la grande hystérie ou hystéro-épilepsie*, 2nd ed. (Paris: Adrien Delahaye & Emile Lecrosnier, 1885), plate 5. Copyright of The University of Manchester.

time of Hippocrates.[53] Paul Richer was the first to visually classify the hysterical attack in an orderly and supposedly universal progression of postures (fig. 28). This stark mapping demonstrated Charcot's and the Salpêtrière School's belief in the principle of the archetype: by dividing the disease into stages and cataloguing and photographing the potential postures of each, they hoped to create a universal diagnostic model. Photography thus proved useful for them not only as a visual means of recording the phases of the hysterical attack but also as a way of validating their own diagnoses, which some claimed were invented—in fact, as noted previously, Charcot responded to such accusations of fraud by stating that he was "absolutely nothing" but a photographer.

In the first half of the 1870s, before the camera had formally entered the Salpêtrière, Désiré-Magloire Bourneville, one of Charcot's most promising collaborators, asked a professional photographer to capture images of the epileptics and hysterics at the hospital. He was soon frustrated by the results. "Often, by the time the photographer [*opérateur*] arrived, everything was over," Bourneville remarked. "In order to realize the goal that we had set for ourselves," he continued, "we needed to have at hand at the Salpêtrière itself a man who knew photography and was devoted enough to be ready to respond to our call each time circumstances demanded it."[54] As Beatriz Pichel puts it, "the camera chased the patient" at the Salpêtrière.[55] Paul Regnard, one of Charcot's *internes*, began to take the photographs that would eventually illustrate the first volume of the *Iconographie photographique de la Salpêtrière* in 1876. The "contingent instance of deviance," to borrow Allan Sekula's phrase, would thereby be captured and put on display for both the international medical readers of the *IPS* and the popular audience that would see reproductions of its images in other sources.[56]

It is not well known that Bourneville and Regnard published an album of photographs of hysterics and epileptics, also entitled *Iconographie photographique de la Salpêtrière*, in 1875, one year *before* the first volume of the *IPS*.[57] This earlier volume does not contain explanatory text, only headings and eighty-seven unretouched photographs; the focus on images would explain why Regnard's name takes precedence over Bourneville's on the title page. The only extant copy of this album of photographs of which I am aware was in Charcot's personal collection, now part of the historical Bibliothèque Charcot collection at the Salpêtrière.[58] For clarity, I will call it the IPS Album, in order to distinguish it from the better-known first volume of the *Iconographie*.

There is a third tome that is critical to this discussion: a handmade album in the Archives of the Assistance Publique–Hôpitaux de Paris (hereafter the Archives Album), most of whose photographs are reproduced in the same order as the IPS Album. Yet the retouchings visible on their surfaces do not make an appearance until the so-called first volume of the *IPS* (which I will refer to as Volume I), where some of these photographs are repeated, sometimes heavily retouched, and accompanied by textual case studies. In the transition from the IPS Album to the widely disseminated Volume I, an important change occurred: instead of being self-evident demonstrations of disease, the photographs became illustrations for the clinical notes. Bourneville and Regnard recount the process in the preface to that first volume: "We had composed an album of a hundred [*sic*] photographs and perhaps we would have stopped ourselves there, if our excellent teacher M. Charcot, who followed our clinical work and our photographic essays with his usual benevolence, had not encouraged us to publish the observations we had gathered in the wards, illustrating them with photographs taken by M. Regnard."[59] Therefore, the Archives Album is a transitional document between the IPS Album and the published first volume of the *Iconographie*—a working document in which Bourneville and Regnard experimented with editing the photographs through retouching (and also cropping), their decisions visible in what was left in or taken out of Volume I. Along with the instructions to the retoucher on the verso of several of the pages in the Archives Album, the state of the prints, made from glass plates using the wet collodion process, situates the Archives Album between the IPS Album and Volume I.[60] For example, a provocative photograph of Mlle. Marcillet, in which the aureole of her breast is just visible next to her contracted hand, is included in all three tomes (figs. 29–31). By the time the first volume of the *IPS* was published, the glass negative had cracked, leaving the trace of a sinuous line running over the patient's face in the top third of the photograph. The prints in the IPS Album and the Archives Album do not display this crack and must, therefore, predate Volume I.

The Archives Album is octavo size, as is the *IPS*. It is divided into four sections: the first on hysterics (which is not labeled), then "Epilepsy/Physiognomy," "Epilepsy/Epileptic Insanity," and "Varia" at the end. It contains seventy-five photographs in total (six of which are repeated), pasted onto hard, thick pages. It is unclear at what

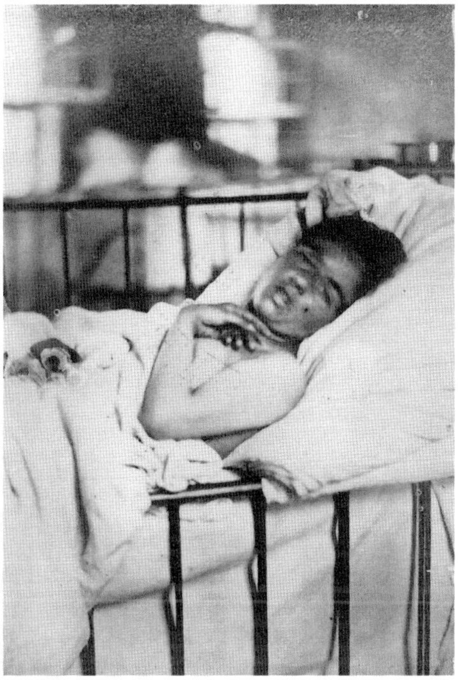

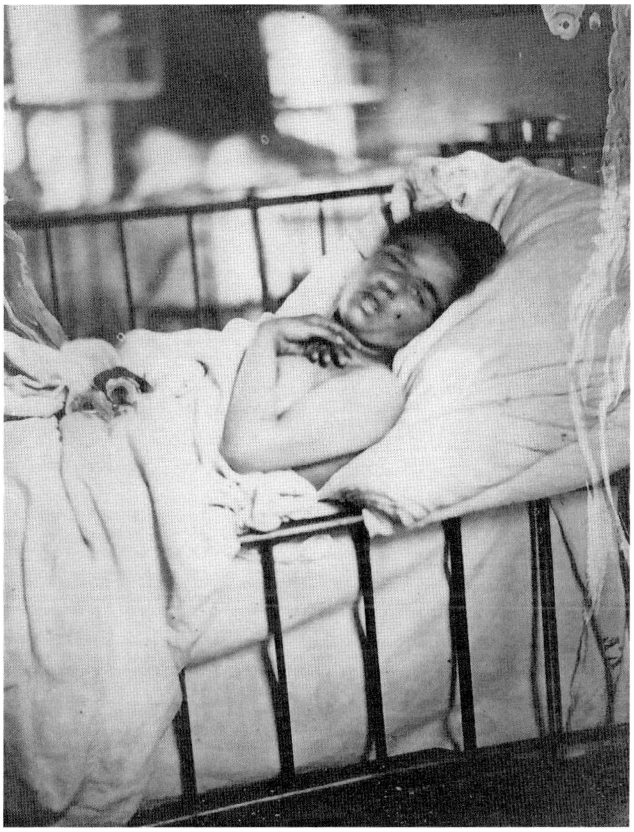

Fig. 29 (above)
Photograph of Mlle. Marcillet from Paul Regnard and [Désiré-Magloire] Bourneville, *Iconographie photographique de la Salpétrière* [*sic*], *Service de M. Charcot* ([Paris], 1875), n.p. Paris, Bibliothèque Charcot. Courtesy of the Bibliothèque Charcot, Bibliothèque de Sorbonne Université. Photo: author.

Fig. 30 (above right)
HYSTERO EPILEPSIE *Marcillet Contracture* (HYSTERO-EPILEPSY *Marcillet Contracture*). Photograph from Album 646 FOSS 5. Paris, Archives de l'Assistance Publique–Hôpitaux de Paris. Courtesy of the Archives de l'Assistance Publique–Hôpitaux de Paris. Photo: author.

Fig. 31 (right)
Hystéro-épilepsie: Contracture permanente (*Hystero-Epilepsy: Permanent Contracture*). Albumen print. From [Désiré-Magloire] Bourneville and P[aul] Regnard, *Iconographie photographique de la Salpétrière* [*sic*], vol. 1 (Paris: Bureau du Progrès médical / Adrien Delahaye, 1877), plate 28. Courtesy of the Wellcome Collection.

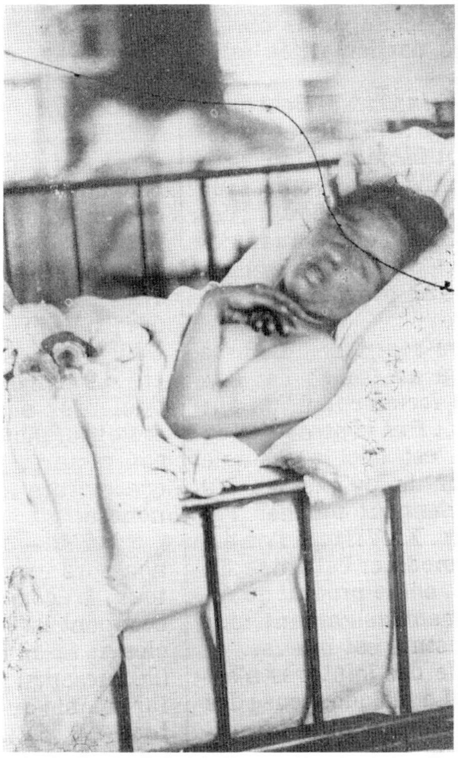

stage the album was bound. Underneath many of the photographs are printed labels with the name of the disorder, the stage of the hysterical attack, and/or the surname of the patient, which indicates that this was indeed a "private" document, as surnames were abbreviated in published case studies. Seven of the pages have handwritten notes on the verso that give instructions to the retoucher. Others have crosses underneath the photographs written in blue pencil and/or numbers that indicate plate numbers in future *IPS* volumes.[61] Photographs that have a red X written in pencil underneath were all included in Volume I; these are mostly images of the hysteric Geneviève Legrand. Images from the Archives Album account for twenty-two of the thirty-nine plates of Volume I of the *Iconographie*—more than half. Some pages have pinholes at their edges and even traces of tacks at their corners, evidence of their informal use at the hospital. With only two exceptions, all of the photographs also appear in the earlier IPS Album. Many of the photographs have been retouched, including some without instructions on their versos.

The photographs in the Archives Album vary significantly in quality. Many were taken outside in order to take advantage of the bright sunlight; we thus see hysterics during an attack lying on the rough cobblestones with bars on the windows behind them.[62] Many are out of focus, with visible cracks in the negatives and stains on the prints. It is not a coincidence that retouching was introduced at the same time as Bourneville's lengthy case histories: suddenly the photographs needed to compete with the written word. The fact that the photographs came first means that they tend to "interrupt" the flow of the text and create moments of disjunction.[63] Some photographs display an uneasy beauty, like the striking image of Thérèse Laugier, an "ordinary hysteric," according to Bourneville (fig. 32).[64] The straight lines of the windowpanes and headboard echo the foreshortened cross of the straitjacket on her chest and contrast with the sinuous folds of the sheet in the foreground. Her face is seen in profile, brightly lit and framed by her long hair, while the edge of the pillow behind her head mirrors the curve of her jaw. Laugier died at the age of twenty-two of pulmonary tuberculosis within a year of this photograph being taken, her autopsy results detailed in the case notes in Volume I of the *IPS*.[65] These photographs therefore also raise questions about agency, ethics, and the unequal power dynamics at play between patient and clinician-photographer, even if the theatricality evident in later photographs, such as those of Augustine in the second volume of the *Iconographie*, are mostly missing here. Joseph Delboeuf reported after his visit to the Salpêtrière that "the young women to whom I have spoken complain about the abuse of their images.... But when we get to the bottom of things, this abuse is more imaginary than real. Who, outside the scientific world, will be interested in these precious case studies with such grim text?"[66]

My goal in this chapter is to work through the issues specifically related to the retouching of these medical photographs. By attending to these material changes, I want to begin to answer Sabine Kriebel, who asks, "How does matter mean? How do the material and physical processes of different photographic practices contribute to the meaning of the image represented? How are politics and culture imbricated in its very form?"[67] This album exposes the pervasive practice of extensively retouching photographs under Charcot's supervision, which belies his declarations of the clinician's objectivity. Instead of attempting to reconcile these tensions, I tease out some of the issues inherent in them.

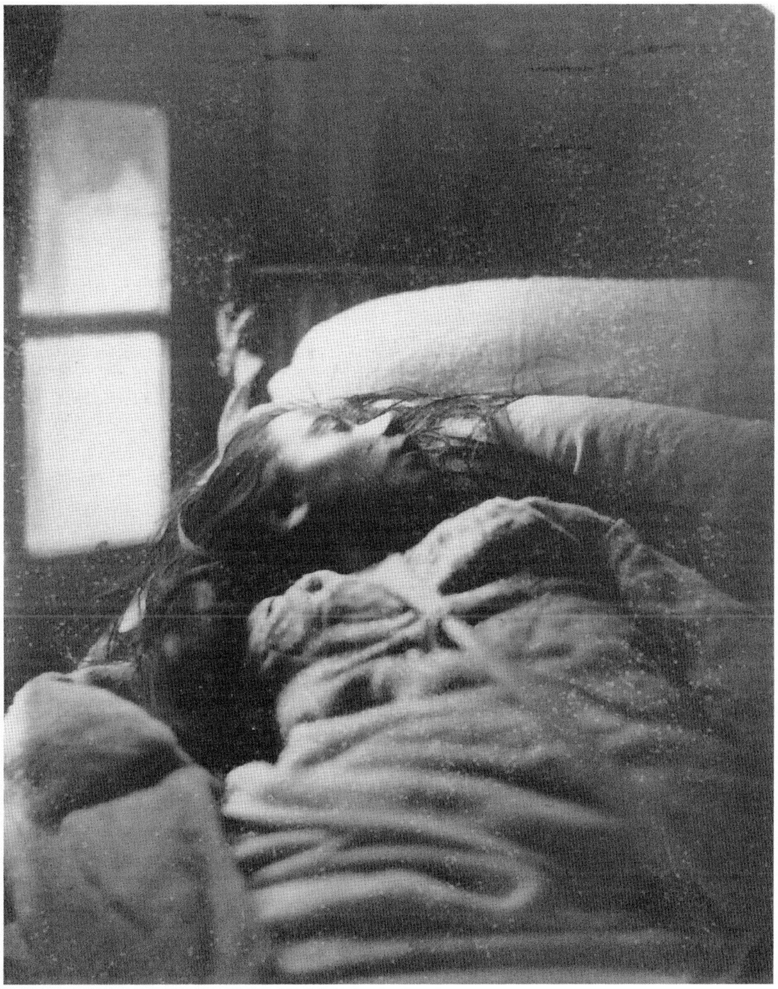

Fig. 32
HYSTERO EPILEPSIE Laugier (*HYSTERO-EPILEPSY Laugier*). Photograph from Album 646 FOSS 5. Paris, Archives de l'Assistance Publique–Hôpitaux de Paris. Courtesy of the Archives de l'Assistance Publique–Hôpitaux de Paris. Photo: author.

An Occluded History

According to photography historian André Gunthert, retouching is "a practice without a history."[68] He continues, "A lying practice, in which the aim is to not appear as such, it is also a shameful practice, since the condition that allows it contains simultaneously the negation of its intervention. . . . Without being strictly speaking secret, retouching displays the special feature of being a practice that is systematically denied."[69] The implications of the manipulation of photographic images were passionately debated from the moment Munich photographer Franz Hampfstängl exhibited a portrait "before" and "after" retouching at the Universal Exposition in Paris in 1855, only sixteen years after the birth of the medium.[70] The newly founded Société française de photographie immediately hosted a heated argument on the subject in the pages of its inaugural *Bulletin*. While Paul Périer argued that the "absolute perfection" of the end result trumped the means, Eugène Durieu, president of the Société, decried the "fetishism" of retouching, claiming that each medium needed to use tools that were appropriate to itself. Retouching was "foreign" to photography, according to Durieu, and called into question the "exactitude" and "sincerity" that gave the photographic print its "particular interest."[71]

Anxiety about retouching was an issue especially for medical photography, as any manipulation could have an impact on its evidential value. In *Mécanisme de la physionomie humaine* (1862), Duchenne de Boulogne wrote that photography was "as faithful as the mirror," for instance, but he added that "in order not to leave any doubt as to the accuracy of the facts shown in the photographs, I wanted no retouching done to them."[72] Yet, according to Martin Kemp, retouching was a widespread practice in the middle of the nineteenth century, especially in anatomical images, to aid legibility or to direct the reader's gaze. He cites the case of Munich anatomist Nicolaus Rüdinger, whose *Atlas des peripherischen Nervensystems des menschlichen Körpers* (Atlas of the peripheral nervous system of the human body) (Munich, 1861) was illustrated with photographs so heavily retouched that they were "virtually handmade prints."[73] In her discussion of astronomical photographs in the Victorian period, Jennifer Tucker argues that retouching was acceptable scientific protocol "under certain conditions, such as the failure to reproduce accurately."[74]

By the 1870s, when the *IPS* volumes were published, retouching was common practice in portrait photography. New lenses introduced in the 1860s were "capable of an unprecedented clarity," which meant that the most minor imperfections emerged as glaring flaws.[75] To paraphrase Charles Baudelaire's caustic take on the photography-loving public, Narcissus rushed to contemplate his image, only to be disappointed with his reflection.[76] One nineteenth-century author warned of the pervasiveness of retouching with this anecdote: "If someone returns his photograph and points out to the photographer that he is sixty and not thirty, that he has wrinkles on his forehead and folds on his chin, as well as hollow cheeks and a flat nose that bears no resemblance to the aquiline nose that the portrait has given him, he is certain to receive the following response: 'Oh! you wanted a portrait that looks like you. You should have told us so. How could we have guessed!'"[77] For example, the wrinkles and harsh shadows visible in the rejected photograph of French writer and activist "Gyp" (the comtesse de Martel) by Paul Nadar from 1891 were removed in the obviously approved portrait on the left (fig. 33). The curve of the sitter's left shoulder was also softened, as were the shadows on her neck and collarbone. The retoucher also adjusted her bodice in order to reduce the size of her bust and removed some stray hairs from her updo. The retouching gives Gyp a more youthful appearance and creates a more polished image. In *A Complete Treatise on the Art of Retouching Photographic Negatives* from 1886, Robert Johnson discussed the professional dilemma facing the retoucher of portraits of middle-aged women: "If you do not make them youthful enough you may offend, and if you do make them youthful you may offend." He concluded that "it is perhaps advisable to err (if at all) in the direction of youth."[78]

The "shameful" practice of retouching can be traced if one looks at texts primarily aimed at amateurs. A book called *Concise Instructions in the Art of Retouching* (1876) by Burrows and Colton, for instance, published contemporaneously with the *IPS*, instructs the amateur on techniques for "hand-work," as retouching was also called in Britain. Once the negative is positioned on the retouching desk, the amateur is urged to "fill in all irregular and transparent spots and lines . . . , giving to these spots and lines the same value as the surrounding portions of the forehead, beginning at the point of highest light."[79] The face could thereby be made smooth and untarnished by blemishes or wrinkles, and the retouching would be imperceptible in the photographic print. A guide by a M. Bech from 1888 recounts that the art of retouching was by then universally understood as the "necessary complement of photography."[80] And, in that same year, C. Klary critiqued the anti-retouching brigade in *L'Art de retoucher les*

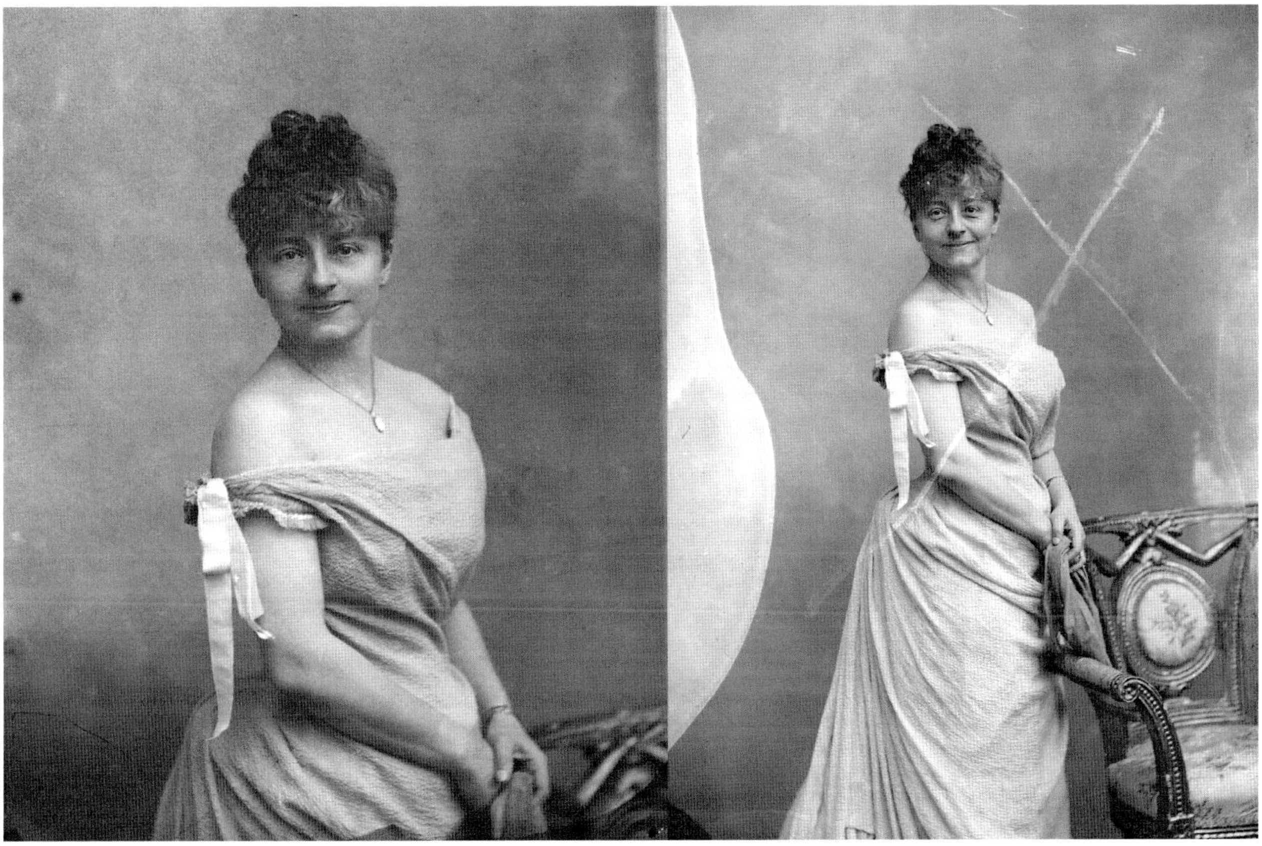

Fig. 33
Paul Nadar, *Marie-Antoinette de Riqueti de Mirabeau, comtesse de Martel (dite Gyp)*, 1891. Charenton-le-Pont, Médiathèque de l'Architecture et du Patrimoine. Inv. NA23811047. Photo © Ministère de la Culture–Médiathèque du Patrimoine, Dist. RMN-Grand Palais / Atelier de Nadar.

négatifs photographiques (The art of retouching photographic negatives) (1888), stating rhetorically that "a photographer accustomed to noticing the different effects produced will immediately see that, in terms of the strength of light and shadow, the darkroom does not always give us the truth."[81] In manipulating the "truth" of the image, retouching, it seems, shifted the photograph from the realm of science to that of art. In fact, in his retouching manual of 1886, Johnson seems to suggest just that in comparing the retouched portrait with a scientific image: "A photograph, to be a likeness of a person, need not be an anatomical diagram of the subject."[82]

Many handbooks on retouching were published in these years, though none specifically about medical photography. One reason for this is that medical photography laid claim to objectivity and truth, which distinguished it from the art of portrait photography, the kind discussed in these manuals. However, medical photography and portrait photography shared common origins. Some of the first medical photographs, notably those from the American Civil War, utilized the conventions of the portrait studio. This is unsurprising, given that doctors would take their patients to portrait photographers to have their picture taken.[83] Soldiers awkwardly displayed their injuries in spaces with ornate furnishings and heavy curtains and sometimes stood in front of embellished mirrors that also revealed wounds on the backs of their bodies. (It is also worth noting that the "collodion" used in the wet-plate process came from medicine—it was derived

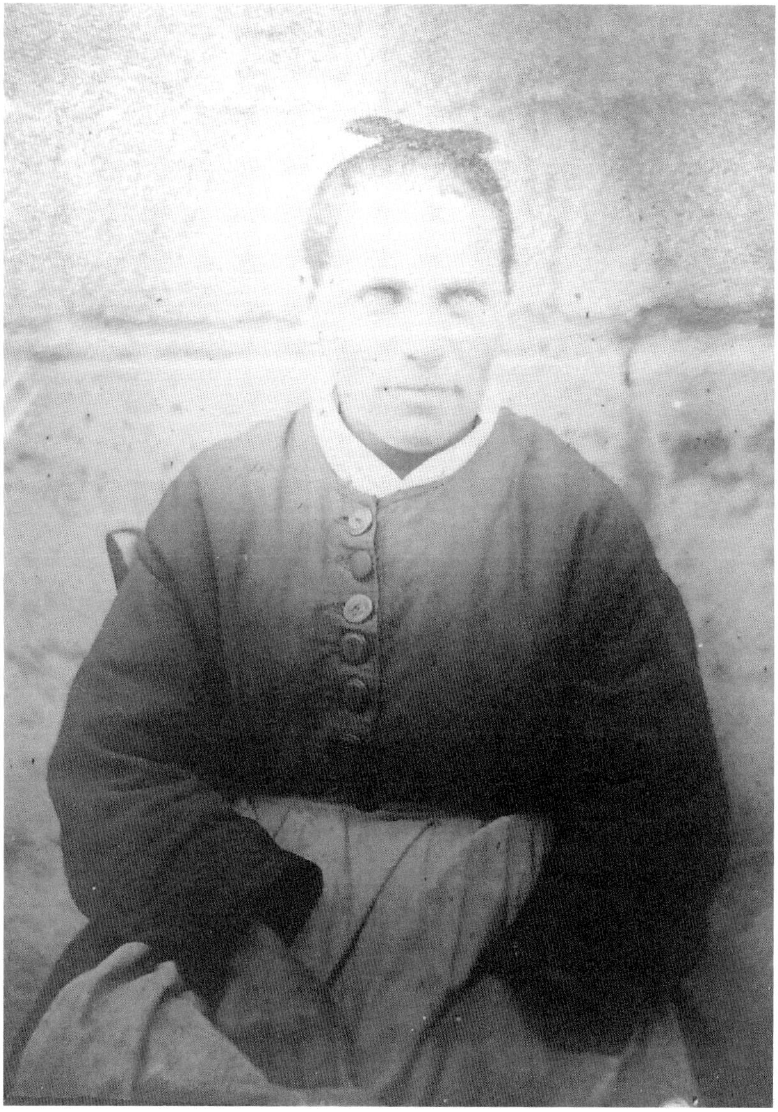

Fig. 34
Photograph from Paul Regnard and [Désiré-Magloire] Bourneville, *Iconographie photographique de la Salpétrière* [sic]. *Service de M. Charcot* ([Paris], 1875), n.p. Paris, Bibliothèque Charcot. Courtesy of the Bibliothèque Charcot, Bibliothèque de Sorbonne Université. Photo: author.

from guncotton, which was a type of dressing for protecting wounds.)[84] The conventions of portrait photography continued to influence medical photography after it left the studio and entered the asylum: Kemp notes that "it was the accepted nature of the conventions that permitted the attentive viewer to determine where postures and expressions departed from the decorous norm."[85]

The Embellished Objective

The individual case studies published in the *Iconographie photographique de la Salpêtrière* always begin with a photograph of the patient displaying "normal physiognomy," a "before" that foreshadows the "after."[86] Kemp's comments are apposite here: in the photograph of an unnamed patient from the IPS Album, the somewhat formal pose seems in keeping with a conventional portrait, but the rough stone wall behind her and the oddly frank—and therefore disquieting—expression are not only unthinkable in a conventional portrait photograph but also seem to predict the dis-ease in the clinical photographs that follow (fig. 34). While the bottom half of her chest, sleeves, and arms are obscured in shadow, her eyes almost disappear into her pale face, which glows in an overexposed aureole. Melissa Miles writes about the methodological usefulness of this "excessive light," which "floods through the camera's aperture, overwhelms the dark chamber within, bounces off its lens and interior surfaces, and leaves a trace of that disruptive movement on the surface of the photograph. The notion that light both bridges and sustains the difference between the 'real,' the camera and the photograph is exposed as a myth, and light becomes the means by which these formerly distinct terms are produced and interconnected."[87] This photograph thus serves as an appropriate entrée into this discussion of retouching at the Salpêtrière, as it reveals the artifice inherent in *every* photograph. I mean "artifice" here in three distinct ways: the "making of something by art or skill"; in its opposition to "nature or a natural phenomenon"; and "a manoeuvre or device intended to deceive."[88] Once we no longer see the photograph as a "transparent envelope,"[89] the ways in which it is constructed—the ways in which light as "an unpredictable force or provocation . . . incites, produces and enables photographic histories, theories and practices"—come to the fore.[90]

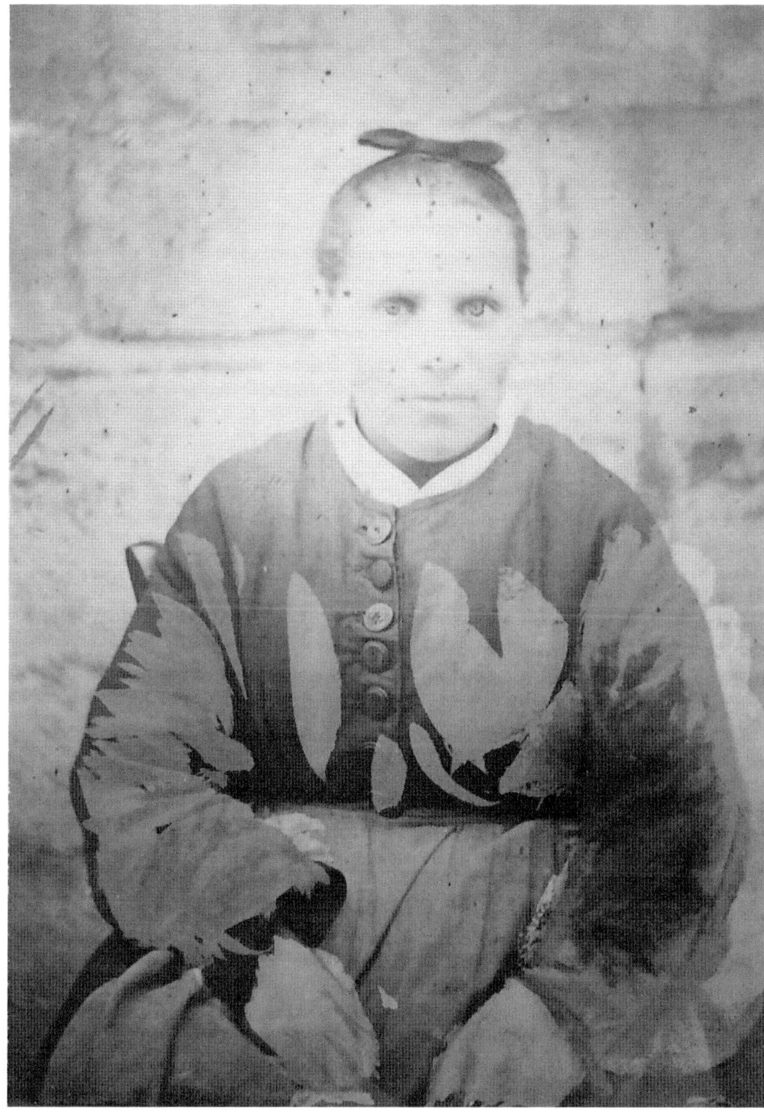

Fig. 35
Photograph from Album 646 FOSS 5. Paris, Archives de l'Assistance Publique–Hôpitaux de Paris. Courtesy of the Archives de l'Assistance Publique–Hôpitaux de Paris. Photo: author.

In the Archives Album, this patient's eyes are especially pronounced: dark semicircles with uneven edges make up the iris and tiny black dots pinpoint the pupils (fig. 35). The obscured hands and sleeves have been lightened to such an extreme that they now appear as bleached-out areas that bleed into the patient's apron and the stone wall behind her. In an attempt to correct the overzealous retouching, her left sleeve has been drawn in, as have her hands. The fingers of her left hand, nesting in her apron, are awkwardly sketched, appearing cartoonlike. The retoucher has inexpertly followed the instructions on the verso of the page: "Lighten the bottom of the clothes and the hands a little / accentuate the eyes in the feeling of the gaze [*le sentiment du regard*]."[91] How does the retouching emphasize the "feeling of the gaze"? And why would the Salpêtrière clinicians have been interested in communicating it in this photograph of the patient before an attack? The retouched eyes certainly make the patient's gaze more direct, but the absence of detail in the rest of her face makes it more disturbing. The demonic blankness of her expression is appropriate—as we know, Charcot theorized that the possessed of the past were the hysterics of the present.

The inexperienced retoucher has disfigured the patient's hands, dress, and face. The large unnatural patches across her body demonstrate that the instruction to "lighten" has been taken too far. Burrows and Colton warned the amateur retoucher about working an unvarnished negative: "Not being thoroughly accustomed to this work, he is constantly making mistakes, or finds when his negative is printed that he has done *too much* upon it, which will have to be removed. Upon the varnish this can be done by reabrasion of the surface . . . ; but upon the unvarnished picture it is not such an easy matter, and in many instances cannot be done."[92] It is possible that in this early example, the

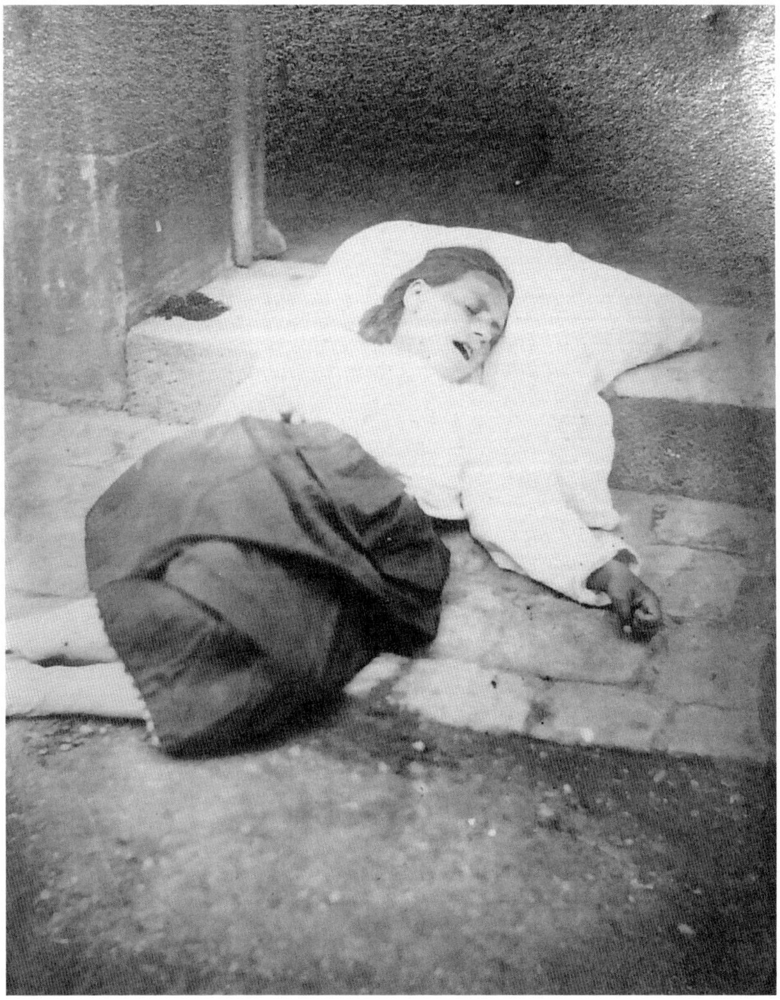

Fig. 36
Photograph from Paul Regnard and [Désiré-Magloire] Bourneville, *Iconographie photographique de la Salpétrière* [*sic*]. *Service de M. Charcot* ([Paris], 1875), n.p. Paris, Bibliothèque Charcot. Courtesy of the Bibliothèque Charcot, Bibliothèque de Sorbonne Université. Photo: author.

negative was unvarnished. The botched redrawing of the patient's hands and left sleeve were clearly an attempt to repair the damage. The hapless retoucher's difficulties with this image likely explain its exclusion from Volume I of the *Iconographie*. Presumably Regnard himself tried his hand at retouching and struggled with the fragile medium. The dubious repairs and improvements point to inexperience, as do the myriad cracks in the glass plates that are visible in these prints.

Another photograph from the IPS Album that did not appear in Volume I of the *Iconographie* shows a patient who seems to be moving into the so-called crucified posture typical of the "passionate attitudes" phase of the hysterical attack (fig. 36). She lies on the ground, a large pillow wedged between her and the hard stone step that supports her upper back, neck, and head. Her left hand, clenched into a fist by a hysterical contracture and looking as stonelike as the slabs it rests on, is the only part of the photograph that is clearly in focus. Her body is oddly foreshortened, the coarse material of her skirt having ridden up to obscure her lower torso. The photographer has awkwardly cut off the patient's stockinged feet at the left edge of the photograph and overexposed her face, her white top, and the pillow; the latter two have no definition. The retoucher has been instructed to "make some folds in the blouse" and has followed the recommendation in Paul Piquepé's *Traité pratique de la retouche* (Practical treatise on retouching, 1881) to reinforce the shadows on light fabrics "without fear."[93] But these manipulations, visible in the photograph in the Archives Album, dematerialize part of her body and make her torso look impossibly short (fig. 37).

For the photograph showing Mlle. Hellouin in the hysterical stage of "lethargy," the instructions read, "retouch the figure in order to remove the black dots / redo the linen [*le linge*] and the hands a little."[94] This was necessary because the photographer's soft focus on the patient's face and the very shallow depth of field resulted in the ghostly appearance of her hands in the foreground of the image (fig. 38). His inexperience also led to a chip in the glass plate on her right hand, an overexposed dot near the photograph's bottom edge, and speckles on the patient's face, marred further by inexpert preliminary retouching. In the "final" retouched photograph in the Archives Album, in which more of the original negative is visible, the instructions were followed—but clearly much more was done (fig. 39). Hellouin's hands and nails are coarsely outlined, effectively effacing the flesh below. The retoucher has removed the dots from the patient's visage and has attempted to improve the definition of her chin, lips, left cheek, closed eyelids, eyebrows, and hair, as well as the edge of the pillow. The lines suggesting creases in the thick fabric that covers her body, perhaps an unfastened straitjacket, are poorly executed and counterproductive. These retouches do more to highlight the photograph's two-dimensionality than create the illusion of a body underneath. Rather than lending it substance, they have eliminated it. Moreover, we can see that the photograph in the Archives Album has crop marks, which reveal that a closer view of the patient was desired. The cropping would have removed the dark space above her head and much of her badly rendered left hand, as well as most of the overexposed dot near the bottom edge. Erased notes litter the page, the traces of editorial decisions made and discarded. Perhaps the awkwardly executed retouching of this image explains why it, too, was excluded from Volume I of the *Iconographie.*

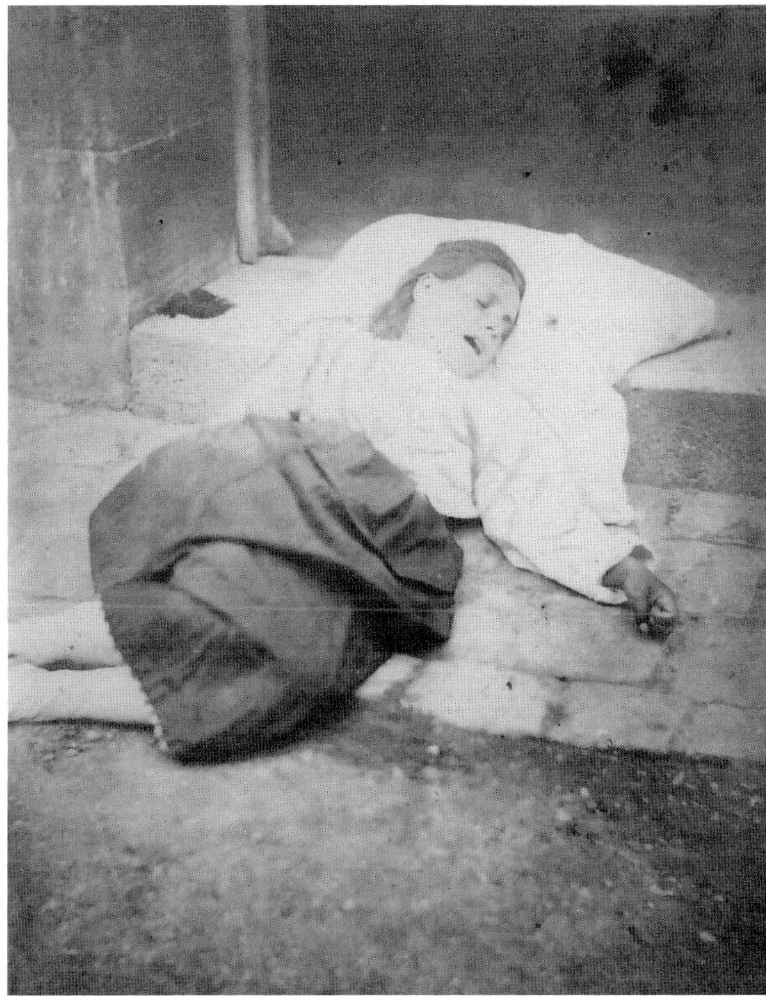

Fig. 37
Photograph from Album 646 FOSS 5. Paris, Archives de l'Assistance Publique–Hôpitaux de Paris. Courtesy of the Archives de l'Assistance Publique–Hôpitaux de Paris. Photo: author.

Though not completely successful, the retouching on Mlle. Etcheverry's portrait is largely subtler and, therefore, more effective (figs. 40 and 41). She sits in a large leather chair—so different from the simpler chairs that appear throughout the three volumes of the *Iconographie* that it suggests Charcot's office—while experiencing a hysterical contracture in her left hand. It is outlined carefully by the retoucher in the Archives Album version and highlighted against the white of the garment that she has draped over her chest to preserve her modesty. The retouching on her right hand and forearm, conversely, is rather inept: whereas in the original image in the IPS Album they are out of focus and partly in shadow, here they have been lightened so that they contrast better with her dark skirt. Unfortunately, they end up contrasting instead with the rest of her arm and body, so that they resemble a prosthesis whose fingers seem to be either missing or fused in a claw-shaped extremity. In the retouched photograph, her

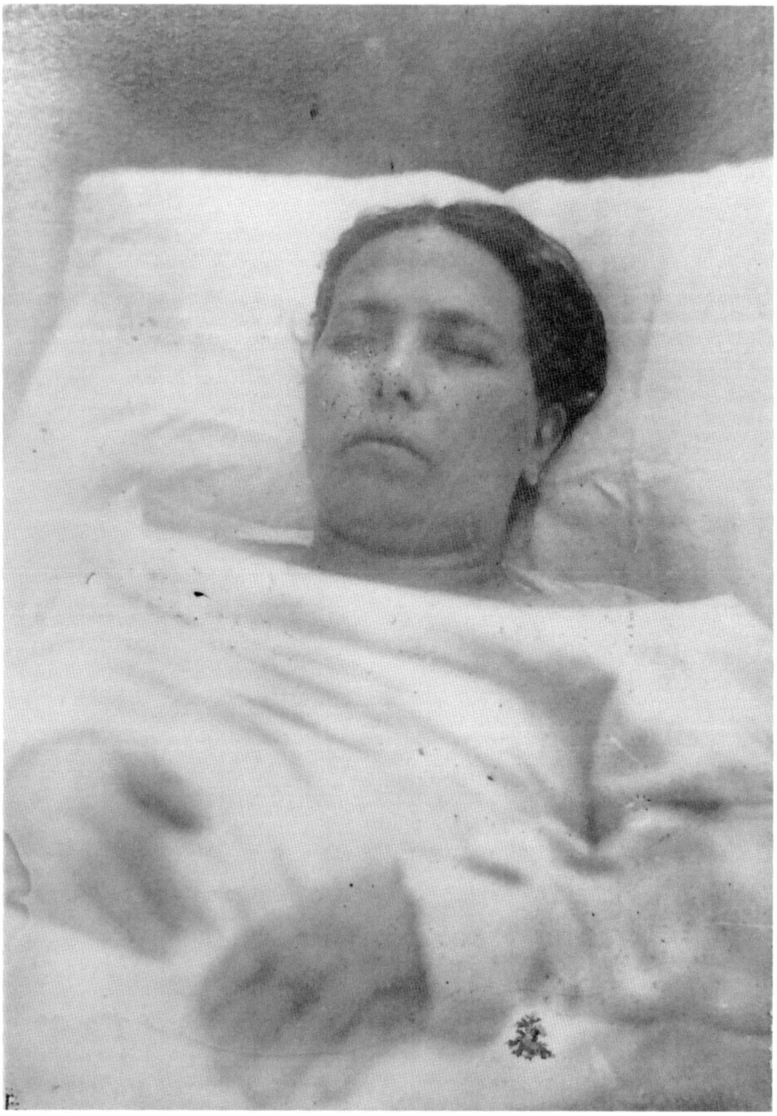

Fig. 38
Photograph of Mlle. Hellouin from Paul Regnard and [Désiré-Magloire] Bourneville, *Iconographie photographique de la Salpétrière* [*sic*]. *Service de M. Charcot* ([Paris], 1875), n.p. Paris, Bibliothèque Charcot. Courtesy of the Bibliothèque Charcot, Bibliothèque de Sorbonne Université. Photo: author.

lips have been lightly colored in, as has her left nostril, which has also been shaded to add volume. Lines help define her eyebrows and eyelids as well as her bonnet at the crown, to restore some of the definition lost in the seconds it took to expose the negative. The retoucher has overcompensated in lightening a dark mark on her face likely left by a speck of dust on the plate; as a result, Etcheverry has simply swapped the black stain on her cheek for a white one. In order to tame the blur of her profile, the contour of her face has been defined with crude dark lines that contrast with the softer sepia tone of the background. The instructions on the verso of the image stipulate, "retouch to make the double of the face disappear / lighten the arm and the right hand, put some creases in the linen."[95] The retouches do, in fact, improve the clarity of the image and remove the distracting blur. In 1864, Alexandre Ken in his *Historic, Artistic, and Scientific Dissertations on Photography* affirmed that "retouches ... are indispensable," adding, "I can sum up the opinion of all photographers in saying that ... the majority of prints obtained demand light corrections that, far from damaging them, only increase their merit."[96] Looking at the photograph without prior knowledge of the retouches, one might think that Etcheverry was able to sit still during the few seconds it took to capture her contracture and that her image was not doubled on the wet glass plate.[97] It appears that in the process of improving the photograph's legibility, though, the retoucher has unintentionally damaged the background, which has been developed unevenly. Waves of white lines behind the patient resemble graphs that might appear in the albums of the Musée Charcot or the "fluidic veil" seen in spirit photographs at the time.[98] In contrast to these seeming traces of the supernatural, there is evidence of the clinician's physical presence in the form of a fingerprint on the plate itself, just above the patient's right elbow. He has, quite literally, left his mark.

Unlike the images discussed thus far, many retouched photographs from the Archives Album *did* appear in Volume I of the *Iconographie*. These include, for example, photographs of the infamous Geneviève Legrand, described as "a patient known to all the doctors who have attended the clinical lessons of M. Charcot or who have visited his department." Her case is discussed, Bourneville and Regnard insist, in order to make known "the sad fate of these unfortunates suffering from chronic hysteria and to show that they deserve much more pity than those who do not know them fully enough are prepared to grant them."[99] The pious Legrand was born in Loudun, where in the seventeenth century a famous witchcraft trial had taken place and a group of Ursuline nuns had subsequently been exorcised; in keeping with Charcot's larger project, the Salpêtrière clinicians fashioned Legrand as a modern-day version of those considered possessed in the past.[100] Her history is unique enough that she is the only patient whose case continues into the second volume of the *Iconographie*.[101] Legrand is pictured in the IPS Album in the last phase of the attack, during which a delirious hysteric would experience hallucinations and visions before returning to the "real world" (fig. 42).[102] She is lying on her back, staring blankly upward. As is often the case with these early photographs, a shallow depth of field has resulted in a limited focal area: in this image, Legrand's face, while the hand on her chest and especially the dark background are rather indistinct. Nebulous areas of light and dark at the left edge of the photograph suggest the presence of another figure—a nurse, perhaps. The retoucher's instructions state: "retouch the face well[,] do [*faire*] the hair / clarify [*éclaircir*] the hand."[103] Indeed, retouching is visible all over the more closely cropped image in the Archives Album—the blurred background details, including the ghostly figure on the left, have been smoothed out and essentially erased so as to prevent distraction, and thick folds have been added to Legrand's garment to hint at the breasts beneath (fig. 43). The retoucher has left the skin of her chest unchanged, creating a somewhat jarring and incongruous patch in the photograph, surrounded by and therefore calling attention to his many interventions, including the painted lines that make her hair look fuller. In the 1890s, *The ABC of Retouching*

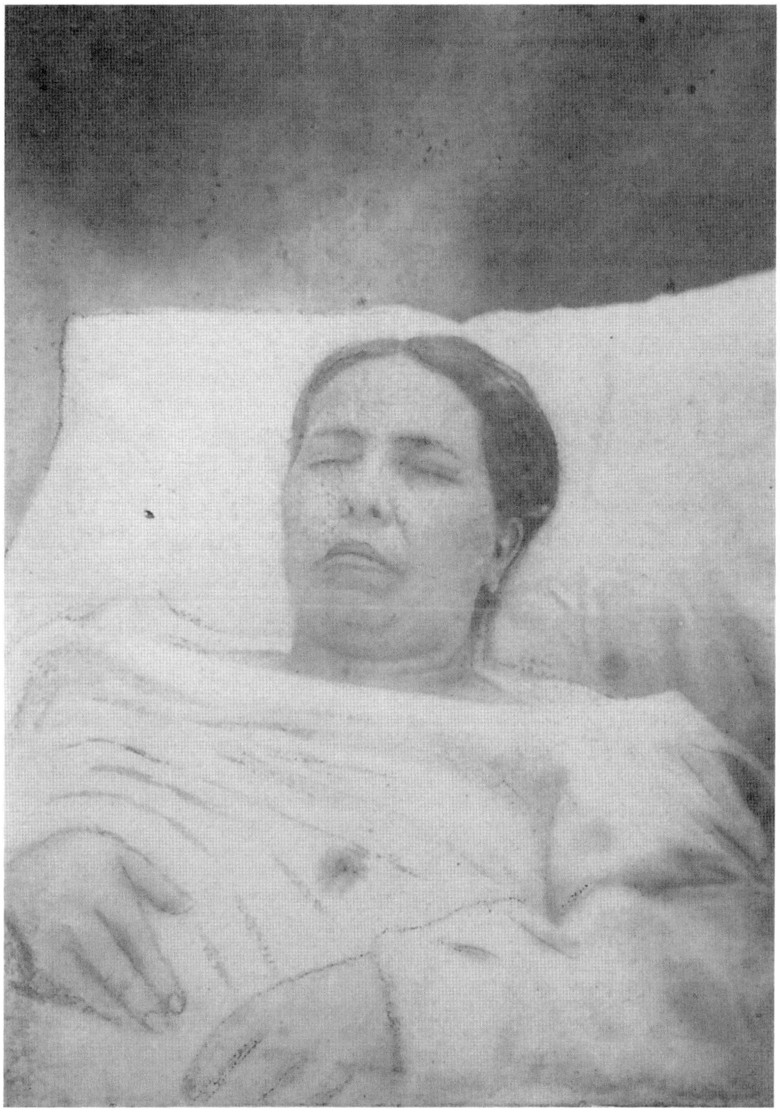

Fig. 39
LETHARGIE *Hellouin* (*Lethargy Hellouin*). Photograph from Album 646 FOSS 5. Paris, Archives de l'Assistance Publique–Hôpitaux de Paris. Courtesy of the Archives de l'Assistance Publique–Hôpitaux de Paris. Photo: author.

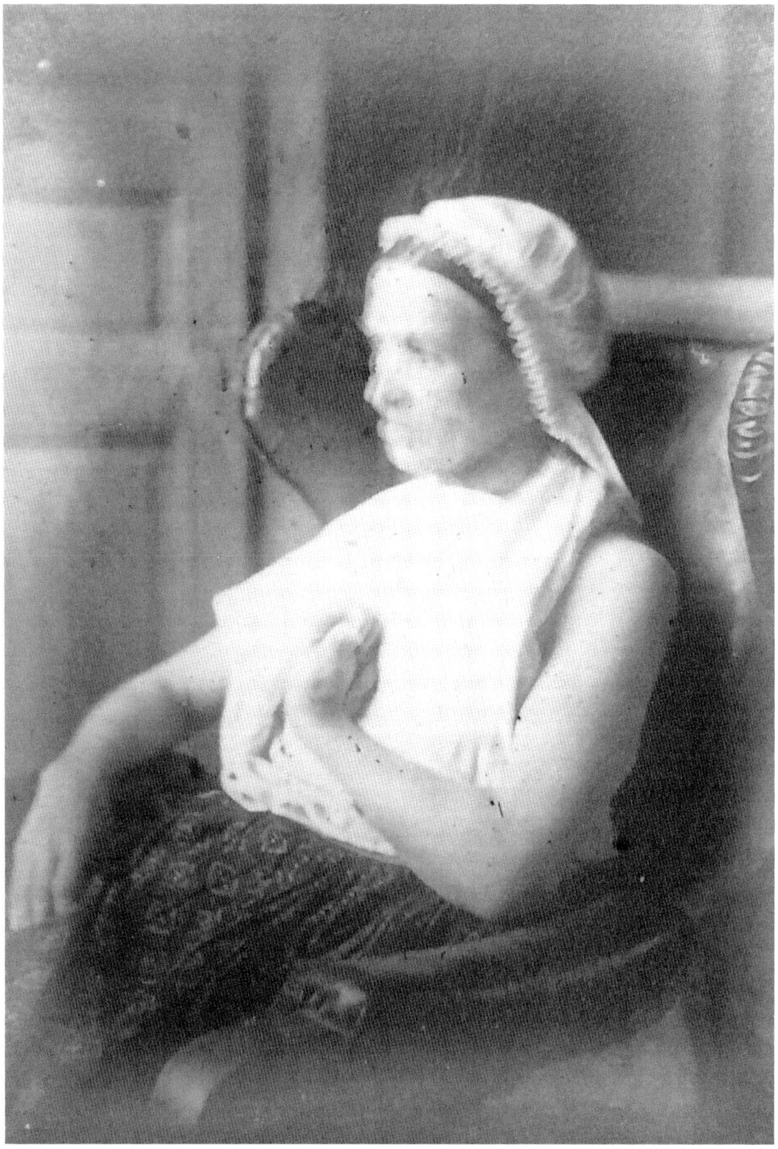

claimed, "The general tone of the hair . . . appears too dark when photographed, and the lights are too strong. Particularly is this so in black hair. . . . Strengthen the half shades with a broad pointed pencil, handling it in the lie of the hair, not aiming at producing lines or hairs, but masses."[104] The retoucher obviously heeded this general advice, but in creating "masses" with broad strokes, he emphasized the hair's dishevelment. Artistic intervention played into contemporary stereotypes of the irrational hysteric here: the retoucher's mediation exaggerated the wildness of her hair and sexualized her by emphasizing her breasts.

The retoucher added lines to Legrand's face—her brow, her eyes and eyelids, her nostrils, her upper lip—as well as the shadows cast by her nose, lower lip, and chin. *The ABC of Retouching* also comments on modeling: "Study earnestly the form of the principal shadows, that from eye to chin, on the shaded side, those under the eyes, nose, and lower lip, and on the neck under the chin. Where these are too dark, strengthen judiciously their details, preserving faithfully all that is beautiful in their shape or *necessary to the likeness*."[105] In the photograph of Legrand, the retoucher clearly encountered some difficulty and inadvertently altered her "likeness." The shape of her face appears rounder and flatter and her cheekbones less prominent. Her eyes have been made deeper, going against Piquepé's advice to leave eyes untouched so as to "not alter their expression."[106] In the retouched image, the direction of Legrand's gaze has been changed—a bit of white has been included near the tear ducts in order to shift her focus slightly. Her Cupid's bow has been penciled in too far to the right so that it is no longer aligned with her now overly large nose. The retoucher also seems to have removed the shadows originally present on Legrand's neck, remaking them instead, creating something strangely thick and giving it an unnatural solidity. Johnson notes in his retouching manual that the "success" of retouching facial features "depends, in a very great measure, on the general experience possessed by the retoucher, as well as his

Fig. 40
Photograph of Mlle. Etcheverry from Paul Regnard and [Désiré-Magloire] Bourneville, *Iconographie photographique de la Salpétrière* [*sic*]. *Service de M. Charcot* ([Paris], 1875), n.p. Paris, Bibliothèque Charcot. Courtesy of the Bibliothèque Charcot, Bibliothèque de Sorbonne Université. Photo: author.

knowledge of what is or is not artistic."[107] Both of these characteristics are lacking in Regnard's work and are evident in the amateurish results of his retouching.

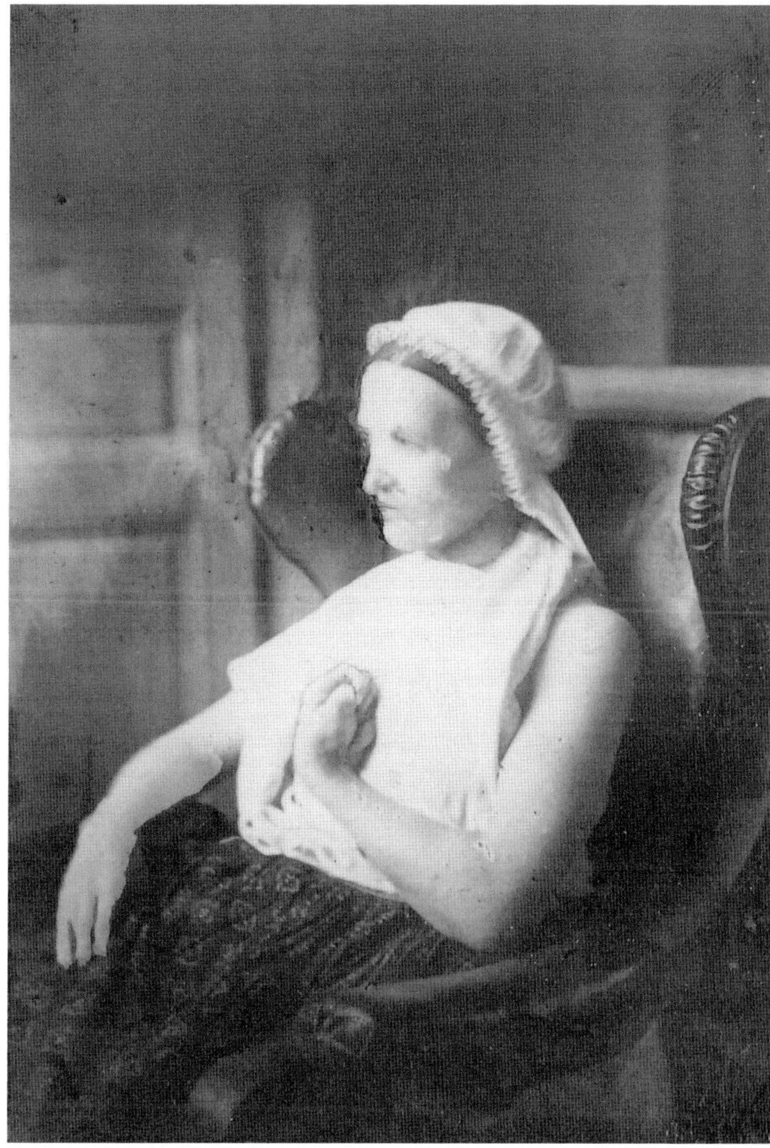

Legrand's seemingly wooden hand is perhaps the most obviously retouched element of the photograph. While *éclaircir*—the verb in the instructions to the retoucher—can mean "to lighten," here it seems to mean "to clarify," because the hand is quite evidently drawn in. Very little of the photographed hand remains; the fingers have been lengthened and the tips have become more pointed. The retouching emphasizes her hand and contradicts the advice given by Burrows and Colton: "The hands, unless nicely formed, in good focus, and well posed, should always be as subdued as possible; and in no instance should either the hand or any accessory be more prominent or attract the eye more than the face."[108] The retoucher seems to want the body to express as much—or, perhaps, as little—as the face, which has, according to the case notes, the look of "profound sadness."[109] Hands were, of course, one of the most obvious signifiers of the hysterical attack, and therefore the advice from Burrows and Colton about hands would not always be relevant for the Salpêtrière clinicians. However, Legrand's hand here does not seem to be fixed in a hysterical contracture, unlike the previous plate in the Archives Album, in which the circular border of the photograph emphasizes the contortion of her hands (fig. 44). There is a second version of the same photograph in the Archives Album. Written underneath it is "Pl. XVIII," which is the plate number of the image in Volume I of the *Iconographie*, although a retouched version was published. Pinholes above and below the image, as well as the circular impression left by a tack almost a hundred and fifty years ago, attest to the functional uses of this album's pages in the day-to-day context of the hospital.

Fig. 41
HYSTERIE Etcheverry Contracture (*HYSTERIA Etcheverry Contracture*). Photograph from Album 646 FOSS 5. Paris, Archives de l'Assistance Publique–Hôpitaux de Paris. Courtesy of the Archives de l'Assistance Publique–Hôpitaux de Paris. Photo: author.

In the case of Mlle. Marcillet, the retoucher has again been rather heavy-handed (figs. 45 and 46). He has attempted to fill in the cracks of the glass plate and to create highlights in the folds of her sleeve in order to add volume. He has also eliminated

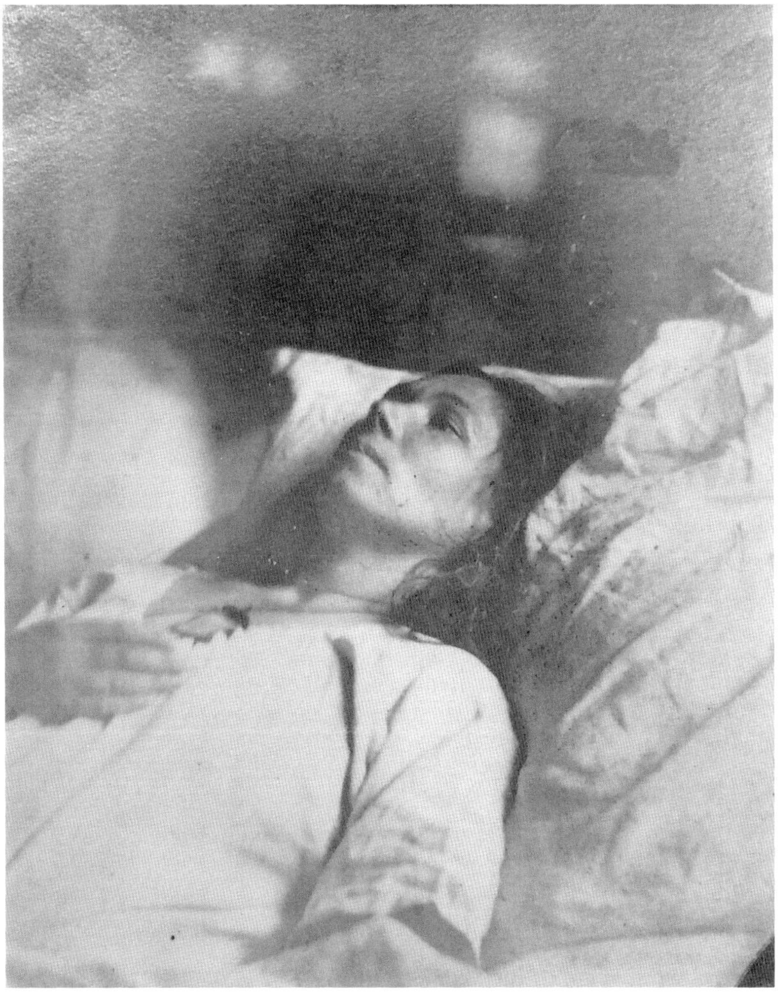

Fig. 42
Photograph of Geneviève Legrand from Paul Regnard and [Désiré-Magloire] Bourneville, *Iconographie photographique de la Salpétrière* [*sic*]. *Service de M. Charcot* ([Paris], 1875), n.p. Paris, Bibliothèque Charcot. Courtesy of the Bibliothèque Charcot, Bibliothèque de Sorbonne Université. Photo: author.

the star-shaped shadow behind her head, evening out the darks and lights. In the process, the contour of her hair against the background has become almost jagged, and the added highlights impart a tousled and unkempt look. According to Johnson's retouching manual, "Those who retouch badly generally proceed in sharpening hair to make lines running in the direction of the growth of the hair," which is exactly the case here.[110] The excessive and ill-considered interventions have seriously exacerbated the minor photographic imperfections on Marcillet's face in the IPS Album version. It has been dramatically discolored, with a mess of light patches all around her face, especially her forehead and her right cheek. Her eyes and mouth, too, have been overworked, with particularly egregious results.

The retoucher must have realized the disastrous effect of his work. This is the only example in the album where the instructions on the verso have been crossed out. They state: "retouch the black lines [*raies*], the face, and fill in the blurred square of the paper / with outlines and background, if possible."[111] The retoucher obviously made another attempt, as a photograph with vastly different—and superior—retouches was published in Volume I (fig. 47). Here, he followed the advice given by Johnson: "If you are dissatisfied with what you have done to a negative, clean it off with turpentine, and commence again, and do not repeat the same faults."[112] The new print is less tightly cropped, revealing more of Marcillet's bedsheets and straitjacket. The crack has been expertly filled in and is almost imperceptible, with the background thoroughly darkened so as to eliminate all detail. It is essentially black in the area immediately surrounding Marcillet's head, creating a sort of nimbus in negative. The darker print better defines her facial features and expression. Most unusually, the published photograph repositions the patient, who now leans sharply to the left; this change in orientation destabilizes Marcillet and makes her mental state seem even more precarious. It is also not as closely cropped, thereby increasing the distance—both physical and psychic—between the viewer and the patient. Bourneville tells us that she is hallucinating, and our greater remove intensifies the impression of her impenetrable interiority. The newly blackened background reinforces this with a note of mystery and foreboding, as we glimpse Marcillet mid-hallucination. The soft shadow around her head has been replaced by the demonic black "halo," but both echo spirit photographs from the second half of the nineteenth century. At the time of these photographs, the accusations of the "invention" of hysteria leveled against Charcot were still in the future, but the manipulations of the photographic process by the clinicians of the Salpêtrière are not dissimilar to those used by the charlatans who claimed to see the dead alongside the living.

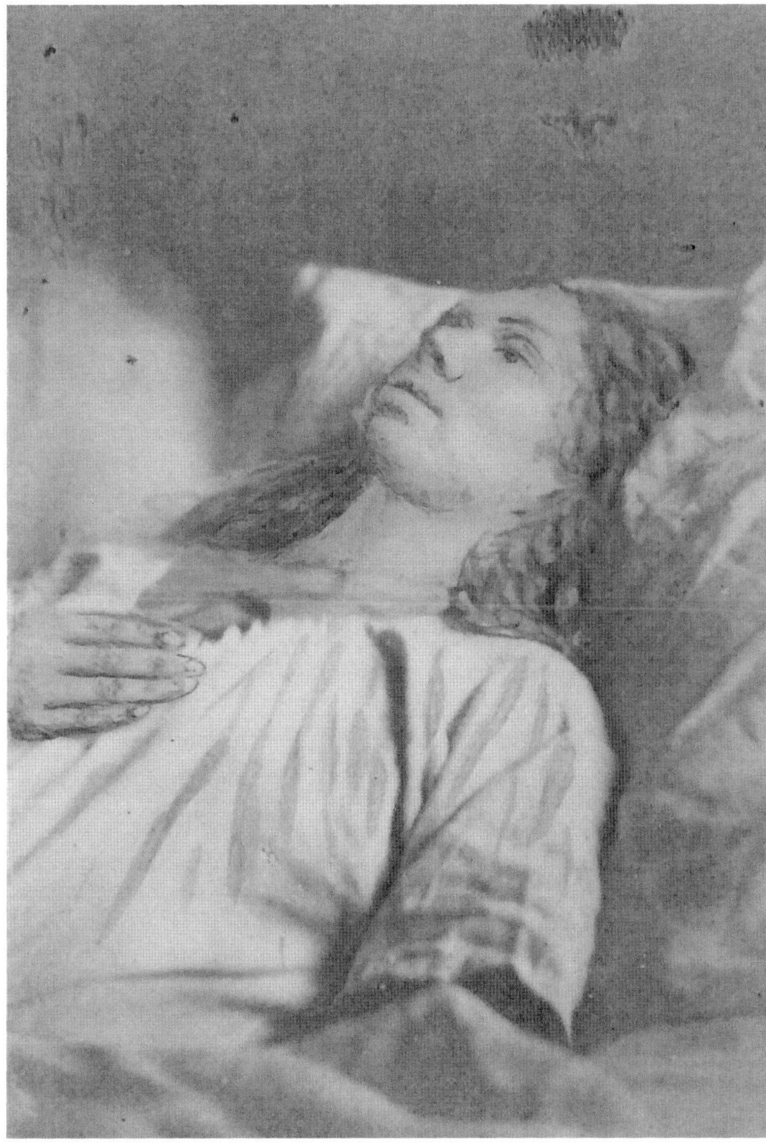

Fig. 43
Photograph of Geneviève Legrand from Album 646 FOSS 5. Paris, Archives de l'Assistance Publique–Hôpitaux de Paris. Courtesy of the Archives de l'Assistance Publique–Hôpitaux de Paris. Photo: author.

The Image of the Hysteric

In the photographs examined in this chapter, we can see that, in some, the retouching has clarified the image: here a blurred profile made distinct, there a hand emphasized and defined to facilitate the observation of bodily contortions and contractures. But for the most part, the retouching has not added to the medical information we are meant to glean, nor has it improved the photograph's legibility. It has not helped to reveal pathology to the viewer: the symptoms of the hysterical attack and the "stigmata of degeneracy" purportedly written on the bodies of these women are not made more apparent.[113] The retouchings have contributed more to connotative meanings than to denotative ones.

Looking at the image of the hysteric, Sander Gilman sees "the movement from the aesthetic to the real, from the artistic to the therapeutic, from the image of the patient to the definition of the patient's reality."[114] But the retouched photographs discussed in this chapter move in the opposite direction: from the "real" to the aesthetic, from the therapeutic to the "artistic," from the "definition of the patient's reality" to the "image" of the patient. This is particularly obvious in a photograph of a patient with epilepsy included in the Archives Album but only retouched for the second volume of the *Iconographie photographique de la Salpêtrière* (figs. 48 and 49). In the published

Fig. 44
HYSTERO-EPILEPSIE. Genevieve [*sic*] *LEGRAND* (*HYSTERO-EPILEPSY. Genevieve* [*sic*] *LEGRAND*). Photograph from Album 646 FOSS 5. Paris, Archives de l'Assistance Publique–Hôpitaux de Paris. Courtesy of the Archives de l'Assistance Publique–Hôpitaux de Paris. Photo: author.

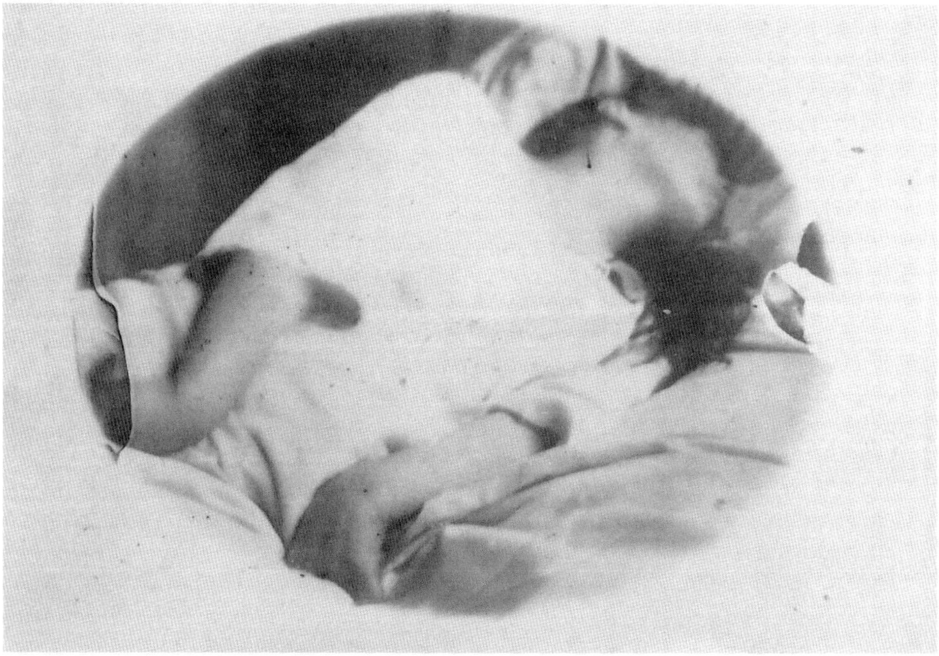

image, the retoucher has darkened the folds and shadows on the patient's dress as well as the contours of her body, making more visible the contracted left hand that overlaps her hips. He has completely erased the stone wall behind her to remove any elements that might distract from her body's address. The patient's facial features, blurred in the original photograph, have been drawn in, giving her a cartoonish appearance. If, as Susan Sontag writes, "there is an aggression implicit in every use of the camera," then retouching has heightened that violence by effacing the individual buried underneath these "corrections."[115] The doctor, photographer, and retoucher's decisions were privileged over the patient's embodied experience, yet her inability to keep still can be read as a resistance to the medical gaze of the clinician made manifest by the camera.[116]

The manipulations evident in the retouched photographs diminish the agency of the Salpêtrière patients by imposing an aestheticizing veil over scenes of medical phenomena. The retouchings call attention to the surface of the photographs, just as the surface of the hysteric's body was the only place where Charcot was able to locate her illness. It is significant that no "before" photographs—images in the "normal state" before the start of a hysterical attack—are retouched. Through retouching, then, the patient in the throes of a hysterical attack or epileptic seizure is doubly lost. Literally, her likeness is often obfuscated or even erased. And theoretically, as Miles argues, "within the ambivalent light of photographic translation, . . . this 'original' presence retreats into the shadows of the photograph where it is accessible only through the photograph's manifold discursive, photo-chemical and material relations."[117]

The struggle that Sontag theorizes as lying at the heart of photography, between "beautification, which comes from the fine arts, and truth-telling, which is measured not only by a notion of value-free truth, a legacy from the sciences, but by a moralized

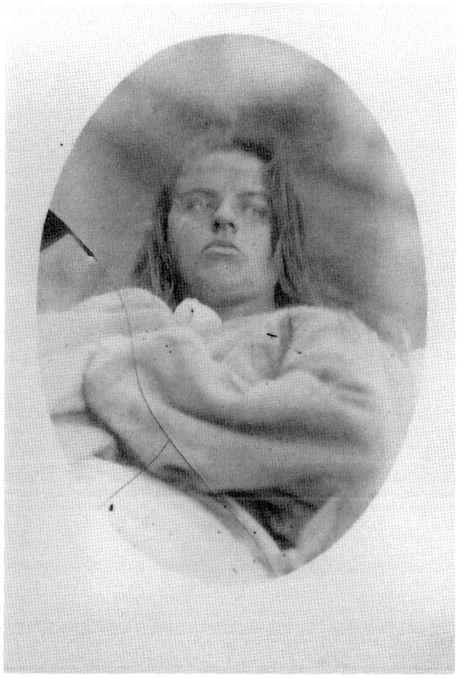

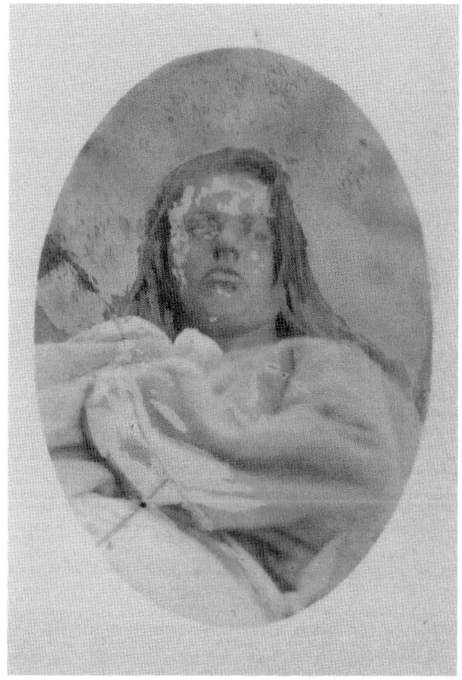

Fig. 45 (above)
Photograph of Mlle. Marcillet from Paul Regnard and [Désiré-Magloire] Bourneville, *Iconographie photographique de la Salpétrière* [*sic*]. *Service de M. Charcot* ([Paris], 1875), n.p. Paris, Bibliothèque Charcot. Courtesy of the Bibliothèque Charcot, Bibliothèque de Sorbonne Université. Photo: author.

Fig. 46 (above right)
Photograph of Mlle. Marcillet from Album 646 FOSS 5. Paris, Archives de l'Assistance Publique–Hôpitaux de Paris. Courtesy of the Archives de l'Assistance Publique–Hôpitaux de Paris. Photo: author.

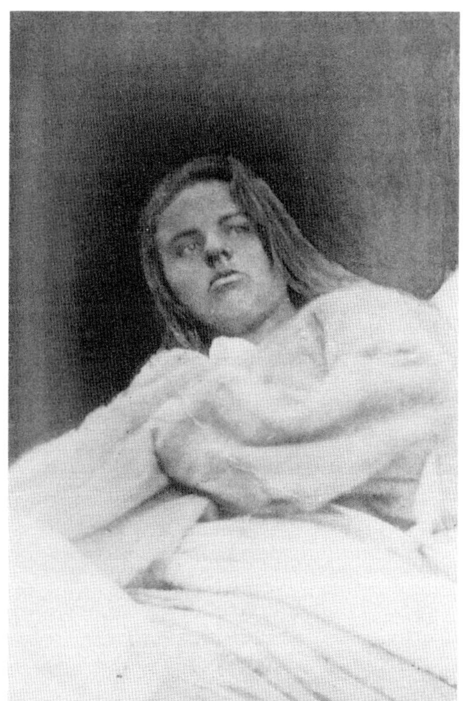

Fig. 47 (right)
Hystéro-épilepsie: Hallucinations. Dédain (*Hystero-Epilepsy: Hallucinations; Disdain*). Albumen print. From [Désiré-Magloire] Bourneville and P[aul] Regnard, *Iconographie photographique de la Salpétrière* [*sic*], vol. 1 (Paris: Bureau du Progrès médical / Adrien Delahaye, 1877), plate 31. Courtesy of the Wellcome Collection.

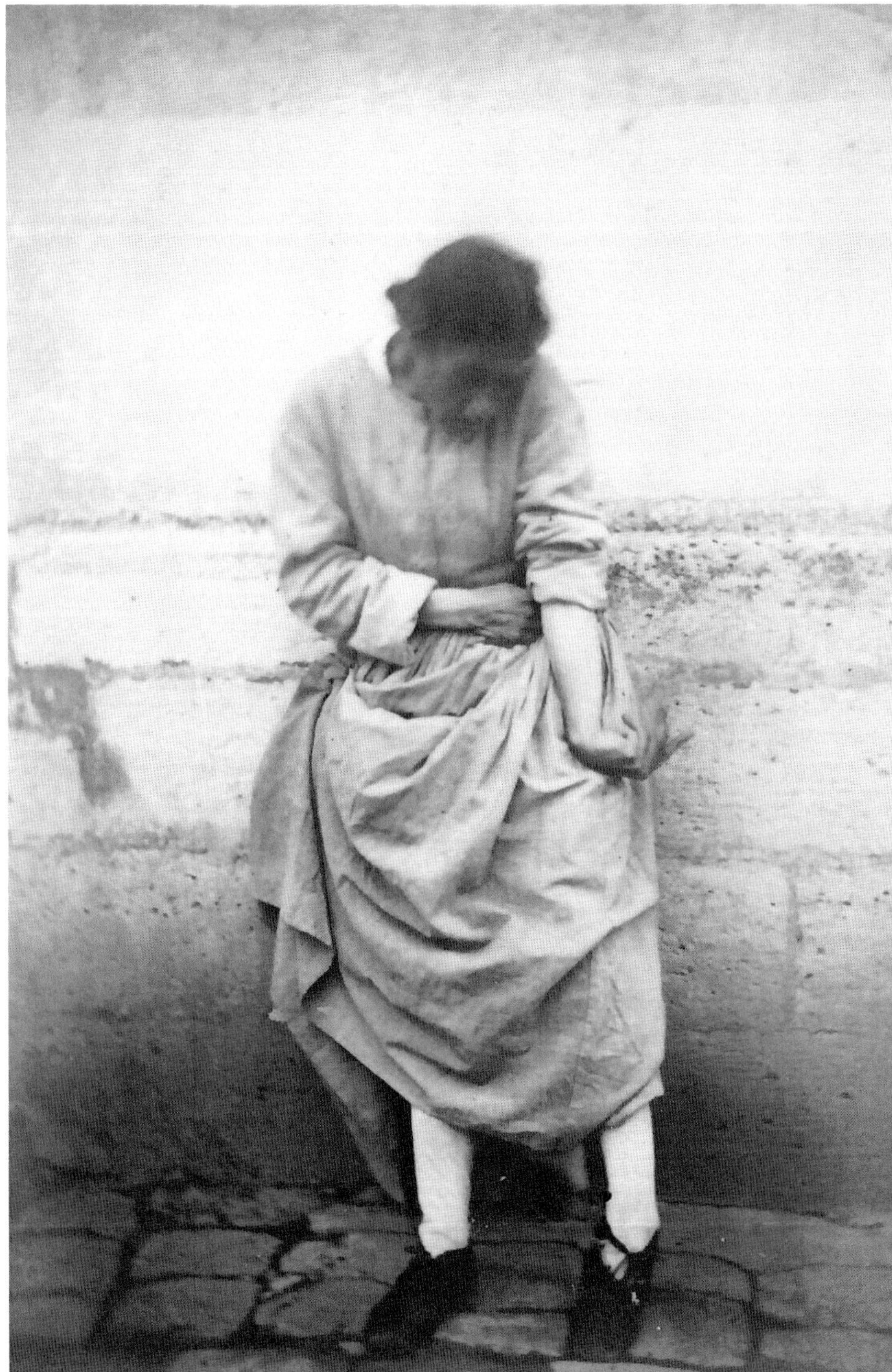

Fig. 48
Photograph of a patient with epilepsy from Album 646 FOSS 5. Paris, Archives de l'Assistance Publique–Hôpitaux de Paris. Courtesy of the Archives de l'Assistance Publique–Hôpitaux de Paris. Photo: author.

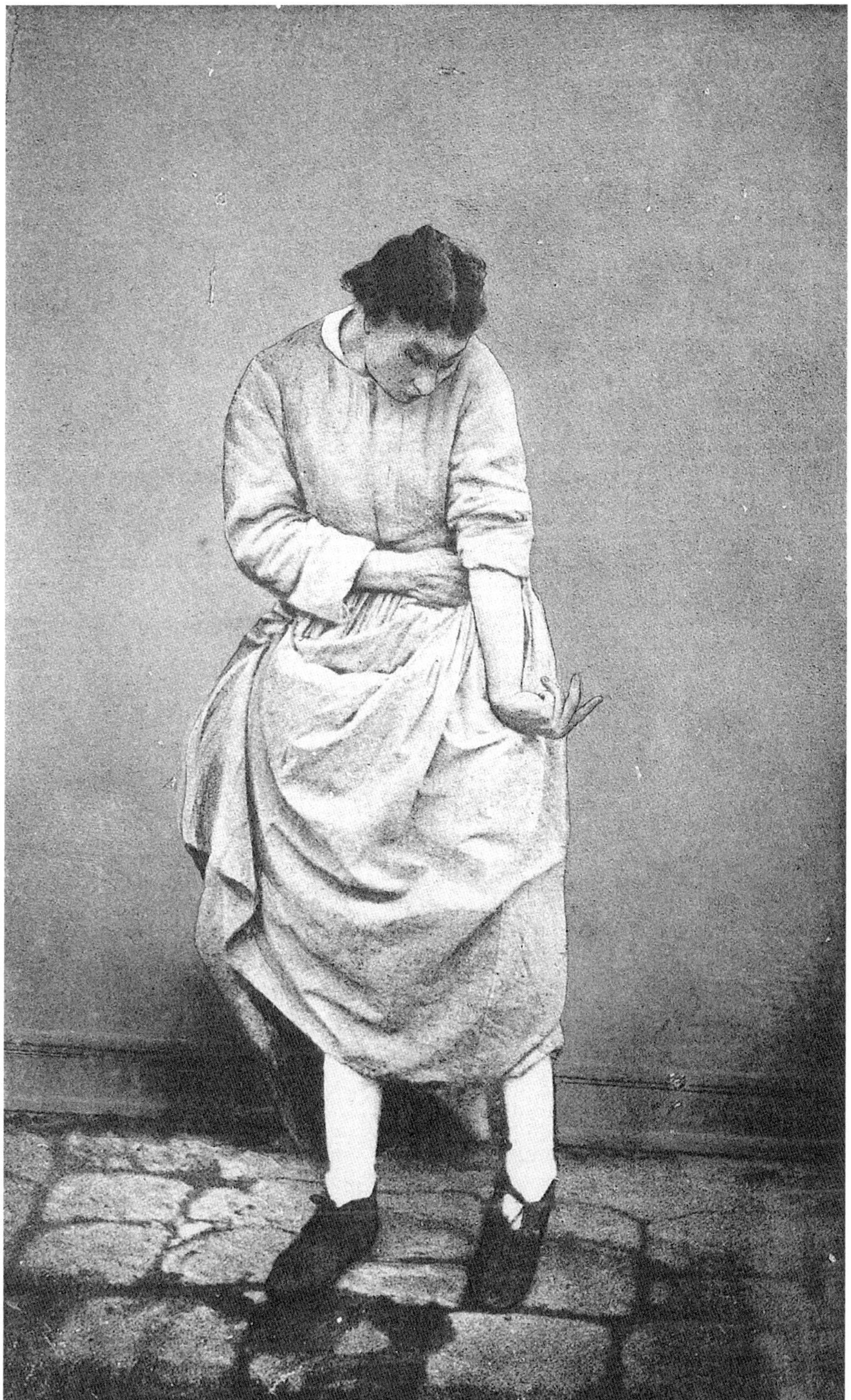

Fig. 49
Épilepsie partielle. Forme vibratoire (*Partial Epilepsy: Vibrational Form*). From [Désiré-Magloire] Bourneville and P[aul] Regnard, *Iconographie photographique de la Salpêtrière*, vol. 2 (Paris: Bureau du Progrès médical / Adrien Delahaye, 1878), plate 8. Courtesy of the Wellcome Collection.

ideal of truth-telling," is enacted on the surface of these retouched photographs.[118] One way for us to understand and accept that these retouched photographs could appear "truthful" to the clinicians of the Salpêtrière would be to nuance our understanding of such a loaded term. In the nineteenth century, many people believed in photography's "truthfulness" and willfully ignored its distortions and misrepresentations.[119] As Alan Trachtenberg puts it, "the conventional idea of photography's infallibility is not a demonstrable truth but a belief, held with the irrational conviction of a myth."[120] German photochemist and photographer Hermann Vogel makes clear that the popular understanding of the word "truth" was far from clear-cut. In an article from the 1860s devoted primarily to an explanation of optical and other errors, he states unequivocally that photographs are not truthful. These errors can be "avoided," he claims, by positioning the camera correctly, with proper lighting, and through "the employment of original and negative retouching." Vogel concludes, "It constitutes the *art* of photography to present the reality true and beautiful."[121] To present "reality true" is an interesting concept. Larousse's *Grand Dictionnaire universel* from the 1860s makes a distinction between "truth" and "reality": "the word 'truth' is nothing more than the conformity of a representation with the thing or reality that is represented."[122] Truth is not the same as that which is real; the word "conformity" hints at the possibility—or even necessity—of mediation between the two.[123] For Vogel, as for Charcot and the Salpêtrière School, retouching was a legitimate and even necessary conduit for that mediation. Far from diluting or diminishing the truthfulness of an image, retouching would in fact correct it, enhance it, make it conform more closely with the "real." Henry Peach Robinson, in his influential book on photography, argued that "it is not the fact of reality that is required, but the truth of imitation that constitutes a veracious picture. Cultivated minds . . . do not require to believe that they are deceived, and that they look on actual nature, when they behold a pictorial representation of it."[124] This theorization requires a more elastic definition of objectivity, one in which artistic intervention can be beneficial or even necessary.

The retouching in the Salpêtrière photographs—sometimes arbitrary and principally aesthetic—clearly exceeds the bounds proposed by none other than Albert Londe in *La Photographie moderne* of 1888 as "[consisting] in principle in removing the flaws that can exist in the sensitive layer [of the negative]. . . . As long as retouching stays within these limits, one cannot reproach it; but when it goes so far as *to modify a resemblance*, which unfortunately happens too often, we believe that it is more often an evil rather than a good."[125] Significantly, in his seminal book on medical photography published five years later, the first treatise to deal with this burgeoning field, Londe notes that retouching "can always alter truth."[126] Clearly, "hand-work" on photographs in the medical realm was a complicated and loaded enterprise. While retouching was widely used in medical photography, by the 1880s scientists in Germany had denounced it in the name of preserving objectivity.[127] We know that in France during the years when the *Iconographie photographique de la Salpêtrière* was published, "the precise limits for retouching were . . . not defined."[128]

Photography seemed to guarantee medicine an "immediate and transparent identity between image and ... referent."[129] This unfulfilled promise of the medium is perhaps most evident in the last image in the Archives Album and the IPS Album: a photograph of a brain, with no caption or text of any kind to help us make sense of it. It can perhaps be understood as an epilogue to all of the pictures in the album, not least the two showing a stooped, elderly, and seemingly dejected woman on the penultimate pages. She likely remained under the gaze of the camera after death. As Erin O'Connor notes, "What haunts the medical photograph is the certainty that there is no object to take, only a subject to erase, only the possibility of metonymy, of surface standing in for depth, of separate faces signifying a set type."[130] The photograph of a brain bears witness to the belief of the Salpêtrière clinicians that illness had to be written somewhere on the body, self-evidently. By closing with this photograph, the Archives Album seems to suggest that all the disorders illustrated within it can be traced back to this organ. It is as revealing of illness as the rest of the photographs—in other words, not at all, telling us more about the beliefs of the clinicians than about any particular pathology. Charcot believed that hysteria was a neurological disorder, but he was frustrated throughout his long career at his inability to find a lesion to support his belief. The cause of hysteria eluded Charcot, and photography's promise of transparency utterly failed him.

THE *ATAXIC VENUS*

3

Between Portrait and Specimen

Life and death do battle in every detail: here it's a woman, there a statue, further on a cadaver.

—HONORÉ DE BALZAC, 1837

In André Brouillet's *A Clinical Lesson at the Salpêtrière, le tout Paris* is enraptured by Charcot's use of hypnosis (see fig. 1). One of his most controversial diagnostic tools, hypnosis was revivified by Charcot in an attempt to better understand hysteria. He even managed to convince the Académie des sciences in 1882 to reverse its past decision to condemn "mesmerism."[1] Charcot believed that the hysteric's increased suggestibility was another neurological manifestation of the disorder.[2] His experiments were not without their detractors, however.[3] While Brouillet's painting hung in the Salon, a critic writing under the pseudonym Théophraste compared the experiments of the Salpêtrière's illustrious doctor with the antics of fairground charlatans who hypnotized gullible young women—the only difference, he wrote, was that hospital patients were not given a choice.[4]

The medical voyeurism evident in Brouillet's painting was equally apparent in Parisian popular attractions, as Théophraste tells us. These included traveling anatomical museums, where casts of diseased body parts and life-size figures revealing their internal organs could be scrutinized by a paying public. In the middle of the century, Alsatian entrepreneur Pierre Spitzner began assembling a significant collection of wax models, as well as anatomical specimens and medical photographs, for a "grand anatomical and ethnological museum" whose motto was "Science! Art! Progress!"[5] This popular institution (which later traveled around Europe) had an obvious pseudoscientific bent, and Spitzner seems to have given himself the title of "Doctor" in order to enhance his credibility. At the museum, groups of Red Cross workers, nurses, veterans, and orphans, in addition to anyone who was willing to buy a ticket, received a "course in public health [*hygiène sociale*]."[6] Spitzner hoped that the syphilitic faces, cirrhotic livers, gangrenous chancres, and other curiosities—cast in wax by some of the most important medical modelers of the day—would shock his audience into leading

Fig. 50 (opposite)
Interior of the Spitzner Collection showing the sculpture of *A Clinical Lesson at the Salpêtrière*. Undated photograph. S. Nayral Collection. Courtesy of S. Nayral.

moral lives. The instructive merit of such displays of skin diseases, fetal abnormalities, and obstetric or eye surgeries, among hundreds of other marvels, is hardly clear, but the promise of edification likely helped attract customers.

A poster for the Spitzner Museum from the early twentieth century includes a perfunctory sketch of Brouillet's painting, captioned simply "Doctor Charcot and Hysteria," exploiting the public fascination with the Salpêtrière.[7] A copy of the painting may also have decorated the exterior walls of its fairground shack.[8] Charcot's fame was so great that Spitzner considered it advantageous to create a life-size wax copy from Brouillet's painting of the neurologist and his retinue: an enlarged detail of the painting's focal figures was rendered in wax and displayed prominently on the inside of the museum, offering Spitzner's customers the frisson of standing in for Charcot's usual audience of doctors and intellectuals (fig. 50).[9] Thus Charcot figuratively presided over the itinerant museum just as he literally presided over the Salpêtrière.

Certain liberties were taken with the waxes. Wittmann's body was tilted frontally, providing a better view for the spectators gawking at her exposed chest and shoulders. The angle of her torso has been rendered more acute, and her neck and head brought almost parallel to the floor, further emphasizing the unnatural contortion of the hysteric's *arc-de-cercle* pose. This slight rearrangement of the wax figures in relation to the painting places Babinski somewhat more to her side than behind her, but the direction of his gaze has not been adjusted accordingly. This has left him staring down at the ground instead of at Wittmann, and so his expression, which we read as compassionate in the painting, inadvertently conveys embarrassment or shame in the wax. Nurse Bottard, her left arm lowered in a gesture of supplication or presentation, no longer looks at Wittmann but at Charcot, who stands behind a small table loaded with medical implements, so that the still life in the background of Brouillet's painting is brought forward in Spitzner's tableau. Most interestingly, in the wax simulacrum, Charcot's orientation has been slightly rotated to become completely frontal. He no longer discourses to the medical and cultural elite of the time—instead, from an elevated platform, he engages visitors to the Spitzner Museum who are learning the effects of illness on the body and acting as voyeurs, engrossed by others' misfortunes. The equivalence between examining portraits and examining patients that I noted in chapter 1 is made explicit in this space, located somewhere between the licked surface of Brouillet's painting and the uncanny gestalt of the wax figures, between the Salon and the *foire*, through the triangulation of gazes, through Charcot's invitation to look.

Charcot's museum, like Spitzner's, invited visitors to gaze at a patient's body reformed in wax. But Charcot's was a remarkable wax of a particular patient, cast from life. Visible in the right foreground of the photograph discussed at length in chapter 1, it is mentioned in most descriptions of the museum (see fig. 4). Charcot's earliest biographer, Paul Peugniez, writes that the museum

> included a great quantity of natural anatomical preparations, specimens of skeleton, arthropathies or bone deformities, the tabetic ossuary; as well as

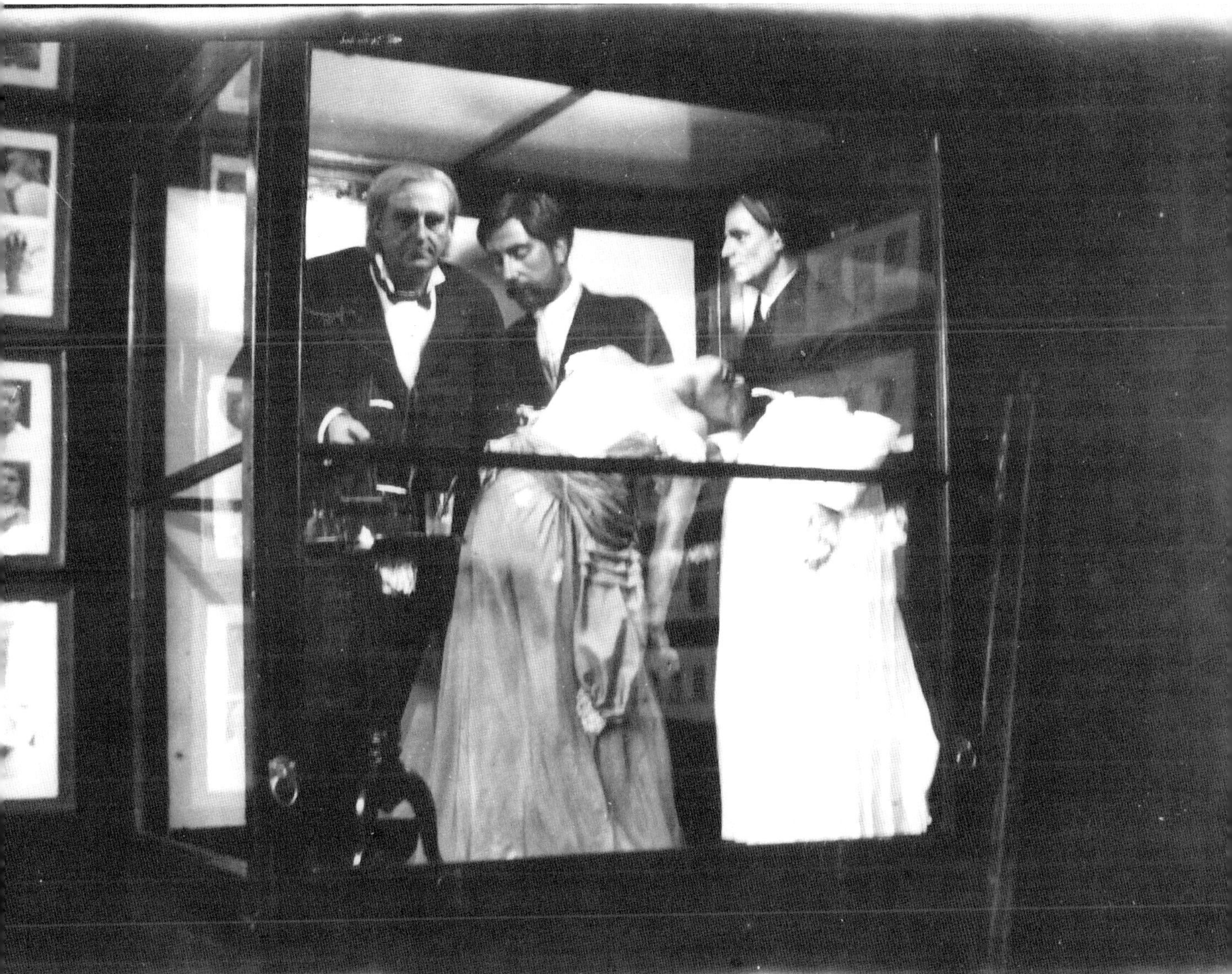

other artificial pieces, molds in wax by Loreau, among others an old tabetic from the hospice showing in nearly all of her joints the distortions described so well by Charcot, cast whole and of a frightening realism: she was called the ataxic Venus; diseased brains, hemispheres affected by classic lesions, an entire pathological anatomy no longer abstract and lifeless as it is in books, but resuscitated, animated, alive, so to speak, throwing into relief the fundamental characters of lesions, teaching us how to see them, leaving memories that no longer fade.[10]

In the left foreground of the photograph, we can see a glass case—the "tabetic ossuary" mentioned above—that includes the actual skeleton of the patient whose postmortem cast Peugniez identified as "the ataxic Venus."[11]

We can assume that the title of *Ataxic Venus* is ironic, since this sculpture is far from beautiful or idealized (fig. 51). It is more than just a striking medical specimen; as Édouard Papet claims, it is "without a doubt the most impressive cast from nature created in the nineteenth century in the medical domain."[12] It is also a portrait of a patient who had locomotor ataxia, which was also known at the time as tabes dorsalis—the reason that the figure is characterized as "tabetic" by Peugniez.[13] A complication of tertiary syphilis, this devastating illness typically resulted in loss of coordination and the degeneration of the joints, among a host of other painful symptoms. It could eventually lead to paralysis and insanity as well as amputations.[14] Yet a layperson's lack of clinical knowledge about locomotor ataxia does not diminish the powerful impact of the deformities that are central to this sculpture's meaning.

The *Ataxic Venus* is a key material remnant of the Salpêtrière School's engagement with the history of art and contemporary artistic practices. As Charcot and Richer would write in *Les Difformes et les malades dans l'art*: "Science and art are nothing more than two manifestations of the same phenomenon, two faces of the same object."[15] A close reading of the *Ataxic Venus* raises many questions about the medical and artistic project of Charcot and the Salpêtrière School. In what ways can the methodological tools and vocabulary of the art historian be instructive here? Can we use the term "portraiture," for example, to describe this medical specimen—an individual who is clearly identifiable, but also meant to represent a "type" and quite literally serve as a "textbook example"? To what degree does the patient's pain figure into its purpose as a "specimen" of the particular disease of locomotor ataxia? Put another way, what is the meaning of the cast, and what is the role of pain in conveying that meaning?

The *Ataxic Venus* exemplifies the "history of disappearance" that, according to Hanneke Grootenboer, characterizes the history of wax sculpture and "can only be captured by recording the surprising capacity of certain wax objects to survive against all odds."[16] This chapter exhumes, as it were, the *Ataxic Venus*, an object once prominently discussed and displayed, provocatively open and exposed, but since enshrouded in protective layers, stowed in a wooden box, and tucked away in museum storage.

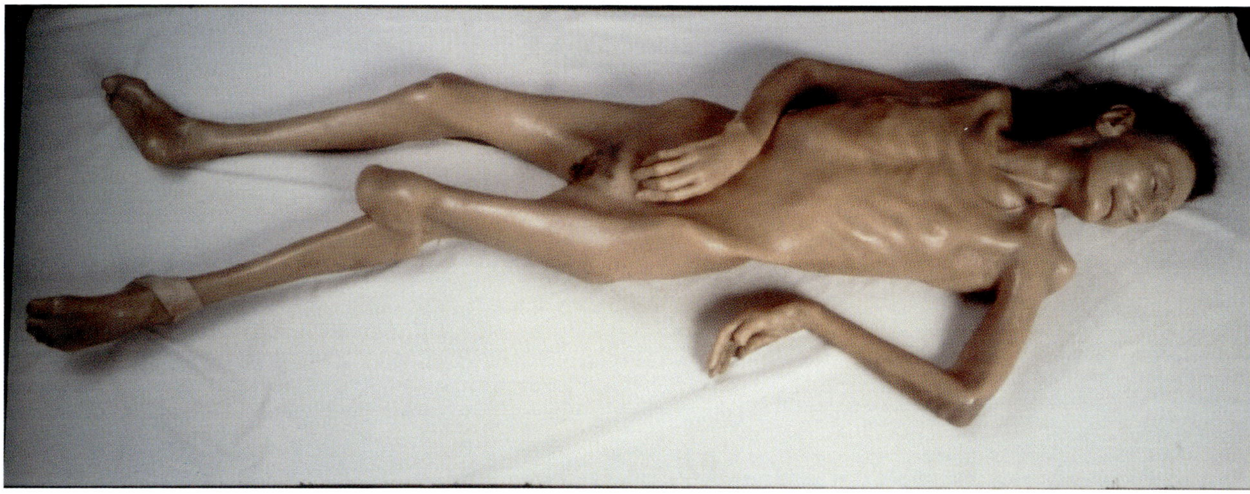

Fig. 51
Loreau, *Venus ataxique (Ataxic Venus)*, ca. 1880. Polychrome wax cast, 158 × 54 cm. Paris, Musée de l'Assistance Publique–Hôpitaux de Paris. Inv. AP 2001.0.4.3.1. Photo: AP-HP/musée–F. Marin.

Charcot's "Wax Lady"

We do not know much about sixty-year-old Berthelot, the Salpêtrière patient whose corpse was cast after death.[17] There are some clues in an important lecture Charcot gave on "Arthropathic Affections" in 1881 at the International Medical Congress in London. He mentions that at the Salpêtrière Berthelot had "been shown for several years" because she was "one of the best existing types . . . of ataxic affections of the joints."[18] Berthelot, then, had participated in Charcot's lectures while alive, as surely as her body was used as a prop after her death. She was his most important case study of this illness, and he described in detail the presence of lesions unsuspected during life and discovered only upon autopsy, as well as the joint atrophy and erosion typical of the disease. Charcot notes that "in the left shoulder-joint the axis of the humerus is seen to be directed toward the coracoid process rather than the glenoid cavity, the shaft terminating above in a pointed extremity, resting on the clavicle. It is evident that here also the head and neck of the humerus have disappeared." And in the knee, "the tibia has slipped backward, the whole of the lower extremity of the femur being in front of the tibia."[19] These are evident in the *Ataxic Venus*: a (literally) disjointed body whose limbs project at unsettling angles. The unnatural protrusions of this bony figure, awkwardly posed like a disused marionette, vie for attention. The left shoulder juts out to meet the tensed neck and pointed chin. The left wrist returns to the risen pelvic bone only to see the hand repelled by it. The left thigh continues the line of the lower arm, but that knee is particularly shocking—its grotesquely distorted form is difficult to look at.[20] The emaciated feet stretch out uncomfortably.[21] The *Ataxic Venus* defies normal physical limitations on the poses and positions the human body is capable of; it seems incapable of walking or even resting. Its deformities would appear to preclude any mobility or comfort. The most poignant element of the cast is at its center, where the right hand lies gently on the pelvis, reminding us that this individual shared our sense of touch and perhaps our predisposition to modesty.

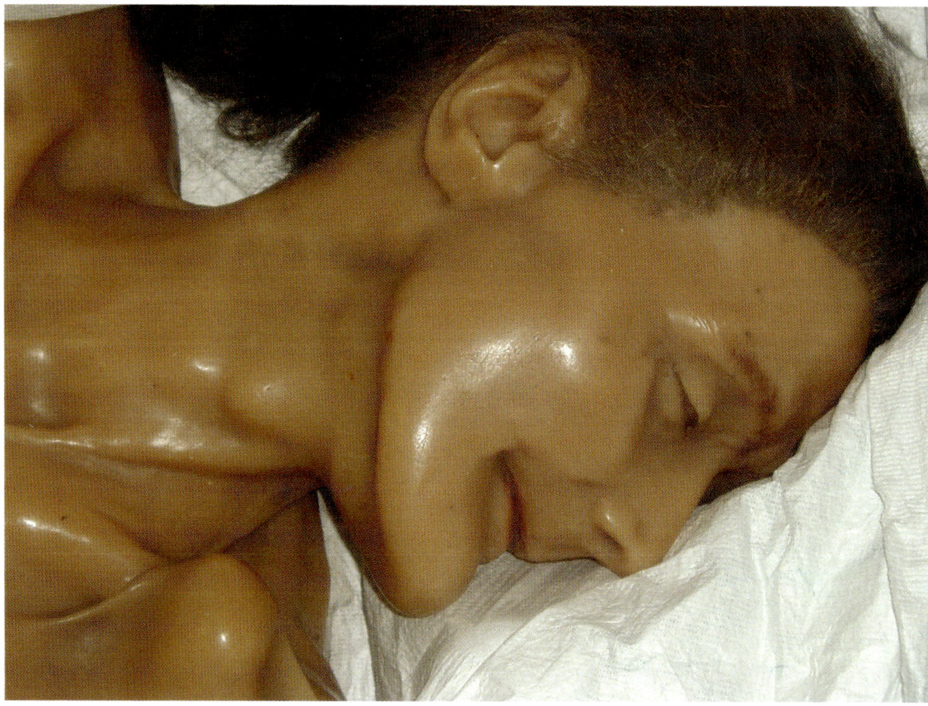

Fig. 52
Loreau, *Venus ataxique* (*Ataxic Venus*), ca. 1880, detail of the head. Polychrome wax cast, 158 × 54 cm. Paris, Musée de l'Assistance Publique–Hôpitaux de Paris. Inv. AP 2001.0.4.3.1. Photo: AP-HP/musée–author.

A close look at the *Ataxic Venus* reveals an uncanny sliver of eye just visible beneath the eyelashes (fig. 52)—she is both awake and asleep, looking simultaneously outward and inward.[22] The reddened lips, too, are ever so slightly open, but they suggest somnolence rather than speech. The body is smooth and unblemished, and its coloring suggests life rather than death or decomposition.[23] The liminal space occupied by the *Ataxic Venus*—with hints of animation emanating from its clearly lifeless form—makes it a compelling medical specimen. Charcot was fully aware of this: he brought this full-body wax cast with him to the International Medical Congress in 1881, along with Berthelot's actual skeleton, microscopic sections of the skeleton, and a photograph of Berthelot while alive.[24] The fact that he traveled with medical specimens begs a comparison with itinerant anatomical collections like the Spitzner Museum. These potent visual aids also certainly heightened the effect of Charcot's lecture at the Congress, during which he even indulged in a moment of self-congratulation, remarking, "This is the first time that a complete skeleton of the kind has been preserved."[25] Given his artistic interests, he was likely gratified by the fact that his lecture was held next door to the Royal Academy of Arts in the Congress's temporary museum at the Geological Society.

Charcot donated specimens of arthropathic joints to various British medical collections, but he also gave a cast of the *Ataxic Venus* to St. Thomas's Hospital in London.[26] He proudly wrote to his wife during the Congress, "My wax lady has made a sensation," indicating that he saw both Berthelot's wax cast and her legacy as his possessions.[27] In this letter, he also claimed, "I have here a veritable triumph."[28] His showmanship paid off: the International Medical Congress concluded, "This disease is, in fact, a distinct pathological entity, and deserves the name, by which it will be known, of 'Charcot's disease.'"[29] (Charcot joint is the nomenclature still used to describe the kind of joint deformity exhibited so effectively by the *Ataxic Venus*, also known as arthropathy, commonly seen today in people with diabetes rather than syphilis.) The pyrotechnics display at the end of the Congress included a spectacular "fire-portrait" of Charcot in the sky above London.[30] Berthelot and her sculptural representation were thus instrumental in establishing the neurologist's European reputation.[31]

It seems that Charcot went to the expense of having a second wax cast made of the *Ataxic Venus*, and, perhaps predictably, it became the star of the Musée Charcot.[32] In fact, it is possible that the cast of Berthelot's body would not have been commissioned in the first place if not for the existence of the museum of pathological anatomy at the Salpêtrière to house it. Almost nothing is known about its creator, a M. Loreau, who was the director of the Salpêtrière's casting studio at the time of Berthelot's death. Charcot mentions him in 1879 when thanking the Assistance Publique for the new pathological anatomy museum at the Salpêtrière "to which is annexed a casting studio, directed by a skilled artist"; the note in the printed version of his speech names Loreau.[33] By 1881, the Assistance Publique noted that Loreau was in charge of the casting and photography studio and was moved to give him a salary and an allowance for expenses incurred as *modeleur* (modeler) and photographer at the hospital because of the "good results" achieved by the casting studio.[34] In making his role permanent, the "appointment decree" also reveals the precarity of the Salpêtrière's casting studio until that point. The impressive wax sculpture must have factored into the Assistance Publique's judgment of "good results."

Loreau's drawings of hypnotized patients illustrate the third volume of the *Iconographie photographique de la Salpêtrière* from 1879 to 1880.[35] These drawings were presumably copied after photographs he took as head of the hospital's photography studio, following Paul Regnard's departure in 1878 and before Albert Londe took over in 1884.[36] However, his role in the casting studio was clearly more important than his work behind the camera and as a draughtsman: Charcot and Richer characterize Loreau as the "modeler of the pathological anatomy museum at the Salpêtrière," even as they thank him for his photographs.[37] Both roles saw Loreau attempting to "reproduce" reality with the indexical media of the cast and the photograph, whose production shared the same studio during much of Loreau's tenure.[38]

Loreau evidently labored long and hard at the ambitious project of creating the full-body cast that would come to be known as the *Ataxic Venus*. It would have necessitated handling Berthelot's (dead) body, becoming intimate with its jagged contours and tender spaces.[39] This body would have already been well known to many at the Salpêtrière. Berthelot spent her last years at the hospital, observed for countless hours by Charcot and other clinicians there. Her likeness was captured in its photography studio while she was still alive (fig. 53). Four photographs pasted onto a blue album page show a mattress placed on the floor and covered in a dark, glossy tarp, with Berthelot's piteous form stretched out on top. In two of them, her back is propped up

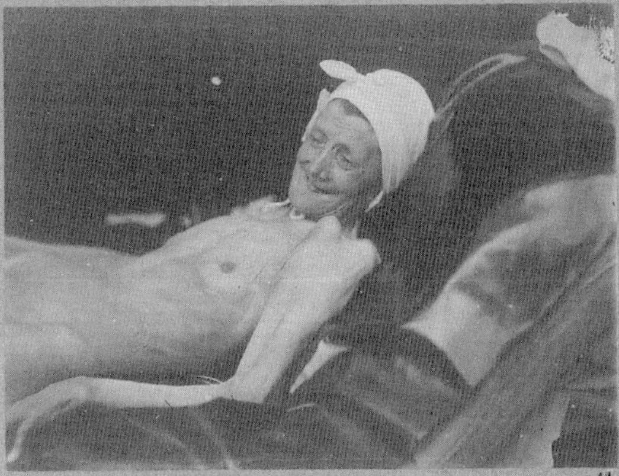

11

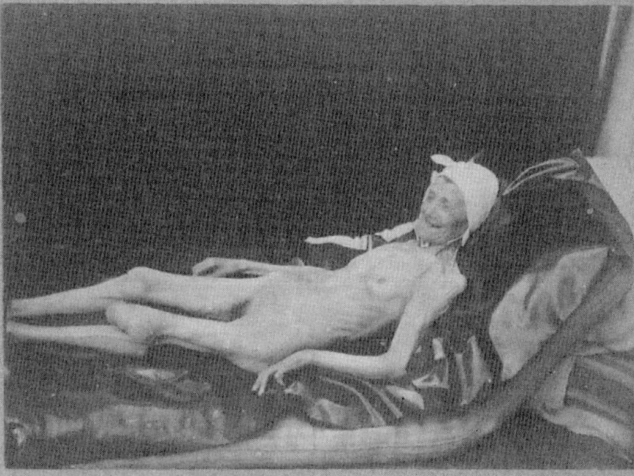

12

Berthelot

arthropathie des ataxiques

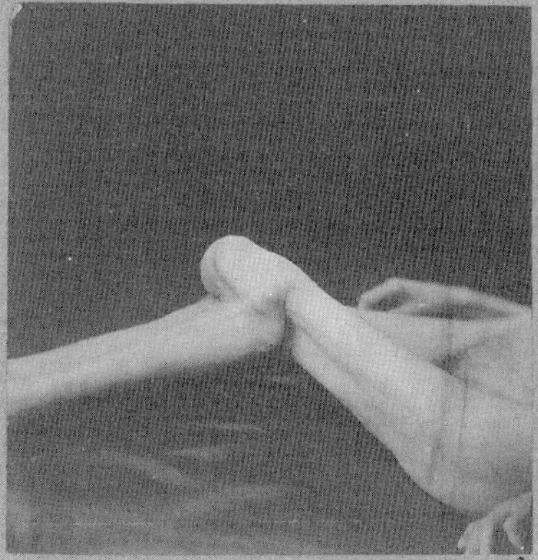

13

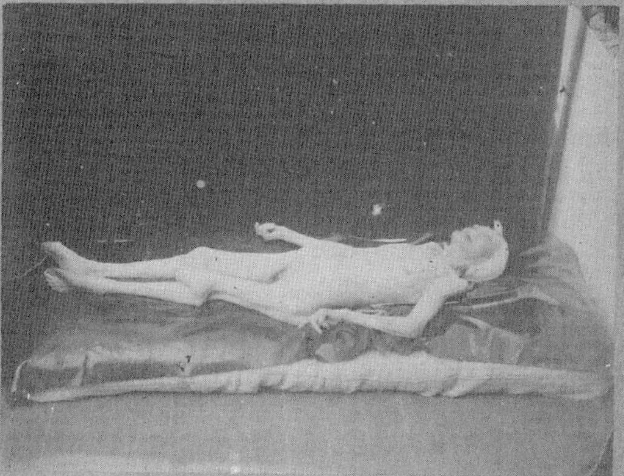

14

and her face is turned to the side and visible to the camera. Her undirected gaze and protruding tongue, along with the blurring of her face in the photo on the top right, which may indicate an inability to remain still, create the impression that she was perhaps not fully aware of what was taking place. In the two details on the left of the album page, we can see her skin pulled taut over her terribly deformed shoulder and knee. The jutting joints and the gaunt yet flaccid flesh elicit a visceral sense of compassion; the images are extremely upsetting. In the photograph on the bottom right, Berthelot's pose bears an unnerving resemblance to that of her doppelganger, the *Ataxic Venus*. It is profoundly affecting to see her living form looking so like the wax cast of her cadaver. Was this position painful for her contorted skeleton? She wears a distressed expression, and it is not unreasonable to imagine an agonized moan escaping her open mouth as the photo was taken. According to another person with locomotor ataxia, sitting up was the only position that could be "endure[d]."[40]

Fig. 53 (opposite)
Venus ataxique (arthropathie des ataxiques) (Ataxic Venus [Ataxic Arthropathy]). Albumen photograph pasted on cardboard. Charcot Album, plate 13. Paris, Musée de l'Assistance Publique–Hôpitaux de Paris. Inv. AP 2003.7.3.49. Photo: AP-HP/musée–F. Marin.

The *Ataxic Venus* is the portrait of an individual *and* the portrait of an illness. Historian of medicine Thomas Schnalke points out that "moulages never failed to tell a second story, the story of how much a body . . . represented features of an individual identity."[41] The relationship between "sitter" and "artist" highlights the cast's engagement with the conventions of portraiture: the *Ataxic Venus* sits on a continuum between individual likeness and "the generality of type"; it conveys something of Berthelot's identity (in this case, as a person with a particular medical condition); and it is the result of a "series of negotiations" (however inequitable) between sitter, artist, and patron.[42] In the case of the *Ataxic Venus*, the patron would have been Charcot himself.[43]

Loreau, as the Assistance Publique noted, was a *modeleur* (a modeler) and not simply a *mouleur* (a maker of moulages, or casts). His creations both demanded and demonstrated artistic—and not just technical—skill. Schnalke notes that around this time the works of expert mold-makers "had convinced physicians that the factor of subjectivity was reduced to a minimum."[44] Yet, like photography, casting gives the illusion of objectivity even as the details betray artistic talent and aesthetic choice. The casting studio at the Salpêtrière likely created hundreds of wax and plaster sculptures, but none of the others that I am aware of shows the level of care and attention to detail evinced by the *Ataxic Venus*.[45] These casts, which focus the attention on the deformity or contortion of a bodily fragment, would have found their way into the museum or the amphitheater to be used as props during Charcot's lectures (see fig. 7). Some surviving examples of Salpêtrière casts are patinated, mimicking the color of skin. Others retain their casting lines, reminding the viewer of the process of their making. One cast hand rests unnaturally on a pillow or mound, a convention more common in plaster casts of hands sold to artists.[46]

Yet it was clear that the sculpture of Berthelot's body was in a different league than the more "mundane" casts that populated the Salpêtrière's museum and amphitheater. While the living patient was often cast in ghostly plaster—the Italian sculptor Antonio Canova remarked that white was associated with the cadaver[47]—paradoxically,

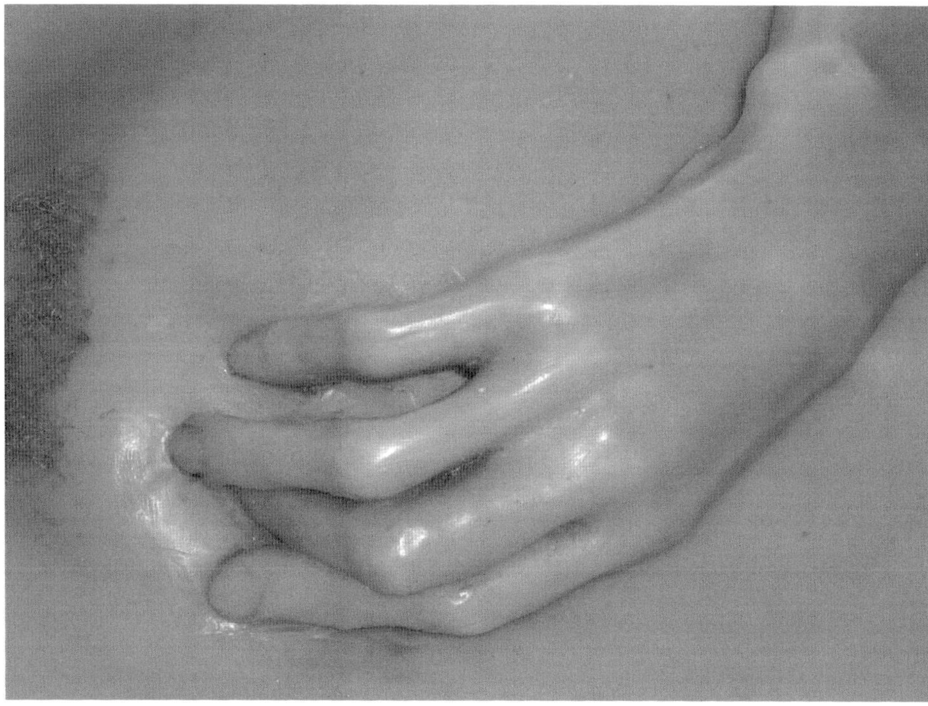

Fig. 54
Loreau, *Venus ataxique* (*Ataxic Venus*), ca. 1880, detail of undercutting around the right hand. Polychrome wax cast, 158 × 54 cm. Paris, Musée de l'Assistance Publique–Hôpitaux de Paris. Inv. AP 2001.0.4.3.1. Photo: AP-HP/musée–author.

Berthelot's dead body was cast in colored wax. Casting the whole body of a dead patient would have been very challenging, and the instability and fragility of both wax and the decomposing body meant that its production came with a certain risk. And it would undoubtedly have been an expensive enterprise. First, Loreau would have taken a "negative" mold from Berthelot's body in either plaster or beef gelatin, then made a "positive" from several layers of wax, colored to match living flesh.[48] The cadaver would have been cast in sections to then be joined together, with the artist diligently effacing the seams.[49] This was a very labor-intensive process, especially given the delicate undercutting evident in parts of the sculpture, such as the area around the right hand (fig. 54). Around this time, physicians at the Hôpital Saint-Louis wrote to the head of the Assistance Publique to say that casting was "reserved for the rarest cases" and that "moulages, because of their cost and the many hours of work that they require, can only be made in a limited number."[50] Charcot likely commissioned the cast of Berthelot's body to establish the casting studio's importance in the eyes of the Assistance Publique and to ensure that a perfect example of "Charcot's disease" would remain in the spotlight.

Wax Flesh

The fact that Charcot and Loreau decided to render the cast of Berthelot's body in colored wax rather than achromatic plaster suggests that it was intended to be the centerpiece of the Musée Charcot. It was not unusual for such anatomical Venuses to be the stars of medical museums—the celebrated Florentine museum of anatomical waxes La Specola foremost among them—as well as fairground anatomical attractions like the Spitzner Museum.[51] Wax has been a medium for sculpture for thousands of years.[52] Colored and molded easily, it is especially well suited to replicating the body, while its material properties are ideal for translation into flesh. Not only can its translucency convincingly replicate the appearance of skin, creating uncanny simulacra that can both attract and repulse the viewer, but metaphorically the medium itself "is tied to the processes of life: birth, metamorphosis, dissolution."[53] As a material, Marina Warner contends, wax can "forestall the corruption of the flesh both literally and figuratively, and as a result, the substance has also provided supple and enduring metaphors for life, for truth, for art"—all of which are in play in the *Ataxic Venus*.[54] Its indexicality especially implies truth, as Warner argues: "Wax takes such an exact impression that it has been used as a stamp of authenticity since the beginning of written documents. . . . This binds it to testimony and to truth, and, as with a life mask or a death mask, it fortifies conviction as well as faith."[55]

This quality made wax especially useful as a medical tool. Wax anatomical modeling began in the seventeenth century with Gaetano Zumbo (1656–1701), whose works form the foundation of La Specola.[56] His move to Paris at the start of the eighteenth century might have led to the creation of a French tradition in medical waxes.[57] However, there was a significant difference between Italian and French anatomical models; the latter were, at least at first, usually only seen by a medical audience instead of the general public.[58] By the end of the nineteenth century, there were probably several thousand anatomical waxes in important Parisian collections, including the Musée Dupuytren and the Hôpital Saint-Louis.[59] Some of the most important artists working in wax moved between medical and artistic circles. Jules Talrich (1826–1904), for example, while *modeleur* for the Faculté de médecine, helped conserve the so-called Wicar Head, a celebrated wax bust of a woman in the Musée Wicar in Lille that was thought at the time to have been sculpted by the circle of Raphael. Talrich also founded his own popular museum on the Boulevard des Capucines decorated in a series of wax *tableaux vivants*.[60]

Creating a wax sculpture requires myriad aesthetic decisions, and Charcot likely played an important role in those made in the reproduction of Berthelot's body. With regard to a contemporaneous collection of wax casts owned by Dr. Jules Péan, Mary Hunter has argued that "the process of detailing the wax model was one that united the *mouleur* with the medical professional, as the medical man directed the *mouleur* on how much color was needed, how much intricate detailing was required and how much hair to insert." She concludes that, in their aesthetic contributions to cast figures, doctors were aligned with sculptors.[61] This union of art and medicine would only have heightened Charcot's identification as an artist. For instance, Charcot and Loreau would have chosen Berthelot's skin tone, since her dead body would not have retained the uniform beige of the *Ataxic Venus*. In addition to tingeing the thin lips with red and coloring the irises, the artist added a reddish-brown stain under incised lines that suggest the hairs of her eyebrows (see fig. 52). On close inspection, the faint

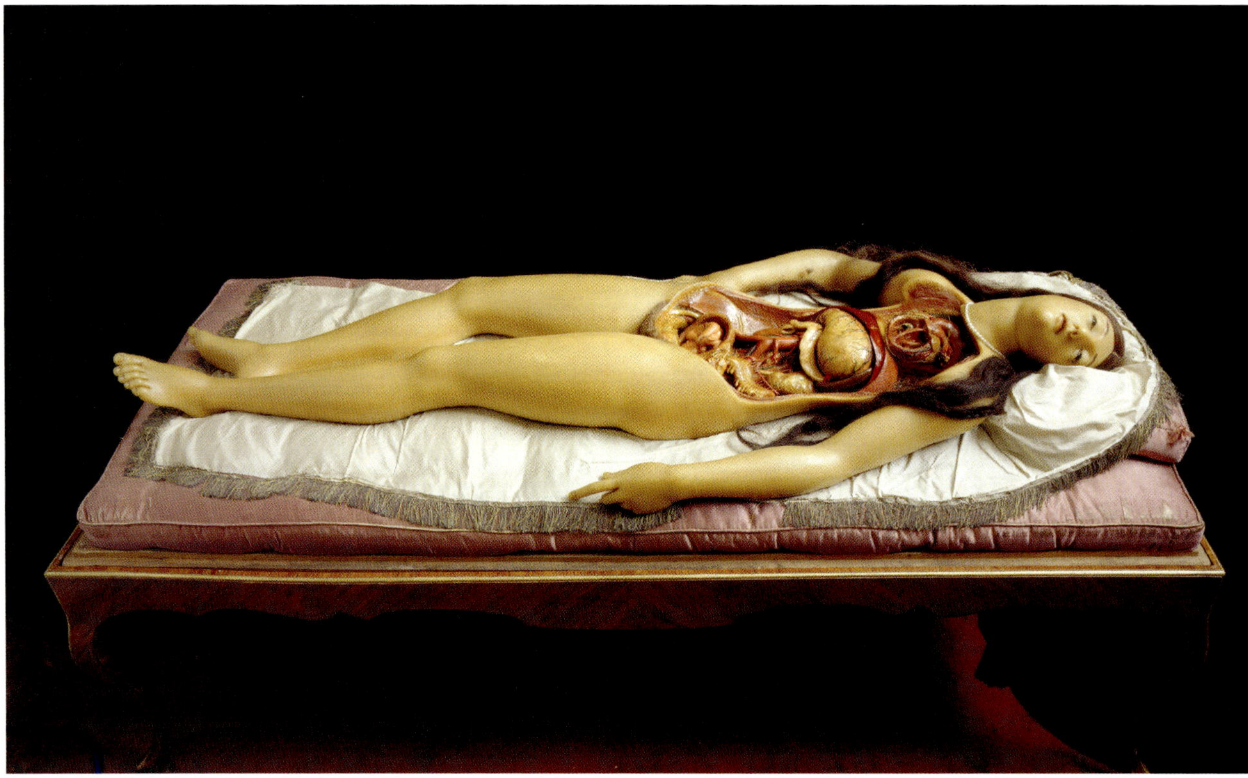

Fig. 55
Clemente Susini, *The Dismantable Venus*, eighteenth century. Wax. Florence, La Specola. Photo: Museo della Specola, Florence, Italy / Bridgeman Images.

marks of the modeler's implements can be discerned all over the body. The parallel lines of a scraping tool run along the fingers that press lightly onto the flesh of the pelvis. They are also visible on the adjacent areas of skin, where the surface has been carefully smoothed over (see fig. 54).[62] In the complicated and delicate process of casting an entire body, the artist works painstakingly to remove evidence of his own hand—and yet traces such as these remain.

While there are hints of color on Berthelot's face, the nipples conspicuously, and oddly, match the flesh of her chest. The eroticism of the recumbent nude, whether clothed as in Madame Tussaud's *Sleeping Beauty* or naked like the Spitzner's anatomical Venus and La Specola's famous eighteenth-century *Venere dei medici* (or, in French, the *Vénus des médecins*) by Clemente Susini (1754–1814), is partially denied to the *Ataxic Venus* (fig. 55). The reproductive fullness of the *Venere dei medici* in particular—a wax sculpture of an idealized, pregnant woman whose body can be peeled back in successive layers to reveal a developing fetus—is repudiated by the desiccated and diseased elderly woman represented in the Musée Charcot.[63] Of course, the trope of the "old woman" had been around for millennia: she represented moral vice and *vanitas* and was depicted as monstrous and decaying. Charles Baudelaire included a poem about "Les Petites Vieilles" ("The Little Old Women") who were "ashamed of existing" in *Les Fleurs du mal* (1857), while physician Joseph-Henri Reveillé-Parise disparagingly described the physical features of the old woman as "quite unsightly" in his *Traité de la vieillesse* (Treatise on old age) from 1853.[64] This anxiety about the aging female body was only heightened by contemporary fears of hereditary degeneration, a theory expounded by Charcot and many others who did not believe that syphilis caused tabes dorsalis.[65] "Sexual excess," a "symptom" of degeneration, was thought to be a possible cause of the disease.[66]

The inclusion of hair on the crown and on the *mons veneris* helps make the wax "as lifelike as possible" and highlights the "individuality of a particular patient."[67] But it also sexualizes this body that is, of course, both culturally produced and socially constructed. The issue of body hair was fraught for nineteenth-century viewers, who reacted with shock to its depiction because it turned an academic nude into a naked woman.[68] As William Ian Miller notes, "Hair shares too much with the erotic, not to play a starring role in the theater troupe of disgust."[69] The *Ataxic Venus*'s sex is visible under a thin tuft of hair that serves more to highlight than to hide it. A viewer's response could vacillate between lust and disgust for an object that could be seen as "repugnant *and* captivating."[70] There is revulsion and fascination in beholding the medical Venus: the easy exposure of the viscera of the *Venere dei medici* signals the breakdown of the "boundaries of self," while the elderly and deformed body of the *Ataxic Venus* shows us the ugliness that was seen as an attribute of female old age in the nineteenth century.[71] Reveillé-Parise's *Traité de la vieillesse* states plainly that "once [a woman's] complexion dulls, her figure thickens, and her beauty fades, one is struck by the advancement of age, and one sees the irreparable ravages of time."[72] The partially shut eyelids allow us to stare with impunity not only at the *Ataxic Venus*'s deformities but also at her raw nakedness. This, in and of itself, constitutes a "violation of norms" that titillates.[73] The aestheticized, sexualized, and medicalized body of the *Ataxic Venus* confirms that, as Michel Foucault astutely noted, *scientia sexualis* functioned in the nineteenth century as an *ars erotica*.[74]

Medical historian Michael Sappol emphasizes the sensuousness of the different materials evident in the medical museum, which provide visual delights and conjure tactile ones as well.[75] It bears repeating that the act of voyeurism is implicit in this space, and perhaps no more so than in the figure of the anatomical Venus: the focus of its body is traditionally its passive fertility. While the typical anatomical Venus exhibits a casual eroticism, the *Ataxic Venus* does not. Nor does Berthelot's cast face display ecstasy; rather, the "imprint of death," the terrible pain of locomotor ataxia, has apparently left its traces.[76] Charcot and Richer comment in *Les Difformes et les malades dans l'art* that "one has seen the anguish of desperation persist [on the face] after death."[77] The photograph taken of Berthelot while alive captures an unexpected grin, likely a sign of the euphoria or mania that was symptomatic of the general paralysis of the insane, also caused by tertiary syphilis (see fig. 53). The photograph recalls art-historical precedents; her pose and the shiny material on which she lies make the photograph of Berthelot a nightmarish pendant to Édouard Manet's *Olympia* (1863, Paris, Musée d'Orsay). Regardless, unlike the idealized anatomical Venus or Manet's modern nude, the face of the *Ataxic Venus* is disfigured. All of Berthelot's teeth were missing, and she had the unfortunate distinction of being the first known case of temporomandibular arthropathy.[78]

Paul Richer noted the fraught relationship between living and lifeless form in a cast, stating in his "Dialogues sur l'art et la science" that "it is a prejudice to believe . . . that the moulage reproduces nature very faithfully. It is sufficient to have seen a mask molded on a living figure to find that it is not. . . . That mask resembles more a dead person than a living one."[79] Wax has an "incestuous bond" with death, according to Roberta Panzanelli.[80] Casting is a way of controlling nature, a literal "getting to grips" with it, with potentially fatal consequences. In attempting to take a full-body cast, the painter Benjamin Haydon almost killed his model when the 250 liters of plaster poured over him began to harden.[81] Paradoxically, the cast body or body part can appear lifeless despite being indexical, especially when the traces of the process—the casting lines—are smoothed over and made to disappear, erasing the artifice. Honoré de Balzac's protagonist in *Le Chef-d'oeuvre inconnu* (1837) made just this point: "Try to mold the hand of your mistress and to place it in front of you, you will find a horrible cadaver without any resemblance."[82] Even a body reproduced with fleshy coloring and realistic details can give the appearance of an individual petrified. This may have contributed to the popularity of certain full-body anatomical waxes, such as the Spitzner's *Sleeping Venus* or Madame Tussaud's *Sleeping Beauty*—beautiful young women whose chests slowly expanded and contracted with the signs of respiration, pretending, momentarily at least, to be alive.[83] The *Ataxic Venus* embodies these paradoxes: the figure is clearly dead, but its coloring suggests life. The body is petrified, yet it radiates pain.

In the Land of Pain

To my knowledge, Berthelot did not leave behind any verbal or written trace, and so we are left only with Charcot's descriptions of her and her illness. Charcot claimed in his talk at the International Medical Congress in 1881 that she had endured the painful symptoms of locomotor ataxia for twenty years, noting that "she had first lightning pains and pains around the waist, disturbances of sight, inco-ordination [*sic*] of movement, but never any gastric attacks." After five years, "the disease showed itself in the left knee, and subsequently walking became impossible. Four years ago, an affection of the left shoulder-joint showed itself; then disease of the right shoulder-joint and of the right hip, and ultimately a disease of the articulation of the right jaw."[84] This description of her symptoms is not accompanied by any documentation of her own words, despite the fact that Charcot would often interview patients in front of his audience and then publish transcripts along with his lessons. Given that the overwhelming majority of the Salpêtrière's long-term patients were poor and working-class women, the absence of her authorial presence is, sadly, to be expected. Berthelot's body and image were reproduced and displayed by Charcot internationally in journals and lectures, but like most of Charcot's other female patients at the Salpêtrière, she was never granted a voice by the physician who treated her until her death.[85] Regardless, her cast "restores all the disquieting and human reality of the deceased model."[86] The *Ataxic Venus* remains a moving material trace of her life.

One of Charcot's patients *did* have the opportunity to put into words, to try to express and perhaps even come to terms with, the symptoms of and pain associated with locomotor ataxia. Alphonse Daudet was one of Charcot's private patients and had the privilege of attending his lectures as an audience member alongside *le tout Paris*.[87] Daudet dedicated his novel *L'Évangéliste: Roman parisien* (1883) to the neurologist. They regularly visited each other's salons, and eventually Daudet moved to a home so close to Charcot's that they could see each other's gardens.[88] His son Léon was one of Charcot's pupils before abandoning his medical studies and becoming a famous writer. By the 1880s, it was clear that Alphonse Daudet had developed locomotor ataxia. Within a few years, Charcot revealed that Daudet was "condemned for life," though he would live for another twelve years.[89] Echoing Charcot's sentiment, Edmond de Goncourt described the lithographic portrait of Daudet by Eugène Carrière (1849–1906) as "Daudet crucified, Daudet at Golgotha [*golgothant*]" (1893, Amsterdam, Van Gogh Museum).[90]

The novelist captured the anguish and hopelessness of the disease in expressive prose compiled for a book that he did not live to see published. Daudet intended to call it *La Doulou* (translated as *In the Land of Pain*, 1930), which was Provençal for "pain." He wrote of "great flames of pain furrowing my body, cutting it to pieces, lighting it up" from the top of his head to the soles of his feet.[91] Daudet complained about some of the typical symptoms: acute pain in the extremities—"a penknife stabbing away beneath the big toenail"—or the feeling that the torso or pelvis was being progressively constricted by a girdle or breastplate until it was no longer possible to breathe.[92] Exasperated at the "varieties of pain," he quoted Charcot: "That's the disease for you."[93] And he lamented in utter exhaustion, "My poor carcass is hollowed out. . . . Pain echoes through it as a voice echoes in a house without furniture or curtains. There are days, long days, when the only part of me that's alive is my pain."[94] At times, words escaped him: "How much I suffered last night, in my heel and in my ribs. Sheer torture . . . there are no words to express it, only howls of pain could do so. Are words actually any use to describe what pain (or passion, for that matter) really feels like? Words only come when everything is over, when things have calmed down. They refer only to memory and are either powerless or untruthful."[95] And while he seems to conclude, like Elaine Scarry, that pain is unrepresentable, his notes for *La Doulou* reveal that he kept trying to find words that could convey pain's power or truth.[96]

Can a visual image succeed where Daudet felt his words fell short? Can it effectively communicate the power and truth of pain? The unnatural contortions of the *Ataxic Venus*—the sharply turned face, the disturbingly angular left arm jutting from a deformed shoulder joint, the gnarled left leg lying stiff and twisted on a table—begin to convey the pain that Daudet also expressed. And while Charcot tells us that Berthelot indeed experienced the excruciating "lightning pains" associated with the illness—pain that could "either nail me to the spot," as Daudet lamented, "or twist me around

Fig. 56 (opposite)
Giovanni Battista Caracciolo, *The Martyrdom of Saint Sebastian*, ca. 1625. Oil on canvas, 202.3 × 113.9 cm. Cambridge, Harvard Art Museums/Fogg Museum, Gift of Herbert Pope, Arthur Pope, Edward W. Forbes and Paul J. Sachs. Photo © President and Fellows of Harvard College, 1924.31.

so that my foot pumps up and down like a knife-grinder's"—the arthropathic joints *did not in themselves* cause pain.[97] In this illness, the joint broke imperceptibly, the area swelled, sometimes cracking could be heard, and then, often, the joint was no longer of any use. Simply turning in bed could cause fractures. Charcot's protégé Charles Féré (1852–1907) hypothesized that Berthelot cracked her pelvis that way, a break not discovered until a postmortem was performed.[98] There is, then, a disconnect between one's empathic discomfort in viewing this cast—I recoil at the sight of those disfigured and damaged joints—and the patient's own lived experience of the pain, which is, of course, unknowable. In other words, my empathy arises from an incongruity: Berthelot's "Charcot joints" did not cause her pain. The cast does communicate pain, but it does so deceptively.

The pain felt when looking at the *Ataxic Venus*'s contorted body is amplified by the ways in which this figure both relies on and departs from precedents, notably the anatomical Venus. The "lineage" of most examples of this type of anatomical model can be traced back to the *Venere dei medici* (see fig. 55). Like the *Ataxic Venus*, the color of its flesh is redolent of life, its lips softly parted, its eyes partially open. But the *Venere dei medici's* expression suggests ecstasy tinged with vague pain. The fantasy of unlocking the mysteries of the female body is here reified and literally placed within man's reach by modeling a woman's body (as opposed to casting it) after having performed countless extensive autopsies.[99] As is visible in the photograph of the Musée Charcot, Berthelot's cast was exhibited below eye level, as if on an examination table, forcing the visitor to identify with the clinician examining a patient or the pathologist encountering a corpse (see fig. 4). The latter is particularly relevant here: one contemporary mentions that the *Ataxic Venus* was kept hidden under a sheet at the Musée Charcot.[100] Even though its internal anatomy was irretrievable—though Berthelot's skeleton hanging nearby could provide the illusion of its knowability—the process of unveiling made literal a metaphor particularly appropriate to anatomical Venuses and, as Ludmilla Jordanova has argued, "equally apt in a sexual and in an intellectual context."[101] And, we might add, in the art-historical context: some artworks were considered so disturbing or pornographic that they, too, were hidden under a veil or behind a curtain.

In the Land of Art

The *Ataxic Venus* powerfully embodies a whole range of artistic traditions. The placement of the right hand on the stomach echoes the *pudica* pose of Venuses from antiquity. In fact, the creator of the *Venere dei medici* was inspired by the Hellenistic *Medici Venus* in the Uffizi Gallery.[102] Perhaps the title *Ataxic Venus* is not only ironic but also intended to elevate this object, about a disfiguring disease, to the level of art. Mythology could certainly furnish both visual precedents—consider the body of the *Dying Niobid* (second century CE, Florence, Uffizi) or of the *Laocoön* (ca. 50–20 BCE, Rome, Vatican Museums), for instance—and metaphors for pain and its effects. Psychiatrist and anthropologist Arthur Kleinman discusses the need to jettison pain "outward into the world in images," concluding that, for him at least, "the language of pain *is* those metaphors."[103] Daudet likened locomotor ataxia's agonizing stiffness to the unexpected transformations found in ancient tales: "I feel like some creature from mythology, whose torso is locked in a box of wood or stone, gradually turning numb and then solid. As the paralysis spreads upward, the sick man changes into a rock or a tree, like those who caught sight of Medusa or some nymph from Ovid's *Metamorphoses*."[104] This is one possible way to "do" pain, as Suzannah Biernoff argues: "to objectify it using metaphor."[105]

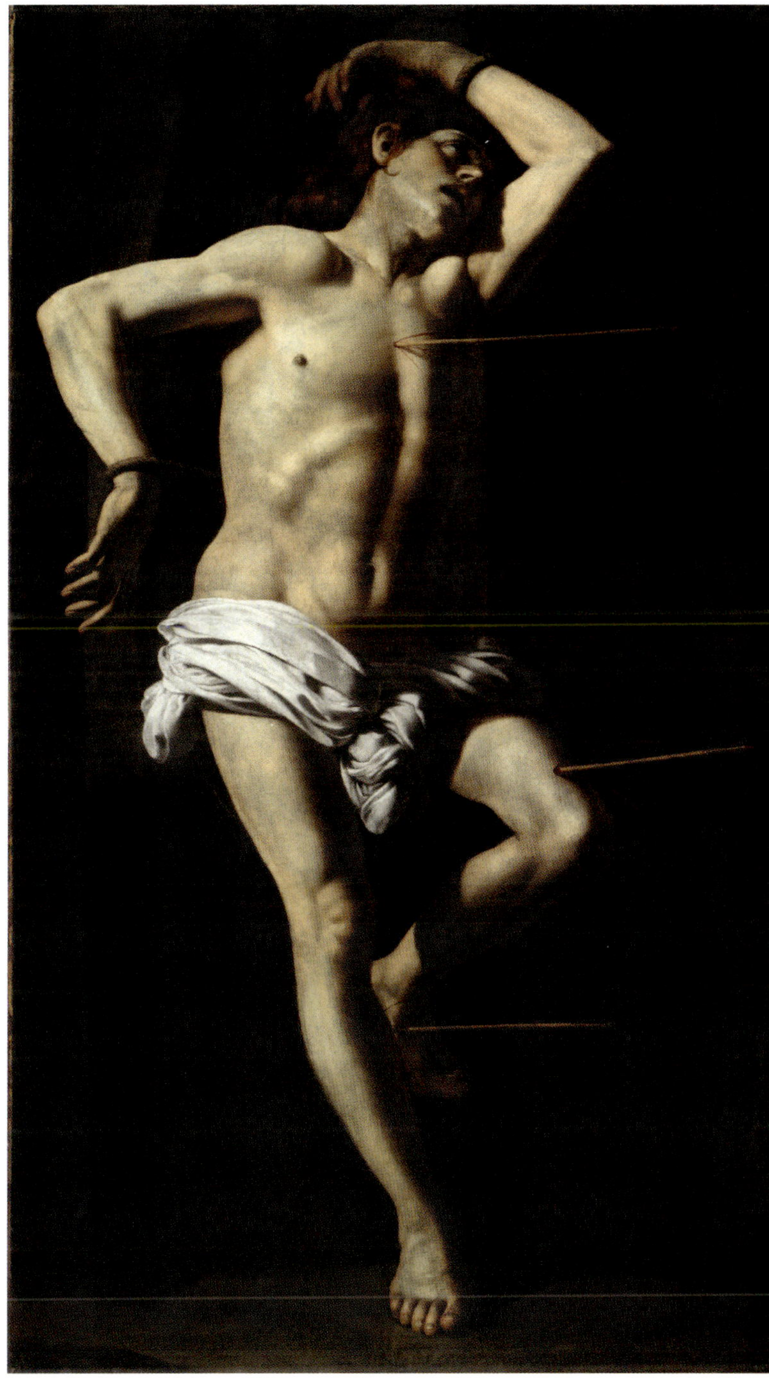

One could look at a number of art-historical precedents specifically as metaphors for pain, metaphors certainly known by the culturally sophisticated and well-traveled Charcot. Christianity, especially, has a "longstanding investment in pain," and the *Ataxic Venus*'s tortured body calls to mind images of martyred saints.[106] Comparing the *Ataxic Venus* to Giovanni Battista Caracciolo's *Martyrdom of Saint Sebastian* from ca. 1625, for example, we see unnaturally twisted limbs, discomfiting countenances, and bodies splayed out for witnessing in strikingly similar poses (fig. 56). Depictions of Saint Sebastian also echo the photographs of hypnotized hysterics in the Salpêtrière's journals in which long metal rods are used to "excite" muscles but give the impression instead of impaling the patient.[107] In both Caracciolo's painting and the *Ataxic Venus*, we cannot see the antagonists. While we can imagine Roman archers shooting at the Christian saint from outside the frame, Berthelot suffers at the hands of an invisible tormentor, one that coursed through her veins and resided in her bones. In the scientific age in which Berthelot lived, there were lessons to be learned, but there was no redemption.

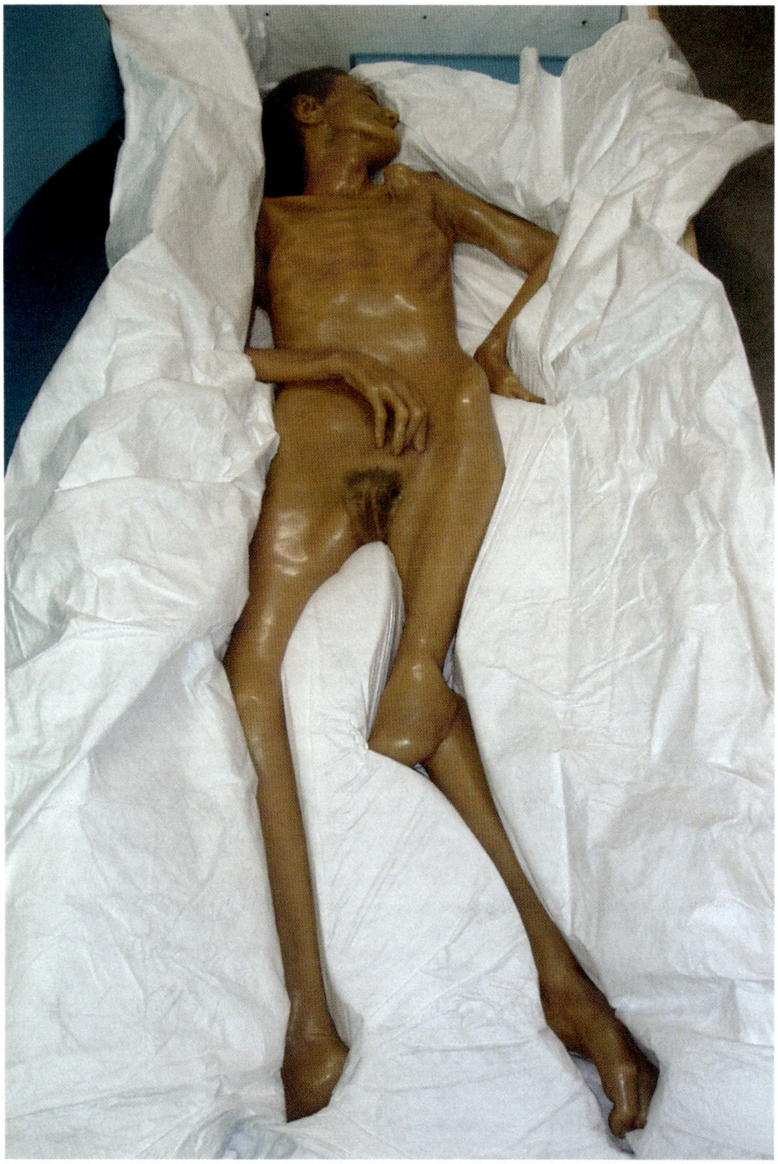

The comparison could be extended to the ultimate martyr, the dead Christ (figs. 57 and 58). In the medieval sculpture by Gregorio Fernández, for instance, the deathly visage is angled awkwardly, the naked body with its lifeless yet oddly taut limbs laid out for viewing. In the case of the *Ataxic Venus*, horrifically deformed joints replace Christ's bloody wounds, yet the hyperrealism of both bodies renders "the horrific death intensely present."[108] Daudet describes the pain from the malady he shared with Berthelot with an apt comparison: "Crucifixion. That's what it was like the other night. The torment of the Cross: violent wrenching of the hands, feet, knees; nerves stretched and pulled to breaking-point. The coarse rope bound tight round the torso, the spear prodding at the ribs. The skin peeling from my hot, parched, fever-crusted lips; to slake my thirst I took a spoonful of iodized bromide, salty and bitter. It was the sponge soaked in vinegar and gall. I then imagined a conversation about Pain between Christ and the two thieves."[109] Daudet's analogy speaks powerfully of the sensations occasioned by the illness. He deploys Christian symbolism that would have been well known to his audience, harnessing the culture's collective awareness of the ultimate example of pain to make his own torment resonate. The Stations of the Cross in every Catholic church were (and still are) intended as a vehicle for communing with Christ through a shared language of embodied pain. Historian Valentin Groebner has written of the importance of *passio* (Latin for passion) for the beholder in relation to both martyrs and Christ: "*Passio* meant identification through narratives of carefully individualized violence." He continues, "A huge historical archive of images and stories represented these pains for an audience of faithful in order to impress, move, and instruct them."[110] (The etymology of the word "patient" itself refers to enduring hardship or having long suffered.)[111] The cast of the Salpêtrière patient was similarly intended to "impress" and "instruct," though Charcot's interest in its ability to "move" was probably slight. Rather than

Fig. 57
Loreau, *Venus ataxique (Ataxic Venus)*, ca. 1880. Polychrome wax cast, 158 × 54 cm. Paris, Musée de l'Assistance Publique–Hôpitaux de Paris. Inv. AP 2001.0.4.3.1. Photo: AP-HP/musée–author.

communicating pain deceptively, as I commented above, the contorted body of the *Ataxic Venus* should be read through the codes of pain that have a long lineage in Christian and classical imagery.[112]

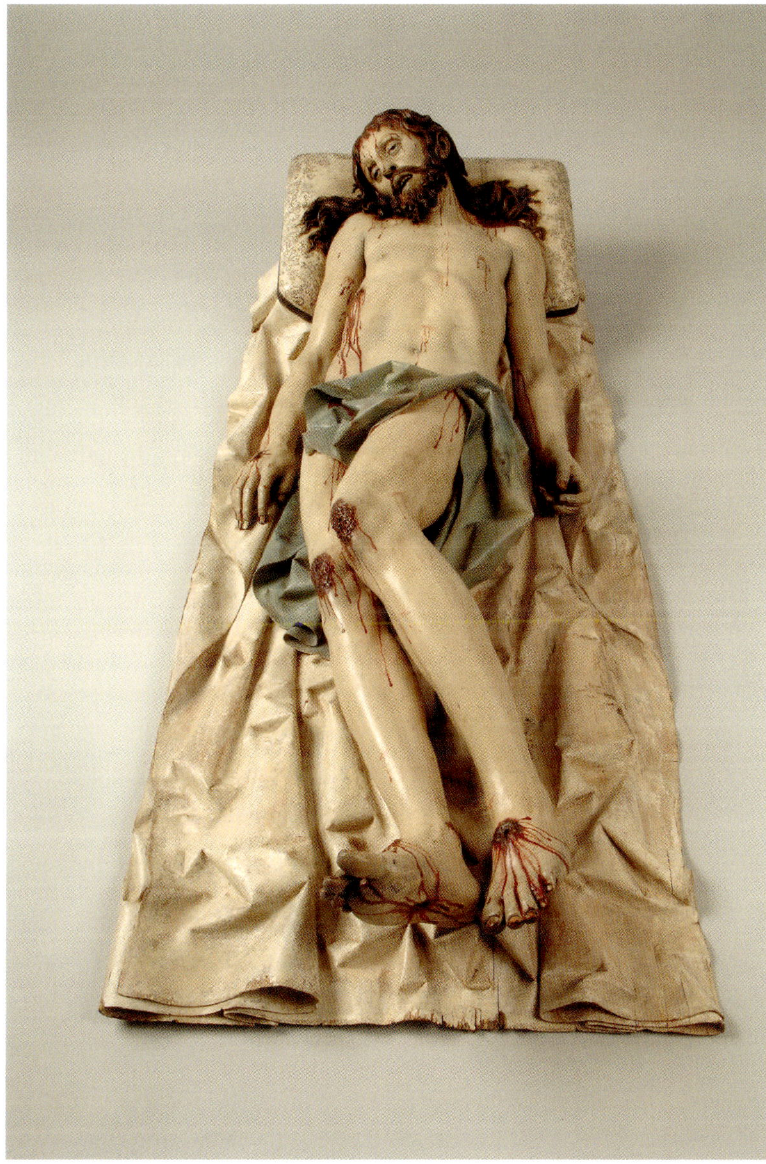

Of course, wax sculptures recall sacred early modern relics and effigies of the dead Christ and his grieving mother, objects that inspired prayer, thus "facilitat[ing] the most noble aims of art."[113] The addition of real hair on the *Ataxic Venus* would have intensified her "relic-like status."[114] Yet the comparison with relics or a crucified Christ only gets us so far. At the Salpêtrière there was an abundance of enervation and pain on faces and bodies, but a distinct dearth of transcendent beauty to manifest their grace. Holly Edwards has noted of images of the suffering Christ that "shrouding our dead in beauty can provide solace and respite from pain."[115] The relics of Berthelot are instead fully secular—just a body, surface replicated here in a wax cast, eviscerated bones displayed there in a vitrine. One of this specimen's roles is precisely *not* to shield the viewer from the disease's attendant deformities, *not* to "provide solace and respite from pain," but instead to enlighten and edify. Moreover, the *Ataxic Venus* is perhaps even intended to provide a modicum of schadenfreude, of titillation at its disturbing sexualization, and of gratification through a knowing recognition of art-historical antecedents.

Fig. 58
Gregorio Fernández, *Dead Christ*, 1625–30. Polychromed wood, horn, glass, and cork, 46 × 191 × 74 cm. Madrid, Museo Nacional del Prado. Photo © Photographic Archive Museo Nacional del Prado.

In *Les Difformes et les malades dans l'art,* Charcot and Richer include a chapter on dead bodies, describing sculptures of kings and queens resting on their earthly remains, or sculpted cadavers serving as *memento mori* on tombs—some of which are, significantly, also portraits. One of the most striking examples they discuss is the *transi* of Catherine de' Medici (ca. 1565–66, Paris, Musée du Louvre) by Girolamo della Robbia (1488–1566), which the authors note was on display in the late nineteenth century in the chapel of the École des beaux-arts, near Charcot's home (fig. 59).[116] Della Robbia imagined the queen, who commissioned the sculpture while still alive, decades in the future,

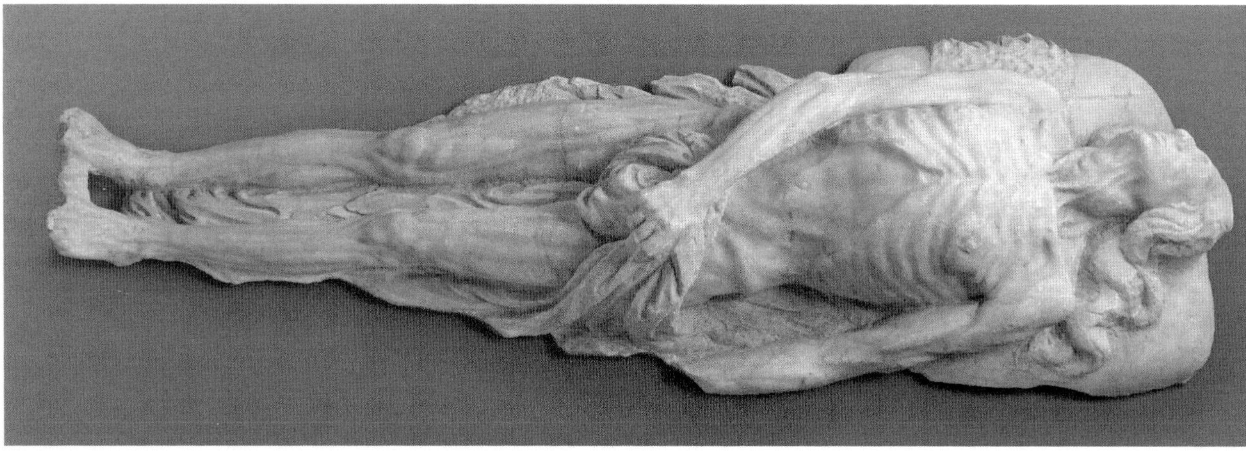

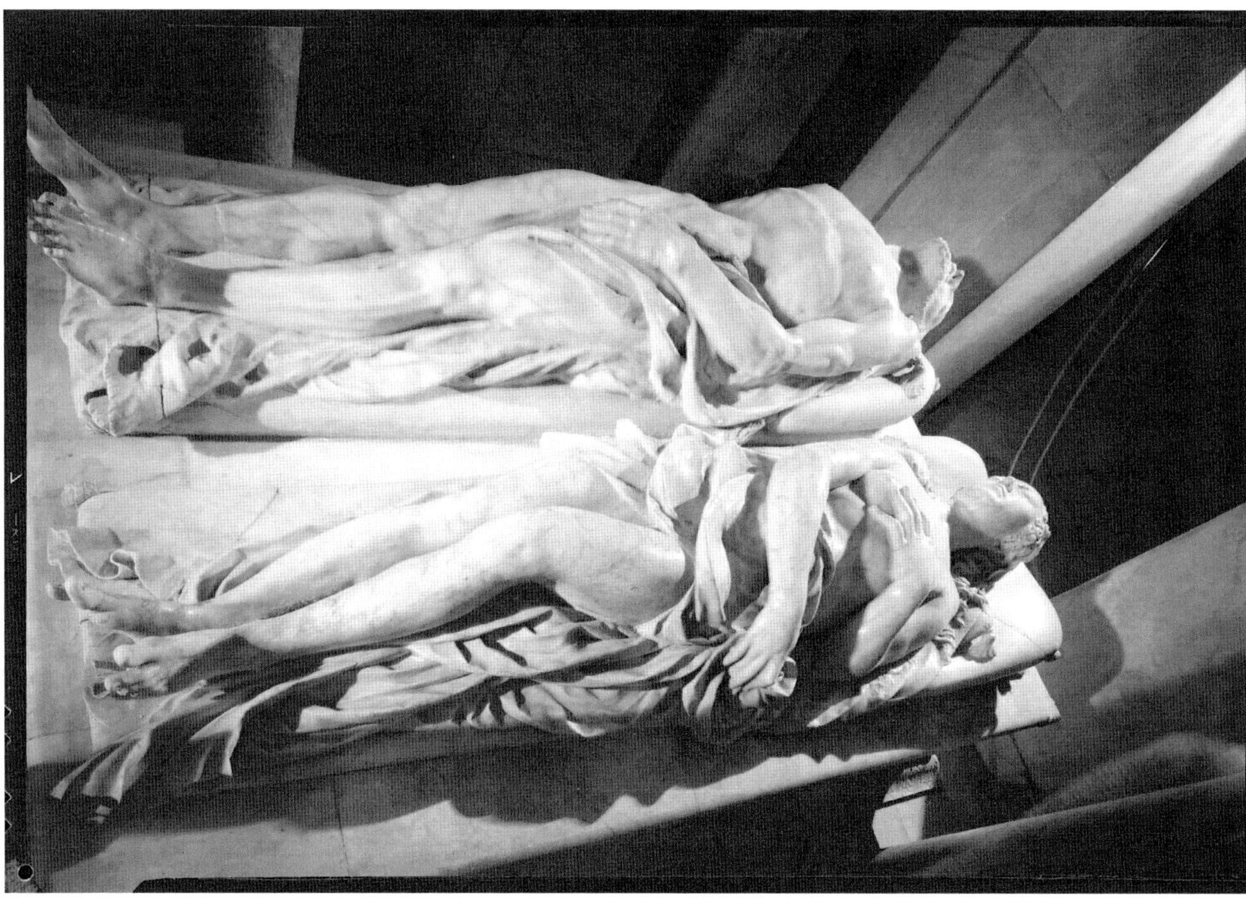

after death and in a state of decomposition (a *transi* is a recumbent tomb effigy of a dead, and sometimes decomposing, body). Recalling Charcot's early claim that the physician is ideally suited to judge the work of the artist, Charcot and Richer perform a clinical examination of this sculpture and conclude that Della Robbia had likely been looking at a male cadaver.[117] Its unadulterated realism was, however, too much for Catherine de' Medici, who was not pleased with the result.[118] In the final version in the Basilica of Saint-Denis, her effigy—created by Germaine Pilon (ca. 1540–1590)—looks more like an idealized *Venus pudica* than Della Robbia's stark reminder of mortality (fig. 60).[119] Nevertheless, both images of corpses are echoed in the *Ataxic Venus*.

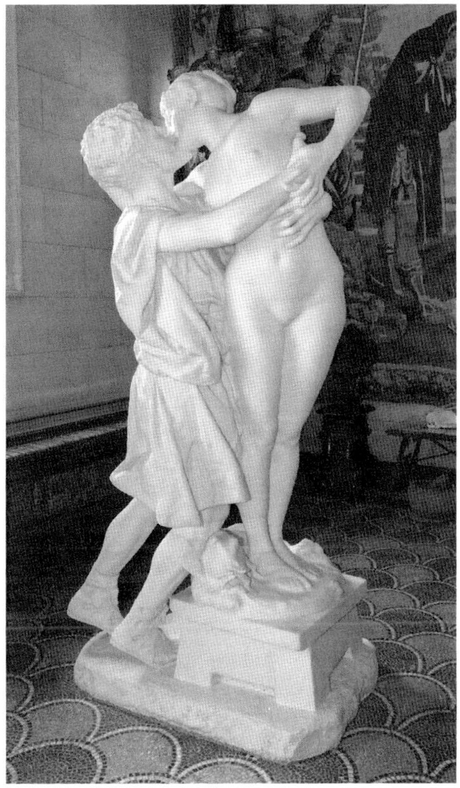

Fig. 59 (opposite top)
Girolamo della Robbia, *Study for the Funerary Effigy of Catherine de Medici*, ca. 1565–66. Paris, Musée du Louvre. Photo © RMN-Grand Palais (musée du Louvre) / Stéphane Maréchalle.

Fig. 60 (opposite bottom)
Germaine Pilon, *Tomb of Henry II and Catherine de Medici*, 1561–73. Saint-Denis, Basilica of Saint-Denis. © RMN–Gestion droit d'auteur René-Jacques. Photo © Ministère de la Culture–Médiathèque du Patrimoine, Dist. RMN-Grand Palais / René-Jacques.

Fig. 61
Jean-Léon Gérôme, *Pygmalion and Galatea*, 1892. Marble. San Simeon, California, Hearst Castle. Photograph by Victoria Garagliano / © Hearst Castle® / CA State Parks.

Wax in the Salon

In the nineteenth century, the realism of polychrome sculptures, including some made or covered in wax, was a source of tension in the Salon.[120] While many critics derided sculptural experiments in polychromy, its adherents were encouraged by the discovery of color on ancient sculpture in the first half of the nineteenth century and of the painted Hellenistic Tanagra figurines in the 1870s.[121] Late in life, Orientalist painter Jean-Léon Gérôme began producing sculptures that demonstrate a wholehearted embrace of polychromy, including tinted marble sculptures like his bust of a fierce-looking Sarah Bernhardt (ca. 1895, Paris, Musée d'Orsay) and the bizarre *Bellona* (1892, Hamilton, Art Gallery of Hamilton), using materials such as bronze, ivory, and even gemstones. Gérôme also utilized pigmented wax on sculptures such as *Corinth* (before 1903, Paris, Musée d'Orsay) and *Pygmalion and Galatea* (1892; fig. 61). The latter, which today is white, was originally covered in colored wax to increase the realism of Gérôme's depiction of a sculpture coming to life, a subject he had already treated multiple times on canvas.[122] As in his painting of *Pygmalion and Galatea* (ca. 1890, New York, Metropolitan Museum of Art), the lower part of Galatea's body in the sculpture was originally left uncolored, so that her transformation from marble to flesh would have been even more striking. The sculpture was contemptuously compared to anatomical waxes upon its exhibition in the Salon of 1892. Art critic Gustave Geffroy, for instance, derided the *Pygmalion and Galatea* in terms redolent of the *Ataxic Venus*:

"It is exactly the opposite of statuary—it is . . . trompe-l'oeil employed in art—it is art denied. The wax figure is near—the horrible effect of dead hair planted in inert matter, the repulsive glass eyes, the flesh of made-up cadavers."[123] Gérôme, dubbed "le père Polychrome,"[124] would surely have known the *Ataxic Venus*, as he was a frequent guest at the Charcot family salon. He may even have been responsible for suggesting Charcot's lessons as a potential subject for a painting to his student, André Brouillet, and could have acted as intermediary.[125]

Of course, the critical debate about realism in sculpture extended beyond simple wax simulacra. In 1881, the same year that Charcot brought the *Ataxic Venus* to London, Edgar Degas showed his small wax *Little Dancer Aged Fourteen* (1879–81, Washington, DC, National Gallery of Art) at the sixth Impressionist exhibition in a glass vitrine, as if it were meant to be exhibited, as one critic brutally noted, in a "museum of zoology, anthropology, [or] physiology."[126] Utilizing contemporary pseudoscientific theories of physiognomy to render the "stigmata of degeneracy" on the dancer's body, as Anthea Callen has perceptively noted, and including real hair and fabric, Degas achieved what was seen by one critic at the time as a "truly modern effort, an essay in realism in sculpture."[127] That he succeeded in this "essay" can be discerned from the comments of Elie de Mont that the little dancer resembled an aborted fetus and should be displayed in a "jar of spirits," or of a "Comtesse Louise" who went so far as to suggest that the sculpture should be placed in the Musée Dupuytren.[128] For Degas, wax was the most suitable material to sculpt modern life. Joris-Karl Huysmans agreed: "Taking up, after M. Henry Cros who uses it to transfer the figurines painted in old missals into sculpture . . . , the process of painted wax, M. Degas has discovered one of the only formulas that could be suitable for sculpture today."[129]

Unsurprisingly, given his appreciation of medieval and Renaissance art, Charcot showed an interest in contemporary wax sculpture through the patronage of the artist who sculpted "the figurines painted in old missals," Henry Cros (1840–1907).[130] As noted in chapter 1, Charcot commissioned Cros to decorate the walls of his museum with sculptures, which seem to have been placed primarily on the wooden beams that supported the ceiling (see fig. 4).[131] The Charcot family also owned at least two polychrome works by Cros: a painted terracotta bust of a woman in Gothic dress from 1882 and a reduced version in *pâte de verre* (glass paste) of *Les Druidesses*, which had been shown in the Salon of 1877.[132] The latter was given pride of place in the Charcot family home when it was incorporated into a piece of furniture that included a mosaic by Mme. Charcot (fig. 62).[133] Charcot's wife and his stepdaughter, Marie Liouville, also sculpted in and with wax.[134] The latter had an important collection of waxes in her own right and won a medal for her art at the Universal Exposition of 1900.[135]

While Cros's polychrome figures had obvious appeal to people who shared Charcot's affinity for medieval and Renaissance art, there was also a growing general interest in wax sculpture among private collectors at the time. These included art critic Philippe Burty, a friend of Degas's, who commissioned Cros to create a copy of the wax Wicar Head, which, as I noted earlier in the chapter, was restored by Talrich.[136]

Burty was a friend of the Charcot family and art advisor to Charcot's wife, and Charcot meanwhile seems to have treated Burty's daughter Madeleine for depression.[137] Burty also appears in Brouillet's painting, standing at the back of the room in front of Richer's drawing. It is likely that Burty introduced Cros to the Charcot family and facilitated the commissioning of works for the Salpêtrière's museum of pathological anatomy.

Cros executed his first wax sculpture in 1867, creating a bust of Charles VII.[138] In the first half of his career, his production concentrated on wax sculptures and bas-reliefs in a medieval vein, such as *Isabeau de Bavière* (1875, Paris, Musée d'Orsay) and *Le Prix du tournoi* (*The Tournament Prize*) (1873, Paris, Musée d'Orsay), as well as portraits. *Le Prix du tournoi*, bought for the Musée du Luxembourg after the Salon of 1873, gives a sense of what the works in the Musée Charcot might have looked like: florid patterns in deep colors, invented scenes, and powerful femmes fatales in elaborate costumes (fig. 63). Jean-Luc Olivié notes that the effect of the relief is "photographic," in that the details of the foreground are sharper than those in the background.[139]

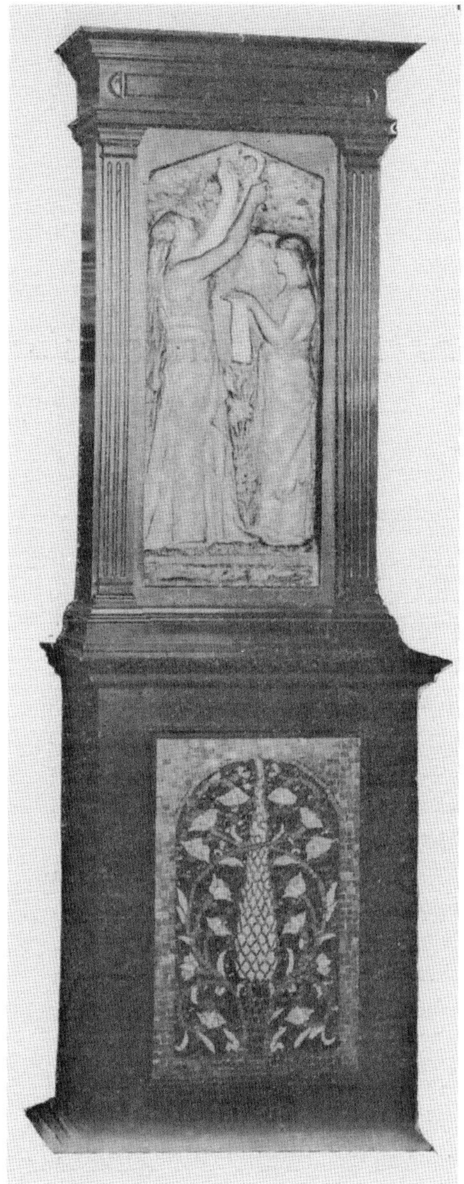

Fig. 62
Furniture from antechamber of Charcot family home with artworks by Henry Cros (above) and Augustine Charcot (below). From Gustave Goetschy, "Les Femmes du monde artistes. Madame Charcot," *Revue des arts décoratifs* 20, no. 1 (1900): 42. Photo © The British Library Board (PP.1803. LAG).

While Cros is mostly forgotten today, he was not an insignificant artist at the time. Auguste Rodin said in 1912 that Cros was "one of the most glorious men of nineteenth-century sculpture."[140] Henry Cros was the son of a philosopher and the brother of poet and inventor Charles Cros and physician Antoine Cros; the latter was the personal doctor of don Pedro II of Brazil, who was also seen by Charcot.[141] The Goncourt brothers described Henry Cros as "a very thin boy, swarthy, bearded, with a worrying fixity in his sunken eyes" and remarked that he was surrounded by "small fragments of wax that look like little pieces of flesh."[142] He was fluent in ancient Greek and Latin, which facilitated his detailed study of past artworks and experiments with lost techniques.[143] His sculptures were exhibited regularly at the Salon and at Universal Expositions.[144] Poet and novelist Jean Aicard wrote in an article on Cros in *La Renaissance littéraire et artistique* of the virtuosity needed to work with wax: "The art of the painter and the art of the sculptor mingle in the art of wax. What skill to melt the correct tones of different colors in a material so slippery, so fleeting!"[145] As an amateur artist himself, making furniture and *objets d'art* with his family at home, Charcot would certainly have been impressed with Cros's technique. Most importantly, Aicard discusses the uncanniness of the material:

> That it is strange in itself, that matter which is neither mineral nor vegetable, which (having been transformed, made, created, by a being animated with breath) must keep something of life itself, a memory of a movement to which color lends a memory of light! . . . This art, which is not the grand, magnificent art that flourishes in epochs of plenitude and health, suits our feverish age, which sleeps little and dreams strangely. . . . Sorcerers understood that this matter, quasi-animal, soft and penetrable as flesh, rendered well the expression of life, but of life devoted to death.[146]

We return here to the liminal state of the *Ataxic Venus*, whose body evokes a series of uncomfortable dualities: the beauty of the anatomical Venus and the dangerous deformities of degeneration; the eroticism of the prone nude and the inescapable infertility and "ugliness" of the elderly woman; the availability of the medicalized body and the containment of a sealed-off cast figure; the portrait of an illness and the portrait of an individual; an uncanny verisimilitude tinged with life and an obvious quietus; Eros and Thanatos.

Painful Impressions

While the *savants-artistes* at the Salpêtrière purported to create an indexical and "objective" representation of disease, the *Ataxic Venus* can also be interpreted through the historical agendas of medical and artistic casting and a vast range of art-historical iconography. Édouard Papet makes the point that the *Ataxic Venus* sits "at the exact boundary of the scientific document, the glossy mannequins of the Spitzner Collection and the colored illusionism of certain studies in sculpture."[147] The history of pain—"the history of what is at once familiar and strange, one's own and another's, individual and collective"—also contributes to the *Ataxic Venus*'s meaning, as does its historical and cultural significance in relation to popular attractions like the Spitzner Museum and other waxworks collections.[148] In this setting, as Marina Warner notes, the "conflicts between instruction and aesthetics, between human empathy and artistic ambition, turn forensic verisimilitude utterly monstrous."[149] Maurice Guillemot stated in the 1880s that the Musée Charcot "leaves a painful impression, like the memory of a museum of horrors, of a gathering of gnomes, monsters, beings who are fantastic, chimeric, nightmarish visions borrowed from Dante's infernal circles or the macabre work of Poe." He singled out the *Ataxic Venus* for its "hideous realism, hideous misery."[150] This description returns us to the cabinet of curiosities, where from the time of the Renaissance anatomical waxes shared vitrines with the bones of giants, fetuses conjoined or missing limbs, and hermaphrodites and "hybrids," among many others classified as "monstrous." By the late nineteenth century, there was a new kind of monster, one created by a different "error of nature": hereditary degeneracy. The *Ataxic Venus* was seen as an embodiment of that most feared malady.

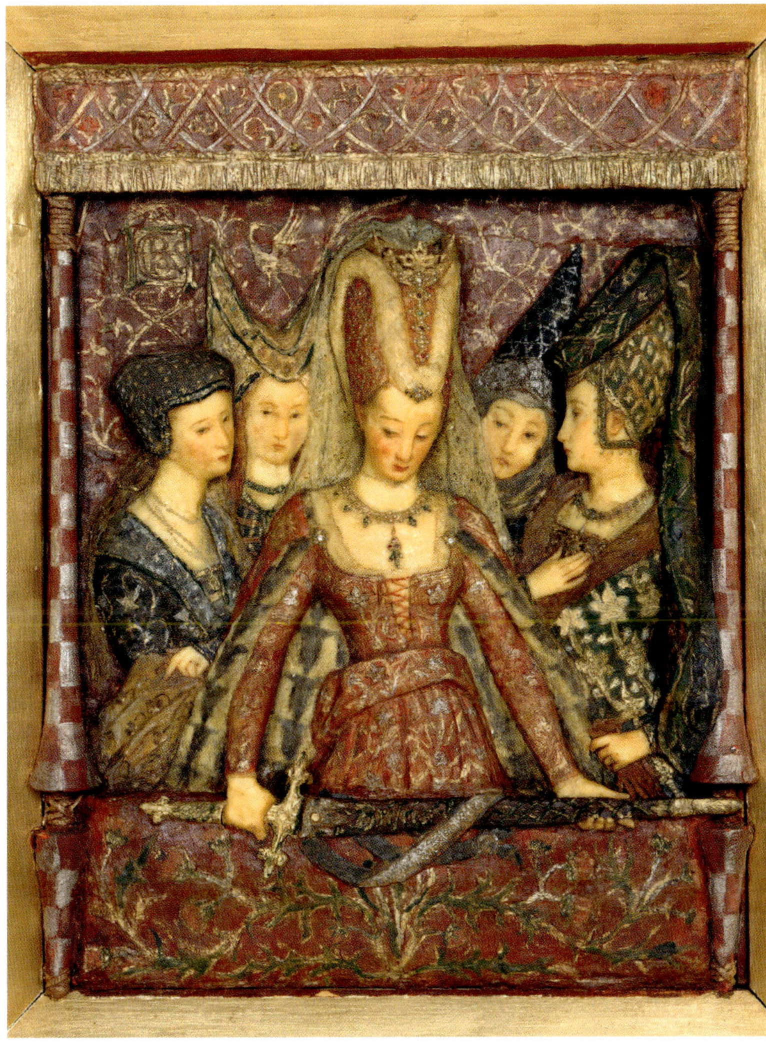

Fig. 63
Henry Cros, *Le Prix du tournoi* (*The Tournament Prize*), 1873. Polychrome wax and pearls on wood, 125 × 109 × 20 cm. Paris, Musée d'Orsay. Photo © RMN-Grand Palais (musée d'Orsay) / Gérard Blot / Christian Jean.

The "realism" and "misery" Guillemot ascribes to the *Ataxic Venus* are equally applicable to the whole of the Musée Charcot and the Salpêtrière in general, where bodies in pain—real, simulacral, and artistically rendered—were on display. The *Ataxic Venus* lies exactly at the point of convergence of the real, simulacral, and artistically rendered: at the slippage, to which I have succumbed, despite my best efforts, between Berthelot (the historical figure who was a patient at the Salpêtrière in the nineteenth century) and the *Ataxic Venus* (the artwork in wax created from a mold taken from that patient's dead body).[151] This slippage is related to both pain and portraiture: the viewer empathizes with the pain because of the recognition that this is a depiction of a human being who has lived and suffered. "The oscillation between art object and human subject, represented so personally, is what gives portraits their extraordinary grasp on our imagination," explains Richard Brilliant.[152] It is too limiting, however, to consider the *Ataxic Venus* merely a portrait of Berthelot; it is also a portrait of a particular debilitating illness and of pain itself. It fluctuates between specificities and generalities. It reminds us that the body is a "composite—of physical form, cultural imagination, social construction, and personal identity."[153] It is a woman, a sculpture, and a cadaver, to paraphrase Balzac's protagonist in *Le Chef-d'oeuvre inconnu*.[154] The *Ataxic Venus* epitomizes the porousness of these categories—history, art history, and medicine, respectively—and demonstrates the complexities of turning medical "evidence" into a "scientific artwork."

Indeed, it is perhaps more accurate to understand this cast as exceeding the limits of the term "portrait," not least through the "realistic" rendering of bodily deformity that flouts the idealization central to traditional portraiture; the word "deformation" comes from *forma* or beauty, while the Latin word *deformis* means ugly.[155] The *Ataxic Venus* implicates not only the patient and the clinician(s)/artist(s) but also the beholder's understanding of and empathy with Western depictions of human suffering. It epitomizes scientific inquiry, but it also evokes Christian faith. It portrays an individual, yet it triggers countless associations in a shared visual culture. The *Ataxic Venus* acts as a medical *memento mori* and shocks us in part through its "mimesis of physical misery."[156] Perhaps ultimately all empathy is deceptive, since we can never truly access another's "real" pain. Daudet attempted to represent his pain through the written word. He concluded that pain was individual, untranslatable: "No general theory about pain. Each patient discovers his own, and the nature of pain varies, like a singer's voice, according to the acoustics of the hall."[157]

PAUL RICHER, SCULPTING PATHOLOGY

4

Art . . . is intimately bound to science; they are but two sides of the same problem, and two different manifestations of the same principle: Truth.

—PAUL RICHER, 1897

Brouillet's *Clinical Lesson* encapsulates the Salpêtrière School's marriage of medicine and art through the visual echo of the *arc-de-cercle* pose in the patient, Blanche Wittmann, at the front of the room and in Richer's "drawing" on the back wall (see fig. 1). These clinicians' exceptional focus on artistic practice within the confines of the hospital was obvious to both specialists and the general public, as is evident from a whimsical image that has been tipped into the British Library's copy of the third volume of the *Iconographie photographique de la Salpêtrière* (*IPS*), across from its frontispiece (fig. 64). Superimposed onto the foreground of this image, a detail of Brouillet's painting clipped from a Salon catalogue, a female nude reclines languorously before the lecturing Charcot.[1] Seemingly unnoticed by the attendees of the lesson, she is perhaps a sort of muse to the clinicians, like the women in Titian's *Fête champêtre* (*Pastoral Concert*) (1508–9, Paris, Musée du Louvre). This odalisque, furthermore, mimics the pose of models in artists' studios all around Paris, visible also in the photographs circulating in those ateliers.[2] Upon close inspection, it became apparent that this picture, which I had assumed was a print, was in fact a collage. It appears that someone has taken the time to cut out the detail of the Brouillet, locate an appropriately sized drawing of a nude, carefully cut it out and glue it—deftly and almost imperceptibly—onto the Salpêtrière scene, and has then pasted the finished product into the journal. We can only assume that this was done by a one-time owner of this particular copy of the *IPS* who, judging from its typical readership, was likely a physician or a serious collector of medical books. Whether the collage was intended to pay homage to the Salpêtrière School's artistic affinities or to lampoon them, we will never know.

This image serves as a fitting entrée into an analysis of the sculptural oeuvre of Paul Richer, who created didactic sculptures during his tenure at the Salpêtrière while also exhibiting realist works at the Paris Salon to advance his artistic career. In the late 1880s, Richer developed a new kind of realist sculpture for the Musée Charcot. As noted

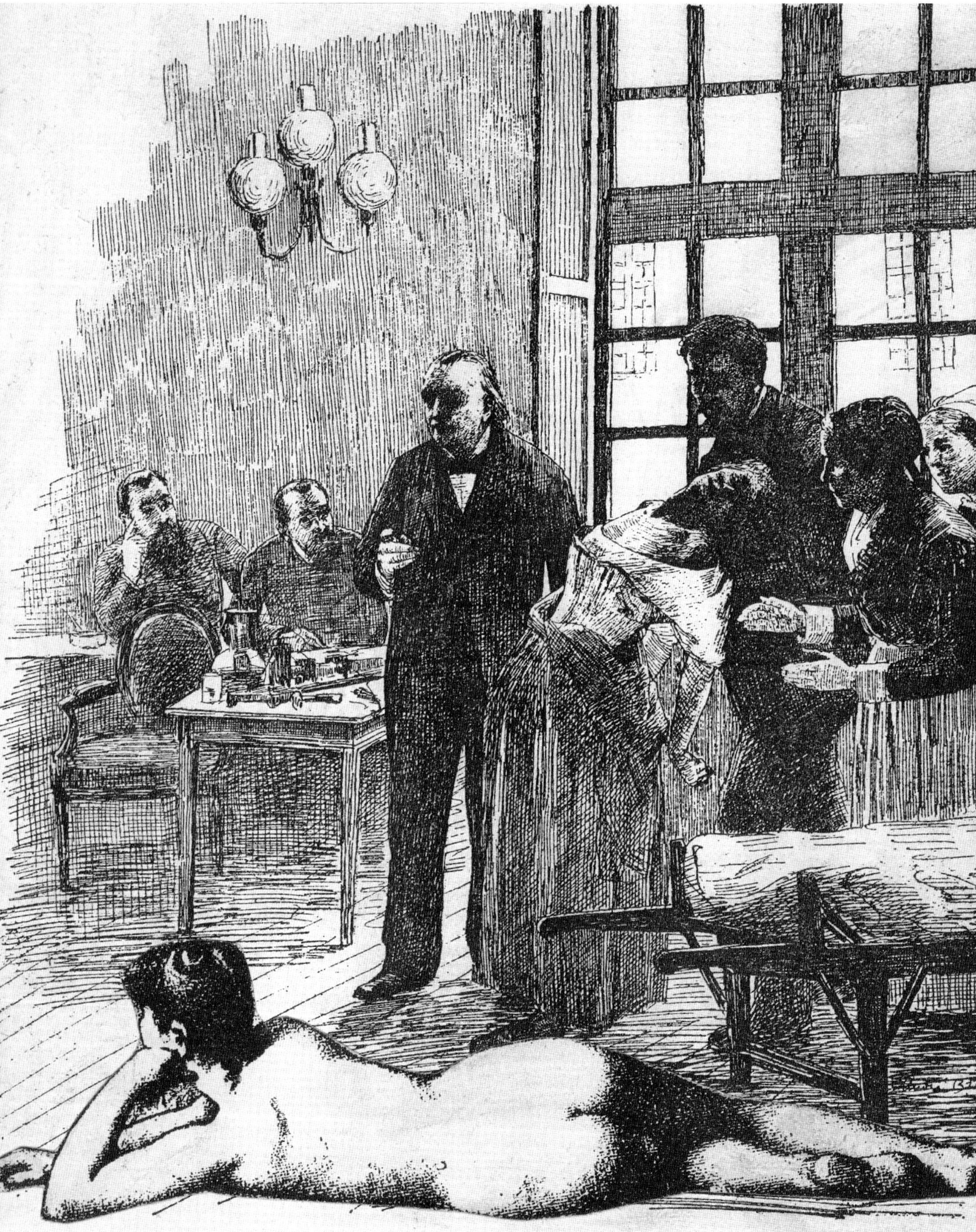

in chapter 1, his sculpture of a woman with labio-glosso-laryngeal paralysis, which was one of four "figural representations of the principal types of nervous pathology," was exhibited in the Musée Charcot (see fig. 4).[3] Other works in this series included a bust of a man with myopathy as well as sculptures depicting patients with juvenile hypothyroidism (*myxoedème infantile*) and Parkinson's disease, seen here in photographs taken by Albert Londe for the *Nouvelle Iconographie de la Salpêtrière* (figs. 65–68). Richer had become head of the Salpêtrière's museum of pathological anatomy in 1882, only a few years after it opened.[4] In an exceptional gesture that attested to the value Charcot placed on his work, Richer was given an atelier on the grounds of the hospital, where he created the sculptures of pathology that are the focus of this chapter.[5]

Fig. 64 (opposite)
Collage from the British Library's copy of the *Iconographie photographique de la Salpêtrière*, vol. 3. Photo © The British Library Board (7660.dd.4).

It was the accuracy of Richer's sculptures that made them exemplary in the eyes of his medical contemporaries. These patient portraits were thought to be objective, "like a photograph in three dimensions"—a testament to their purported truthfulness.[6] Paradoxically, they also provided an alternative to mechanical media such as photography and casting by permitting the clinician's intervention in not only controlling and animating the sitter but also emphasizing the patient's symptoms. Here was a new kind of medical specimen: the "scientific artwork," as Richer's sculptures were called by a colleague, suggesting a hybrid of the indexical and the artistic, the objective and the subjective.[7] Richer's sculptures of pathology were products of a conscious dialogue between scientific and artistic "selves," to paraphrase Daston and Galison, by a doctor who published books on artistic anatomy and exhibited "high" art at the Paris Salon.[8] As the epigraph to this chapter attests, Richer claimed that science and art, both being versions of "truth," were one and the same.[9] His sculptures embody the contemporary medical understanding of pathology rendered via the conventions of art.

Living Anatomy

The fortuitous moment when Charcot lauded the illustrations of hands in Meillet's thesis would mark the beginning of Richer's distinguished, if since somewhat overlooked, career (see chapter 1).[10] It situated him in the fields of both medicine and art, which he would work hard to combine over the course of his long professional life. He was eventually elected to the Académie de médecine as well as the Académie des beaux-arts, the first doctor ever to receive this honor.[11] In the first half of his career, as resident artist at the Salpêtrière and Charcot's collaborator, Richer diagnosed and depicted the physical effects of neurological disorders. His 1881 book *Études cliniques sur la grande hystérie ou hystéro-épilepsie* (Clinical studies on hysteria or hystero-epilepsy) caused a "sensation," principally because of its celebrated illustrations, which helped establish for the first time a visual vocabulary for the manifestations of the hysterical attack (see fig. 28).[12] Its illustrations had wide-ranging medical and cultural influence.[13] In addition to nurturing Richer's evident artistic talents, Charcot also entrusted him with the role of *chef*

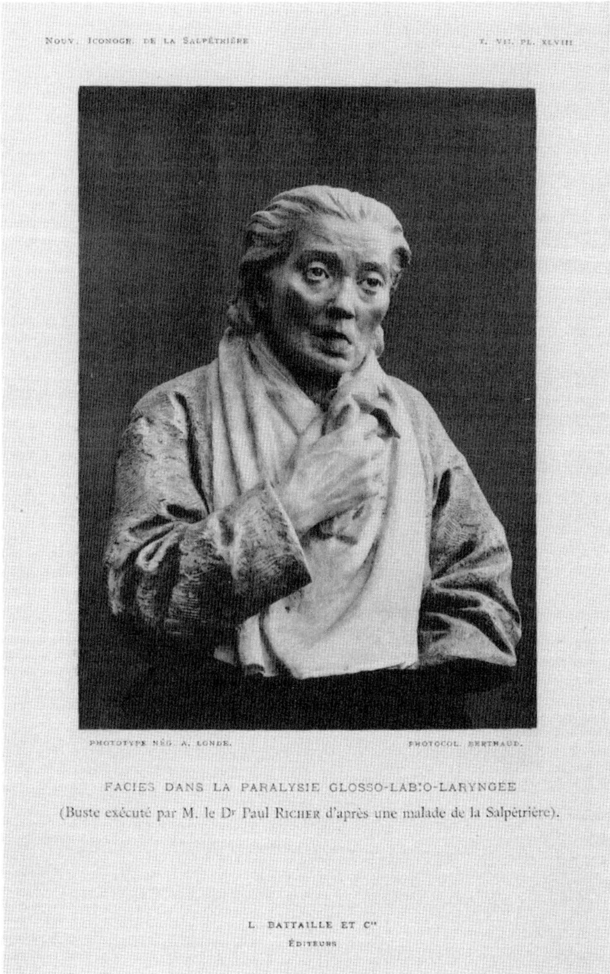

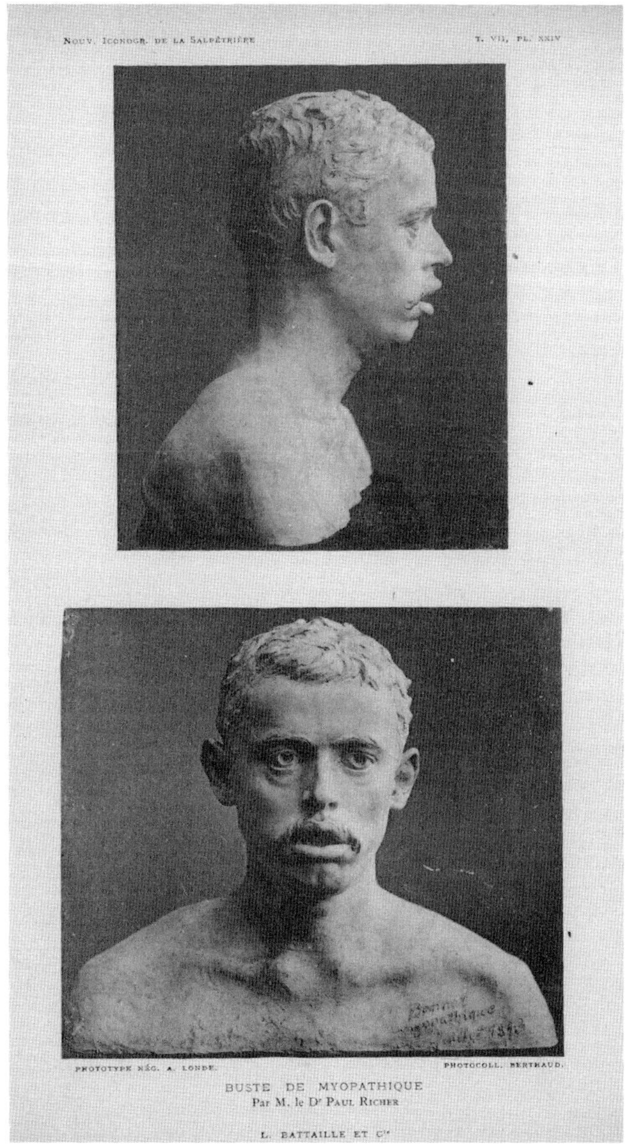

Fig. 65
Facies dans la paralysie glosso-labio-laryngée. (Buste exécuté par M. le Dr Paul Richer d'après une malade de la Salpêtrière) (Facies of Labio-Glosso-Laryngeal Paralysis. [Bust by Dr Paul Richer after a patient at the Salpêtrière]). From Henry Meige, "La Facies dans la paralysie glosso-labio laryngée [*sic*]," *Nouvelle Iconographie de la Salpêtrière* 7 (1894): plate 48. Courtesy of the Wellcome Collection.

Fig. 66
Buste de myopathique par M. le Dr Paul Richer (*Bust of a Man with Myopathy by Dr. Paul Richer*). From Henry Meige, "Les Amyotrophiques dans l'art," *Nouvelle Iconographie de la Salpêtrière* 7 (1894): plate 24. Courtesy of the Wellcome Collection.

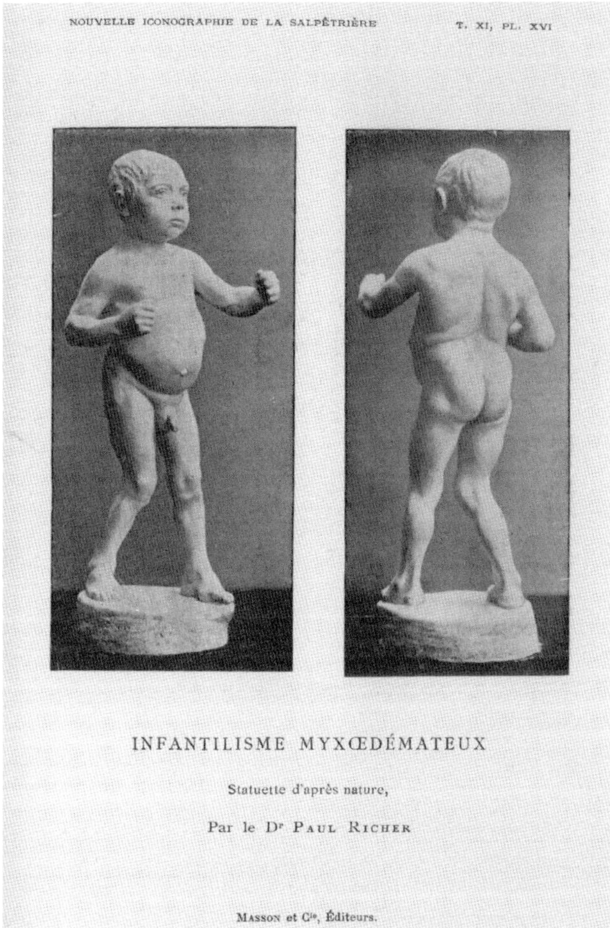

Fig. 67
Infantilisme myxoedémateux. Statuette d'aprés nature, par le Dr Paul Richer (Juvenile Hypothyroidism. Statuette from Life by Dr. Paul Richer). From Henry Meige, "Sur une statuette représentant l'infantilisme myxoedémateux," *Nouvelle Iconographie de la Salpêtrière* 11 (1898): plate 16. Courtesy of the Wellcome Collection.

Fig. 68
Attitude et facies dans la maladie de Parkinson. Statuette de M. le Dr Paul Richer, d'après une malade de la Salpêtrière (Attitude and Facies of Parkinson's Disease. Statuette by Dr. Paul Richer, After a Patient at the Salpêtrière). From Paul Richer and Henry Meige, "Étude morphologique sur la Maladie de Parkinson," *Nouvelle Iconographie de la Salpêtrière* 8 (1895): plates 56–58. Courtesy of the Wellcome Collection.

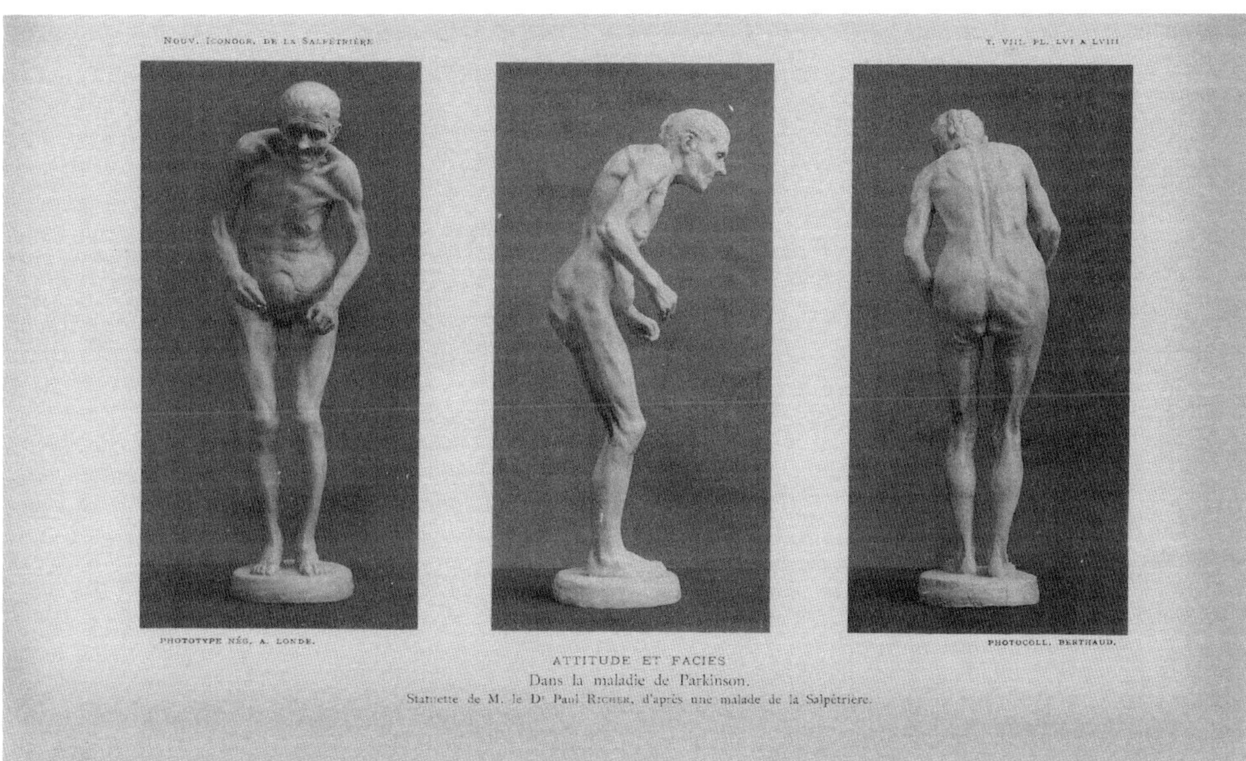

du laboratoire in 1882, and he thereby became head of the Salpêtrière's clinic for the study of nervous diseases and museum of pathological anatomy.[14]

Chapter 1 included a discussion of Richer's sketches of the body in the unpublished albums of the Musée Charcot, which place observations of the living patient next to details of the autopsied cadaver and attempt to make explicit the links between inner pathology and its exterior manifestations. Observing the living pathological body was as critical to Charcot's anatomo-clinical method as examining postmortem remains. By close scrutiny of the body's exterior forms, he was able to make innovative diagnoses; autopsies would later confirm (or disprove) his hypotheses. Richer's work was critical to these studies and included a book published in 1881 that exclusively comprised annotated images of dissected brains.[15]

On October 30, 1888, Charcot examined a male patient who appeared to have sciatica. After a visual examination of the naked patient and a review of his medical history, Charcot determined that instead he had traumatic neurasthenia and hysteria. This affirmed for him the medical need to examine "the nude":

> In reality, . . . we physicians should know *the nude* as well and even better than painters do. A flaw in drawing by a painter or sculptor is serious, no doubt, from the point of view of art, but all in all, from a practical point of view, it has no major consequences. But what would you say about a physician or surgeon who takes, as happens too often, a normal bump or contour for an abnormality or vice versa? . . . This digression may be enough to highlight once again the need for the physician, and for the surgeon, to attach a great importance to the medico-surgical study of the NUDE.[16]

Charcot's invocation of fine art is in character: he often turned to artworks to confirm his diagnoses and to prove the persistence of the disorders he identified at the Salpêtrière, as his two books with Richer make clear. His pretensions to art are hinted at here by the reference to the fine art category of the "nude"—that is, the idealized human body. Charcot further compared the hospital with an atelier: he assured his audience that the naked patient was comfortable because the examination room was "properly heated, as a painter's studio would be."[17] This calls to mind the collage of a nude woman pasted onto the print of Brouillet's painting, reclining comfortably at one of Charcot's lessons.

It is likely that Charcot formulated his lecture that October day with Richer's work in mind. Immediately following his pronouncements on the nude, Charcot announced a book by Richer with large plates made "from life" that would show "art and science walking hand in hand," most likely his *Anatomie artistique* published in 1890.[18] At the outset of this seminal text, which is still in print today, Richer defines his terms: "Artistic anatomy, or anatomy applied to the fine arts, is the science of exterior forms and the relationships that exist between them and the deeper structures."[19] This volume includes over one hundred plates of a male figure by Richer in the "unarmed soldier" pose—standing straight with arms at the side and palms facing forward—along with a discussion of osteology, myology, and morphology.[20] One of the book's epigraphs is telling: "There are many more people who look than who read."[21] Richer asserts that his text is only an "accompaniment" to the plates, in which the skeletal structure is progressively clothed with muscles and then skin.[22] Viewing the living body was paramount for Richer's theories about both art and medicine. In the introduction, Richer notes that, as Charcot had indicated in his lesson, the illustrations were done "from life." In this instance, however, his "après nature" might be qualified with "after a fashion": the body displayed on the book's pages is in fact a Frankenstein-like amalgamation of two models. The torso is copied from one, and the limbs from another.[23] As I have already mentioned, Richer contended in his "Dialogues sur l'art et la science" that "the photographer will always be inferior to the illustrator."[24] Drawing, unlike photography, allowed Richer to manipulate the end result for clarity and emphasis.

In his "role as informant," Richer addresses his text specifically to physicians and surgeons, emphasizing, like Charcot, "the undeniable usefulness of an exact and precise knowledge of normal exterior forms for the diagnosis of deformities brought on by disease."[25] In a noteworthy critique, Richer then goes on to contest the primacy of the cadaver in the study of medicine:

> Dissection, which shows us all the hidden springs of the human machine, only does so on the condition that, in so doing, it destroys exterior forms. . . . It would be hoped, then, that in all our anatomical amphitheaters the study of the live model should have its place beside the study of the cadaver, which it would happily complement. Indeed, the anatomy of forms can only be studied in the living. It has as its foundation, it is true, the understanding that the cadaver provides, but it animates, it invigorates this initial knowledge by means of which it reconstitutes the living man. Its process is synthesis; its means is the observation of the nude; its goal is to discover the multiple sources of the living form and to set them down in a description; it asks therefore to be studied in itself and for itself, and it supplies knowledge that simple anatomy alone cannot give.[26]

The study of "living anatomy," therefore, is as necessary as dissection to an understanding of the body. Richer says that the two are complementary: in effect, dissection furnishes the "beginning" of knowledge, and the study of the living body completes it. But he makes a point of stating that "living anatomy" should also be studied for its own sake, that only in knowing the animated form can the understanding of the cadaver be brought to life. As in Charcot's lesson, here too it is the observation of the nude that is the key to the comprehensive discovery of anatomy. While the artist and doctor are set in opposition to each other at the start of this strongly worded assessment, the implication by the end is that they are both gaining knowledge through the same means and achieving the same ends. Richer comments in a later article that, by emphasizing the study of the living, artistic anatomy provides an unexpected but important service to its "older sibling," medical anatomy.[27]

Richer practiced what he preached. As his series of pathological sculptures demonstrates, at the Salpêtrière he studied the living pathological body to better understand illness while analyzing the healthy body for the benefit of both physicians and artists. His research on morphology included working with his colleague at the hospital Albert Londe, who took photographs of athletes, soldiers, and circus performers in the "unarmed soldier" pose and in motion.[28] In 1888 Richer co-founded the *Nouvelle Iconographie de la Salpêtrière,* in which he published article after article, year after year, testing his ideas on anatomy.[29] As noted in chapter 1, the *Nouvelle Iconographie* also included articles on a wide variety of neurological disorders and "medico-artistic" studies like those that constitute Charcot and Richer's books on the possessed, the deformed, and the ill in art. In the early 1890s, Richer published *Canon des proportions du corps humain* (Canon of the proportions of the human body), in which he used "anthropometric statistics" to conclude that the height of an "average" (*moyenne*) man was seven and a half heads; he also created a sculpture to illustrate these ideas (1892, Paris, École nationale supérieure des beaux-arts).[30] The fact that this book was intended for both doctors and artists was underlined by Georges Gilles de la Tourette (1857–1904), another member of the Salpêtrière School, who wrote that it served as an important reference for sculptors and "all those who, in order to assess pathological deformities of the skeleton and soft tissue, need to know the normal proportions of the human body."[31] The intense and detailed examination of the living body was of fundamental importance to Richer's medical and artistic practice. As he stated late in life, "Anatomy helped me to understand sculpture, sculpture to understand anatomy."[32] It led him to create sculptures for both a medical audience and the Paris Salon.

Laborers at the Salon

In 1887, Richer exhibited his first sculpture in the same Salon that featured Brouillet's painting. It was a small statue of one of the models who posed for the illustrations in his *Anatomie artistique.* The sculpture of "a magnificent athlete," which does not seem to survive either in its original form or in an illustration, did not make an impression on Salon critics, who were instead taken with realist works such as Emmanuel Frémiet's sensational *Gorille enlevant une femme* (*Gorilla Carrying Off A Woman*) (1887, Nantes, Musée d'arts de Nantes).[33] Richer comments in his unpublished autobiography that the desire to sculpt the athlete was almost beyond his control and that he was "haunted" by the need to sculpt a life-size figure during his next annual holiday.[34] He discusses at length the process of creating that next sculpture, *Moissonneur* (*Harvester*) (1888, location unknown), emphasizing his autodidacticism: "I was completely ignorant of the proper technique."[35] He began by making a small study and then an armature, which he says was "ten times too weak," so he asked a local locksmith to create iron buttresses (*arcs-boutants*) for his frame.[36] However, in order to create a lighter sculpture, Richer decided to add straw to his armature. Unfortunately, after a few weeks he noticed that the sculpture was covered with shoots—the seeds in the straw had begun to germinate as a result of the heat and humidity. "If I had not put it right," Richer writes, "my statue would have soon become a veritable wheat field."[37] He salvaged the work by casting it in plaster.

Richer took his figure to the sculptor Paul Gasq (1860–1944) for his professional opinion, and he responded, "How curious it would be if you did not become one of our great sculptors!" In Richer's account, Gasq "summed up his opinion of my work by this simple phrase: 'it is a very good preparation,' meaning that it only lacked the science of modeling that was then taught at schools of fine art."[38] Despite lacking "the science of modeling," Richer's *Harvester* was admitted to the Salon.

In discussing this submission, art historian and critic Paul Mantz, after first noting Richer's contribution to medicine, argued that his sculpture revealed that he was "more of an amateur than a professional." Mantz continued, "He stripped a Norman peasant and copied him with great concern for the exact form and movement. But nature does not provide everything: statuary needs a complement, which is art."[39]

Mantz had kinder words the following year about Richer's *Faucheur* (*Reaper*) (1889, Chartres, musée des Beaux-Arts); he devoted half a page to it out of the fourteen he wrote on more than a thousand sculptures at the Salon that year. He proclaimed that the *Reaper* was "a figure taken from the realities of rural life.... The torso is nude, which has allowed the author to show the many studies he has made from living forms. Compared to the *Harvester* of last year, the *Reaper* reveals a new progress."[40] A photograph shows the model beside the sculpture as Richer works on it (fig. 69). The young man is naked to the waist and holds a pole that keeps his left arm in place during the long session of posing, a prop that would become the reaper's scythe in the finished work. The conceit is that the peasant has taken a break from his hard labor and is wiping the sweat from his brow with the back of his hand. The sculpture Richer caresses is larger and more obviously muscular than the model, while his contrapposto is more pronounced. The sculpted face also appears more regular and conventionally handsome. Richer is showing a "simple" break in the day of the reaper, but his sculpture presents a heroic figure. Remove the belted trousers and boots as well as the contemporary moustache, and the figure could easily be interpreted as an ancient athlete. Within three years of submitting his first work to the Salon, Richer received an honorable mention for the *Reaper*.[41] This was an impressive trajectory for a self-taught sculptor.

Richer's artworks, however, were always discussed in relation to his practice at the Salpêtrière. Mantz felt it was impossible to separate the two: "How could we, in writing the name of M. Richer, forget that the sculptor-doctor is more than ever interested in instructing us?" He comments that Richer's just-released book with Charcot, *Les Difformes et les malades dans l'art*, reveals "the same curiosity of spirit and the same science" as their earlier book, *Les Démoniaques dans l'art*.[42] The author of another article from the time noted that Richer the doctor "doubles as an artist."[43] Critics consistently

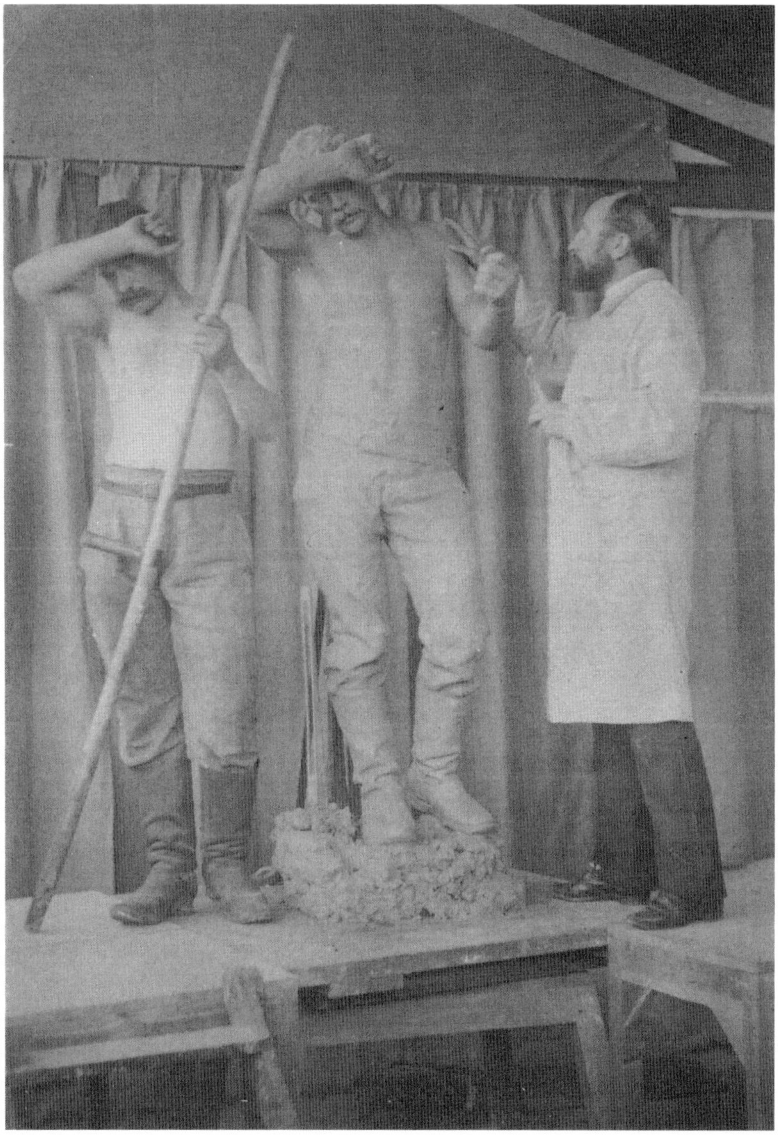

viewed his art through the prism of his medical career. Regardless, the *Reaper* was bought by the state, a purchase that Richer later attributed to the sculptor Jules Dalou (1838–1902), who might have been a member of the Salon jury that year.[44] Medical historian and zoologist Raphaël Blanchard wrote that the sculpture's sincerity had "seduced" Dalou.[45]

Richer and Dalou

According to Richer, he and Dalou met at the Charcot family home *after* the 1889 Salon,[46] which is odd given that Dalou attended Charcot's lectures in the Salpêtrière amphitheater and sculpted a portrait of the neurologist in 1884 (Paris, Petit Palais, musée des Beaux-arts de la Ville de Paris). Exhibited in the Salon that same year, the bust shows Charcot wearing his academic robes, but the focus is on his sensitively rendered, downcast visage. Charcot had been elected to the Académie des Sciences of the Institut de France in late 1883, which probably occasioned the commission for the portrait. Then already a well-known naturalist sculptor, Dalou had just returned from a decade of exile in England, where he had fled to avoid prison or execution for his involvement in founding the Courbet-led Fédération des Artistes and for his role as curator in charge of protecting objects at the Louvre during the Commune.[47] In the 1870s and 1880s, Dalou received portrait commissions from wealthy patrons and depicted workers as well. His sculptures of "noble" rural laborers paid homage to the dignity of the class from which he himself emerged.[48]

Fig. 69
Paul Richer Sculpting a Live Model, undated photograph. Inv. Ph18079. Paris, École nationale supérieure des Beaux-Arts. Photo © Beaux-Arts de Paris, Dist. RMN-Grand Palais / image Beaux-arts de Paris.

Dalou and Richer developed a close relationship that would last until the former's death in 1902; Richer owned several of his *carnets* and two drawings of Dalou's daughter.[49] After Dalou suffered a serious stroke, Richer attended doctor's visits with him and was one of the executors of his will.[50] Remarkably, Richer seems to have had a significant impact on the artistic practice of his more experienced mentor. "Dalou received from Paul Richer even more than he taught him," wrote art historian Louis Hourticq,

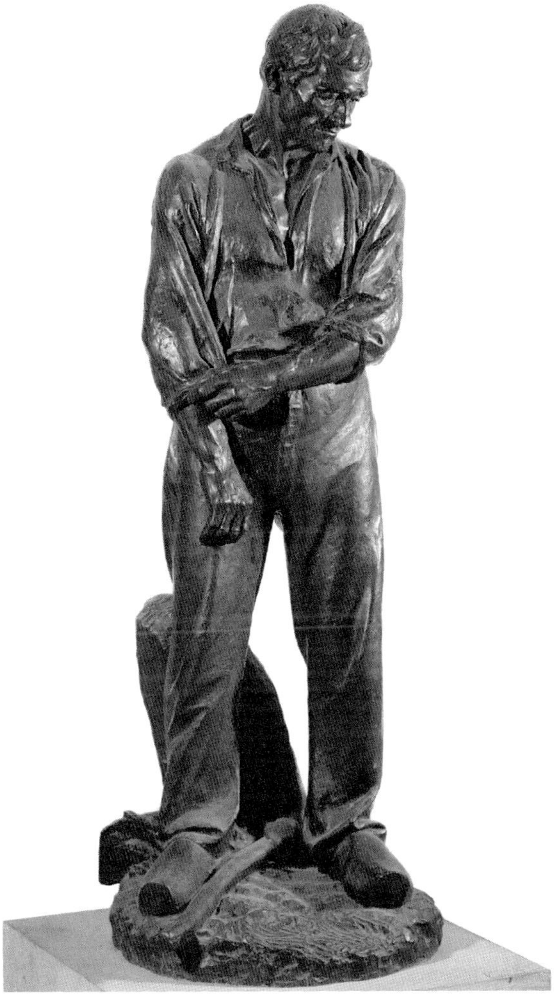

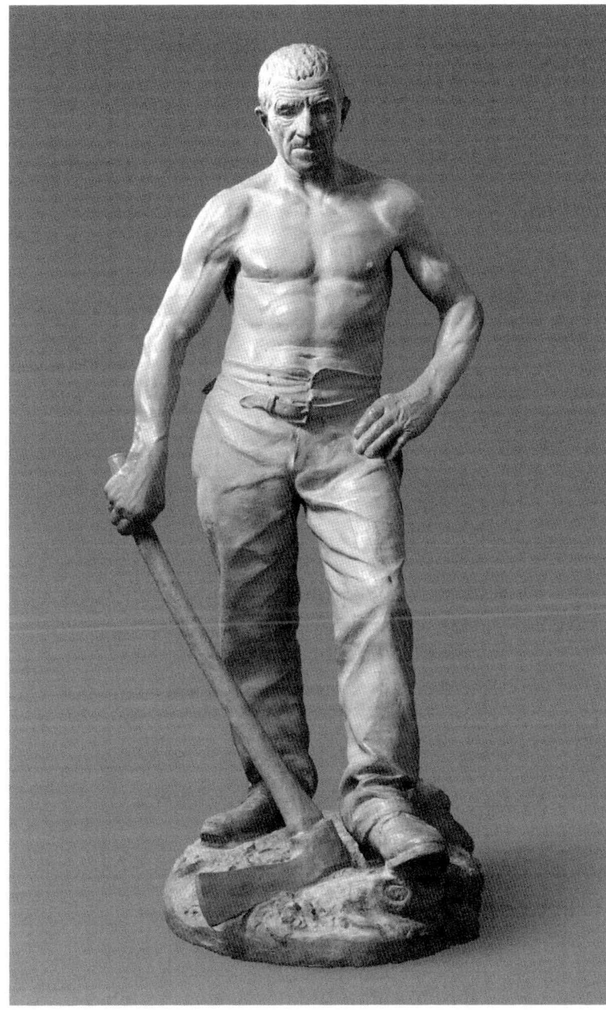

who argued that Richer probably had a huge influence on Dalou's focus on the worker in his last decade.[51] Dalou created countless studies for an unrealized *Monument aux ouvriers* (*Monument to Workers*) from 1889 until his death, inspired, at least in part, by Richer's sculptures of laborers. At the very end of the century, they even shared a model who became Dalou's celebrated *Grand Paysan* (*Large Worker*) (ca. 1899) and Richer's *Bûcheron* (*Lumberjack*) (1899) (figs. 70 and 71).[52] The latter's sculpture, which received a third-class medal at the Salon of 1900, would be reproduced in stoneware by the Manufacture nationale de Sèvres.[53] The two sculptors' artistic visions were obviously in sympathy, given their investment in naturalism and the considerable attention paid to the laborer in their sculpted oeuvres.[54] Yet there are significant differences in these sculptures crafted from the same model. As Andrew Eschelbacher points out, Dalou "interpret[ed] in order to produce an artistic ideal," highlighting "the difference between science and art."[55]

Dalou no doubt nurtured and aided the development of Richer's natural talent as a sculptor,[56] and his London works, which combined genre and portraiture, may have

Fig. 70
Jules Dalou, *Grand Paysan* (*Large Worker*), 1899–1902. Bronze, 197 × 70 × 68 cm. Paris, Musée d'Orsay. Inv. RF 2999. Photo © Photo Josse / Bridgeman Images.

Fig. 71
Paul Richer, *Le Bûcheron* (*Lumberjack*). Limoges, musée national Adrien Dubouché. Photo © RMN-Grand Palais (Limoges, Cité de la céramique) / Tony Querrec.

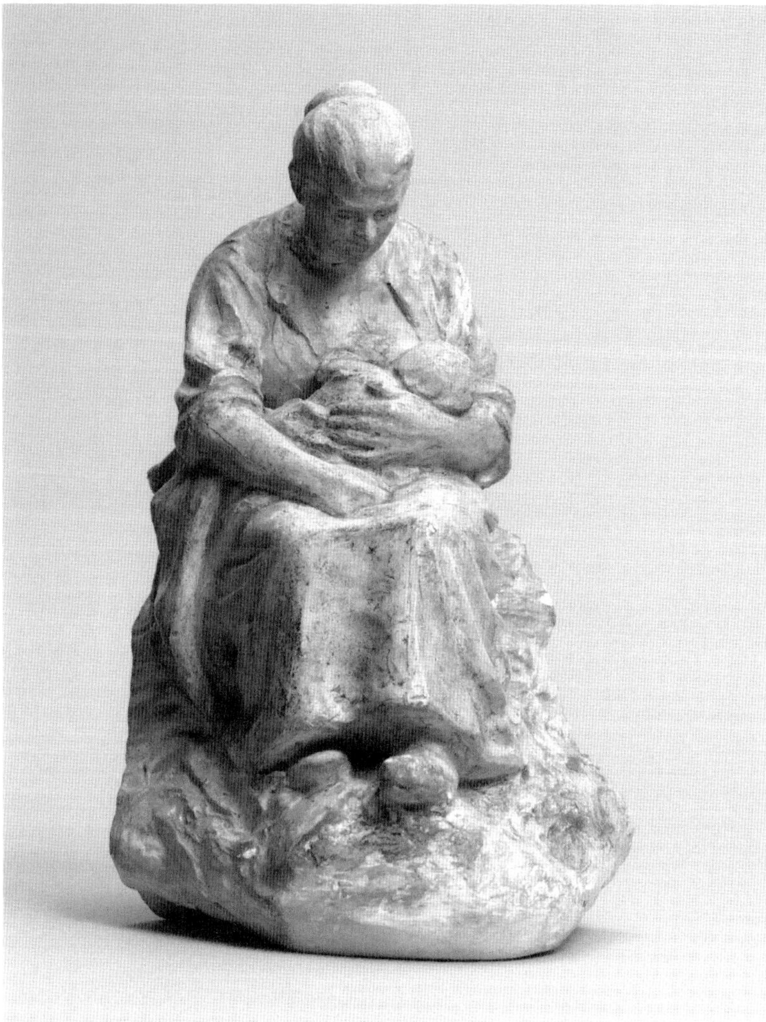

Fig. 72
Paul Richer, *Femme allaitant (Nursing Woman)*, between 1885 and 1900. Plaster, 18 × 9.8 × 11.6 cm. Paris, Musée d'Orsay. Inv. RF 2348. Photo © RMN-Grand Palais (musée d'Orsay) / Hervé Lewandowski.

inspired the project of pathological portraits that Richer began in the late 1880s. In exile, Dalou created a series of sculptures of upper-class, middle-class, and peasant women in banal scenes, such as reading or breastfeeding. *The Hon. Mrs. George Howard (later Countess of Carlisle)* (1872, York, The Castle Howard Collection), for example, depicts Georgiana Howard in bohemian dress with an open book on her lap. It was exhibited at the Royal Academy of Arts in 1873 alongside Dalou's *Peasant Woman Nursing a Baby* (1873, London, Victoria and Albert Museum);[57] the woman in this composition wears a scarf on her head and *sabots* on her feet and sits on an overturned woven basket. Richer's similarly themed *Femme allaitant (Nursing Woman)* (between 1885 and 1900) was one of his only sculptures of peasants to feature a woman as its subject (fig. 72). Cassandra Albinson argues that Dalou's crafting of "sanitized [and] generalized" figures of different classes reveals the radical underpinnings of his sculptural project: "He sought to represent women of different social classes as worthy of equal respect and equally worthy of the visual concentration of the viewer."[58]

Richer submitted to the Salon naturalist sculptures that attempted to express the nobility of the peasant, including *Semeur* (*Sower*), *Forgeron* (*Blacksmith*), *Terrassier* (*Digger*), *Bûcheron* (*Lumberjack*), and *Moissonneur* (*Harvester*) in 1892, all created during his holidays in the countryside.[59] Despite decades of submissions to the Salon and a long career at the École des beaux-arts, Richer claims in his unpublished autobiography, "All these artworks served as amusements for me and did not make me forget my scientific work."[60] The period when he was producing these sculptures overlapped with the making of his pathological portraits at the Salpêtrière (see figs. 65–68), sculptures that he would have seen as quite the opposite of a mere "amusement." The most significant trait shared by Dalou and Richer in their respective sculptural output was not their common interest in peasants and laborers. Rather, it is the fact that both men's sculptures constitute a bold updating of conventional sculptural norms. Dalou fused portraiture and genre; Richer, portraiture and medical specimen.

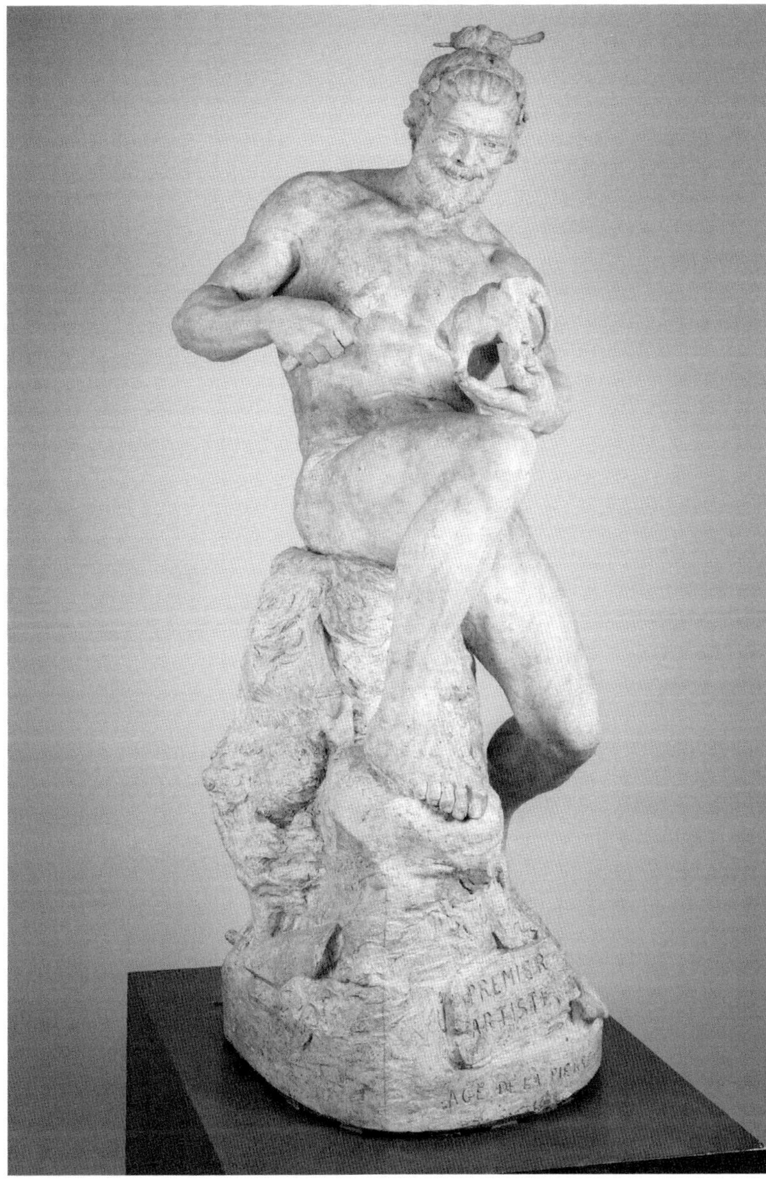

Fig. 73
Paul Richer, *Le Premier artiste* (*The First Artist*), ca. 1890. Le Puy-en-Velay, Musée Crozatier. Photo courtesy of the Musée Crozatier © Luc Olivier.

Richer began incorporating "science" in his sculptural practice with *Le Premier artiste* (*The First Artist*) (ca. 1890), which depicts a caveman sitting on a rock and carving a woolly mammoth (fig. 73). In 1890, he exhibited this life-size figure at the Salon des artistes français, and later a bronze cast was installed outside the Muséum national d'Histoire naturelle in the Jardin des Plantes. Putting into practice his exhortation from *Anatomie artistique*, Richer built up the head of *The First Artist* directly from a cast of a Cro-Magnon man's skull, "the most beautiful and the most complete of those found" in the Vézère Valley in southwestern France.[61] In an article published the next year, Richer wondered, "This man, this first artist whose venerable works, across a long succession of ages, have come down to us, can we re-create him? Does he resemble contemporary men? What were his physical characteristics? What was his physiognomy? Recent scientific discoveries allow us, to a certain extent, to satisfy our rightful curiosity."[62] Unlike other "realistic" treatments of prehistoric man that were in vogue at the time, such as the sculptures of Frémiet, in *The First Artist* "all forms and proportions that in a human head depend on the bone structure can thus be regarded as strictly accurate."[63] "As for the rest," Richer continues, "the soft tissue, it was quite necessary to contrive them, but even here the skeleton, to a certain extent, determined the morphology."[64] A femur found in the same cave as the skull was the basis for the body.[65]

Having started with such material evidence, he optimistically believed that this sculpture was more "truthful" than any other of prehistoric man. Most of the elements of the sculpture were arrived at "scientifically," according to Richer: the hairstyle was conceived by looking at buried remains and "contemporary savages," while the carvings on the rock were copied from archaeological finds.[66] The virile body presented more difficulties. Richer writes that it was "conceived without any specialized research and simply

Fig. 74 (opposite)
Photograph of a Salpêtrière patient with "pseudo-bulbaire," 1894. Paris, Bibliothèque Charcot. Courtesy of the Bibliothèque Charcot, Bibliothèque de Sorbonne Université. Photo: author.

within the general notions of a robust and strongly built type." He notes: "There is no excess fat that would be an obstacle to the agility of his movements."[67] These details are conveyed as if they are self-evident, as if Richer's medical and anatomical training had made these decisions inevitable, even as *The First Artist* mimics Richer's own act of artistic creation. This prehistoric man looks happily at the sculpture of a woolly mammoth that he holds in his right hand, carved with the implement he grips in his left. His face "betrays the surprise and joy that he gets from his first study [of the mammoth]."[68] From inanimate matter, *The First Artist* crafts life, just as Richer takes the skull, symbol of death *par excellence*, and vivifies it by clothing it in muscles, fascia, and skin.

This attempt to animate the figure can also be seen in the pathological portraits that Richer created in his Salpêtrière atelier. In busts of patients with labio-glosso-laryngeal paralysis and myopathy, as well as full-body sculptures of patients with juvenile hypothyroidism and Parkinson's disease, Richer created a new kind of medical specimen, where the minute observation of the pathological body by a *savant-artiste* was meant to aid the diagnosis of disease (see figs. 65–68). A colleague at the Salpêtrière wrote that they were "pathological representations where the artistic execution is second only to the precision of the medical observation."[69]

The seventh volume of the *Nouvelle Iconographie de la Salpêtrière* from 1894 includes two articles about Richer's pathological portraits written by Henry Meige, his colleague at the Salpêtrière and successor at the École des beaux-arts.[70] *Facies dans la paralysie glosso-labio-laryngée* (*Facies in Labio-Glosso-Laryngeal Paralysis*) (1888), a life-size sculpture in tinted plaster "after a patient at the Salpêtrière," illustrates an article by Meige on the facies (or typical facial expression) of the disorder (see fig. 65).[71] Now also known as progressive bulbar palsy, this degenerative and ultimately fatal neurological condition is characterized by progressive paralysis of the cranial nerves and involves the lips, tongue, mouth, pharynx, and larynx. One of its many symptoms is the inability to stop drooling, which Richer represents by portraying the patient with a folded *alèze* (mattress pad) around her neck, which she clutches in the hand she holds to her mouth.[72]

The viewer's focus is drawn to the sculpture's finely modeled face and hand, which reveal delicately rendered veins underneath the skin. The hair has been pushed back to fully reveal the visage, and a couple of unruly locks on the left side of the head lend a sense of immediacy and "reality" to the portrait. Richer has depicted a wrinkled forehead, heavy-lidded bulging eyes, sunken cheeks, and an asymmetrical open mouth. At the center of the composition, the hand clutches the *alèze*, hinting at the patient's agency in tending to her symptoms. This gesture is typical of the condition: it is mentioned in clinical observations and is visible in a photograph of a Salpêtrière patient from 1894, which has a caption that specifies the illness (*pseudo-bulbaire*) and patient's name (Th. Halipré) (fig. 74).[73] Her face is framed by a dark bonnet and the white *alèze* that encircles her neck and tucks into her apron, whose long vertical folds rhyme with the borders of the photograph and the card on which it is pasted. The dark sleeves, bent at the elbows, direct our eyes toward her hands as they lift a corner of the *alèze* to her mouth. She wears an expression very similar to the sculpture's: eyes wide open, brow knitted, lips parted. In fact, it seems likely that this photograph was used specifically as a point of comparison for the sculpture, as a photograph of the sculpture was also printed and mounted onto the same kind of card.[74] Their common gesture traditionally connotes misery or despair in art-historical sources. In the painting *La Veuve* (*The Widow*) (ca. 1865, Paris, Musée d'Orsay) by Évariste Vital Luminais, for instance, a grief-stricken member of the widow's entourage similarly holds a handkerchief to her mouth, as do some of the mourning women in Gustave Courbet's *Un enterrement à Ornans* (*Burial at Ornans*) (1849–50, Paris, Musée d'Orsay). Charged with meaning from art-historical conventions and antecedents, the gesture accentuates the distressed expression of these Salpêtrière patients.

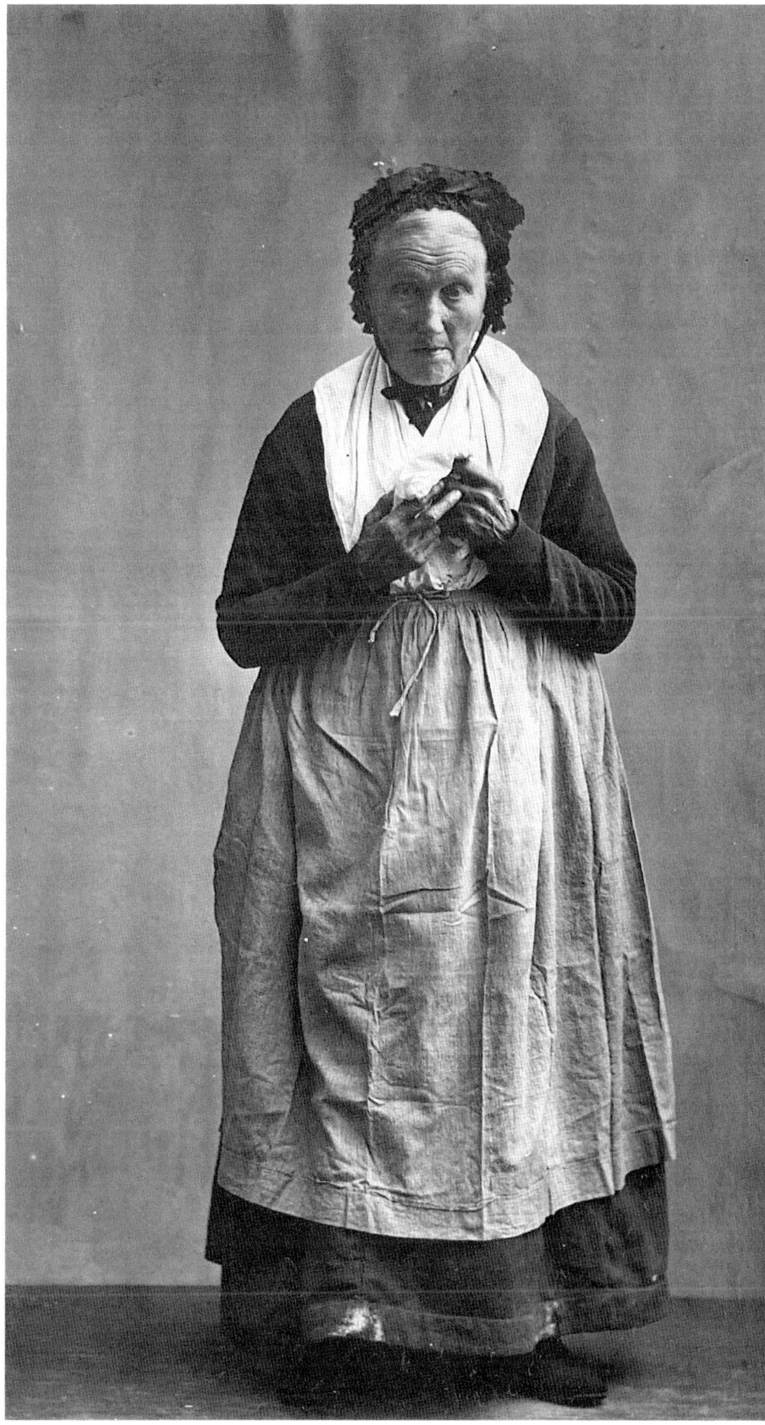

A side view of the white plaster version of this sculpture reveals that the thick folds of the *alèze* overhang the plinth on which the torso rests, helping to create a convincing three-dimensional figure (fig. 75). Richer has taken the unusual step of sculpting the bottom edge of the torso at an angle; the front of the plinth is approximately twice as high as the back. This unique internal plinth lends a sense of forward or upward movement to the figure, as if she were approaching us. Hatching animates and differentiates the elements of the sculpture. While the skin is smooth, the *alèze*, clothes, and plinth are covered in the marks of the sculptor's tool, which are particularly visible in the tinted plaster version (fig. 76). The clothes are more deeply incised than the *alèze*, with sets of thick, almost parallel lines at various angles that are echoed in the hatch marks on the plinth. They bespeak the human touch of the clinician who made the work, the subtle differentiation of textures showing us his artistry and ultimately the artificiality of his vision.

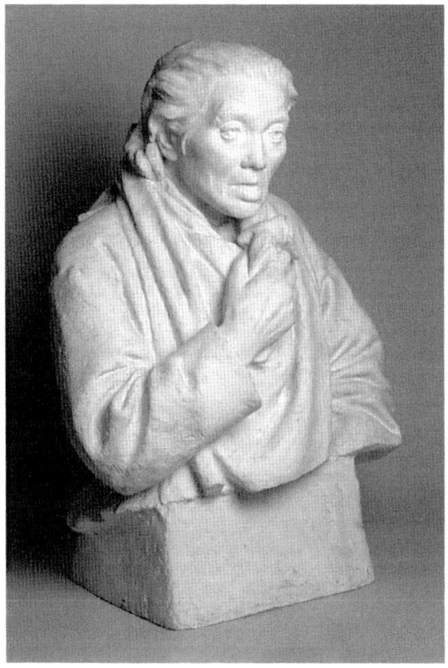

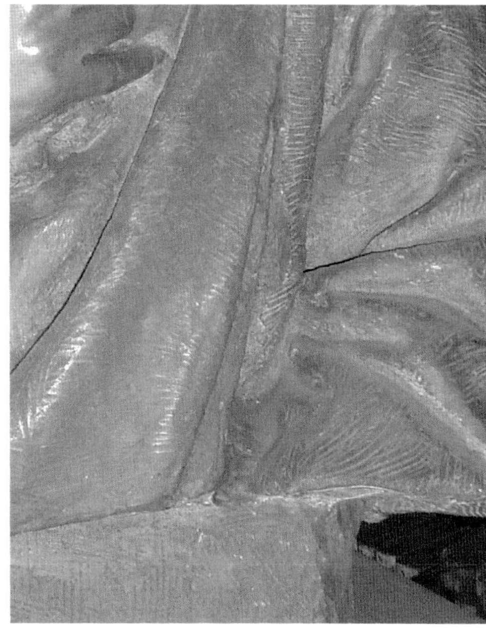

Fig. 75
Paul Richer, *Femme atteinte de paralysie glosso-labio-laryngée* (*Woman with Labio-Glosso-Laryngeal Paralysis*), end of the nineteenth century [1888]. Plaster sculpture after cast clay original, 77.8 × 55 × 39.5 cm. Paris, Musée de l'Assistance Publique–Hôpitaux de Paris. Inv. AP 2344. Photo: AP-HP/musée–F. Marin.

Fig. 76
Paul Richer, *Paralysie glosso-labio-laryngée* (*Woman with Labio-Glosso-Laryngeal Paralysis*), end of the nineteenth century [1888], detail showing incisions from the sculptor's tool. Pink plaster, 77 × 55 × 39 cm. Paris, Musée de l'Assistance Publique–Hôpitaux de Paris. Inv. AP 2003.7.9.3. Photo: AP-HP/ musée–author.

The photographic illustration (a photocollotype) in the *Nouvelle Iconographie de la Salpêtrière* seems to show the tinted plaster version of the sculpture (see figs. 65 and 76).[75] Its color bears a striking resemblance to terracotta, recalling the traditional clay *bozzetto* or sculptural sketch and thereby suggesting, intentionally or unintentionally, an artistic lineage for this new kind of artwork. The camera is almost at eye level with the figure and slightly to its proper right. The lighting has cast into shadow the right cheek and jaw, obscuring the asymmetry of the bottom half of the face. The bright light almost washes out the hand, but one can just make out the veins seemingly beneath its surface and the shadows that define the knuckles. Similarly, the marks of the sculptor's tool on the *alèze* have disappeared in the slightly overexposed image, emphasizing its thick, heavy folds. Only the deeply incised lines on the top remain to add a bit of rough texture to the work. The photograph imbues the figure with a lifelike quality. A hint of luster that seems to quicken the eyes is particularly striking—and may indicate that this photograph has been retouched. The dark cloth covering the plinth deceptively suggests a voluminous skirt and the existence of a left hand.

Richer produced a drawing of this same patient that appears to have been done from life (fig. 77). It is dated May 4, 1888, less than three months after Charcot made this illness the topic of one of his important *leçons du mardi*, in which he examined a fifty-seven-year-old man who had completely lost the ability to speak, could no longer eat or drink normally, and had to keep a handkerchief to his mouth at all times because of his constant drooling.[76] After a detailed examination, Charcot asked the patient to leave the room and declared that the man was "lost," with less than a year to live.[77] Then, in an extraordinary discourse, he explained his role:

> [All treatments] will be powerless to slow the progressive march of the illness in which bulbar death will be the last word: it is sad to say, but that is how it is: For the doctor, it is not about knowing if that is sad, it is about knowing if that is true; that the patient lives in the illusion to the end, that is very good; that is human, that must be, but the doctor, is this his role? It seems we are sometimes reproached for our persistent studies of important nervous diseases that were until now often incurable; What is the use? One would almost say that this is not medicine. Medicine *being the art of healing,* can you picture this: "my friend, I am a doctor, it is true, but unfortunately, I can do nothing for you: you belong to the category of the wretched whom we do not care about!!!" Come, gentlemen, our duty is not this: let us seek, in spite of everything, always seek; it is still the best way to discover and perhaps, thanks to our efforts, tomorrow's verdict will not be today's verdict?[78]

This powerful speech, advocating the fundamental import of medical research, exemplifies Charcot's belief in "truth" above all. It resonates with Richer's search for "truth" through his artistic renderings. The epigraph to Richer's book *Physiologie artistique de l'homme en mouvement* (Artistic physiology of man in motion) (1895) cites Ingres's dictum: "One must find the secret of beauty through truth." Richer, explaining the quotation in his text, equates the "study of the truth" with science.[79]

Charcot's discourse, therefore, may have inspired Richer to sketch a patient at the Salpêtrière who had the same terminal illness and then create a sculpture of her only a short time later. His carefully rendered ink drawing shows many of the details depicted in the sculpture, suggesting that the drawing likely served as its model. In the sculpture, deep furrows in the brow on her proper right near the hairline mimic the hatch lines of Richer's pen; the cresting of the drawn patient's hair on her proper right is also evident in the sculpture; the position of the right hand is almost identical; the drawing's cursory outline of the left hand is barely noticeable, and the hand is completely omitted from the sculpture. Moreover, the lowest portion of the patient's body is drawn at the same "angle" as the sculpted body's placement on the internal plinth. In other words, in the drawing, the back of the patient's clothes can be seen "below" her garments at the front. An attempt at a faithful reproduction in sculpture may have been what led to the unusual shape of the plinth.

The sculpture diverges from the drawing too, of course. It has more pronounced folds in the *alèze,* and the right hand is less animated and more correctly proportioned—in the drawing, it is oversized, dwarfing the indistinct wisp of the left hand. But the face is the site of the most significant changes. The woman in the sculpture appears older, her face wider, the protruding lower lip fuller. The eyes, especially, have been emphasized—they bulge under the rims of thick and heavy lids. When I look into the irises and deeply cut pupils, underlined by the "whites" of the eyes, I am overwhelmed by the pathos of their sorrow and hopelessness (see fig. 65).

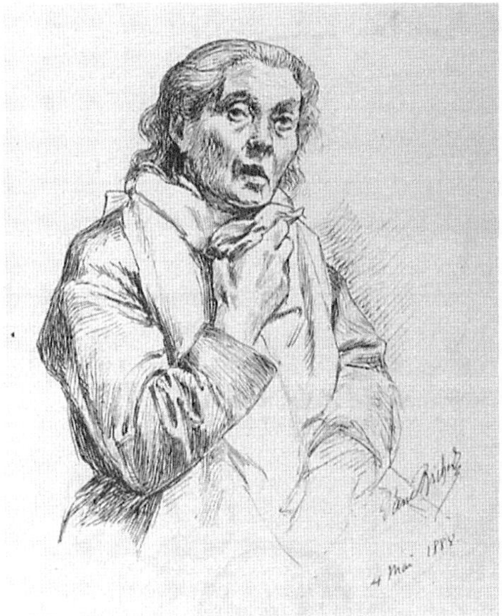

Fig. 77
Paul Richer, *Malade atteinte de paralysie glosso-labio-laryngée* (*Woman with Labio-Glosso-Laryngeal Paralysis*), May 4, 1888. Pen and ink. Private collection.

This work, like all of Richer's sculptures of pathology, clearly engages with the conventions of portraiture, discussed in detail in chapter 3. Indeed, this is almost a modern *portrait parlant*, descended from the speaking Enlightenment busts that were meant to capture an individual's spirit. Yet in Richer's sculpture, the open mouth vacillates between the intimation of an intellectual interiority and the simple portrayal of a pathological symptom. Meige notes that the "gaping" mouth and the "flaccid" lips prevent those with labio-glosso-laryngeal paralysis from laughing or kissing.[80] The detailed features and despairing expression, hinting at an interiority we can only divine, seem to be in tension with the prerogative of the Salpêtrière School to identify specific symptoms that then bolster and conform to an archetype of disease. Richer's didactic sculpture attempts to turn the individual, whose physiognomic traces make up this portrait, into a "type" in order to help train doctors to recognize these facial symptoms.

Facies of Labio-Glosso-Laryngeal Paralysis represents temporality arrested, a "snapshot" of the patient in the inexorable advancement of the condition. Florence Chantoury-Lacombe has characterized Flemish painter Giusto Sustermans's portraits of Grand Duke Ferdinando II de' Medici (1626, Florence, Palazzo Pitti) stricken with smallpox as "[running] counter to the very principle of the portrait, which is to present the individual's enduring appearance, whereas [Sustermans] chose to represent the impression of a moment." She continues that "it is not the portrait of Ferdinando II de' Medici which is shown but rather the portrait of smallpox."[81] As in Richer's sculptures, the pathology is meant to obscure the patient, just as the "type" is meant to mask the individual. However, in *Facies of Labio-Glosso-Laryngeal Paralysis* the patient is not effaced by the disease that ravages her brain. It is impossible to ignore the affecting portrait of this Salpêtrière patient or her individual agency.

In a sculpture five years later, the art-historical conventions of portraiture played a more obvious role. *Buste de myopathique* (*Bust of a Man with Myopathy*) (1893) is another patient portrait by Richer, and, like the *Facies of Labio-Glosso-Laryngeal Paralysis*, it was probably life-size.[82] Photographs of it illustrate a study by Henry Meige of amyotrophy in art from 1894 in the *Nouvelle Iconographie* (see fig. 66).[83] It presents a brief history of the medical understanding of this progressive condition, in which the muscles atrophy, and asserts that there are few others that change the morphology of the face and body as much as myopathy, which is a generic term for any disease of the muscles.[84] He then outlines a brief history of its artistic representation, arguing that artists like Raphael and Charles Le Brun created "mediocre" representations of amyotrophy. The prominent lips and "exaggerated opening" of the eye of the man seeking alms in Raphael's tapestry cartoon *The Healing of the Lame Man (Acts 3:1–8)* (1515–16, London, Royal Collection Trust), for example, could indicate either myopathy or rickets, he argues.[85] In contrast, Meige claims, in the bust Richer has "not only rendered, with a scrupulous accuracy, all the interesting features of the face, neck and shoulders; but also that he understood the raison d'être of all the morphological modifications caused by the illness."[86] Richer's medical knowledge, therefore, ensures that his work is a more accurate or "truthful" representation of the disease than any attempted by his artistic ancestors. Significantly, Meige's article begins with a quotation by Charcot from his early article on the sculpture of Aesop, in which he asserts that only doctors can decide whether an anatomical imperfection in a work of art is the result of "nature or the chisel" (see the introduction).[87]

Richer's sitter was Henri Bonnet, a man in his late twenties who had what was known at the time as the Landouzy-Dejerine type of myopathy, now called facioscapulohumeral muscular dystrophy.[88] Symptoms usually appear before the age of twenty, and the muscles of the face, shoulders, and upper arms are the first to show signs of weakness and then atrophy progressively.[89] As a child, Bonnet noticed that his lips were overlarge and that he could not whistle or sing.[90] By the age of ten, he could not close his eyes completely and played "being blind" with his friends.[91] Before entering the Salpêtrière in 1890, he worked first as a hotel porter, but his weakening muscles forced him to change jobs and become a rural postman. Eventually this too had to be abandoned because of his illness.[92] A photograph of Bonnet alone illustrates the sixth volume of the *Nouvelle Iconographie* (fig. 78). In a photograph published in the journal the next year, Bonnet's nude body appears alongside two others with the same malady (fig. 79); readers could thereby judge the accuracy of Richer's sculpture, published in the same volume (see fig. 66).[93] In the photograph, the patients with myopathy stand on a low platform in front of a simple backdrop, their stance and atrophied limbs indicating their illness. Their chests, too, reveal subtle deformities.[94] Bonnet, on the far right, has an especially asymmetrical posture and uneven shoulders. While the muscles in his neck remained strong, there was "considerable atrophy" of those in his chest and back, where some no longer functioned.[95] In an article on the position of the myopathic body while standing and walking, Richer notes that Bonnet had an atrophied gluteal muscle on his right side, which meant that his pelvis fell to the left.[96]

Bonnet's face is the only one of the three patients in the photograph that betrays another symptom of myopathy. Neurologist Louis Landouzy described it in detail: "The mouth is enlarged, the lips, slightly set apart, almost always asymmetrical, appear thick, prominent. Sometimes the lower lip . . . appears to be drooping, pulled down, almost turned inside out." According to Landouzy, the physiognomy of people with myopathy was, to sum up, "strange, bizarre, inert, cold, sorrowful, and a bit silly," while

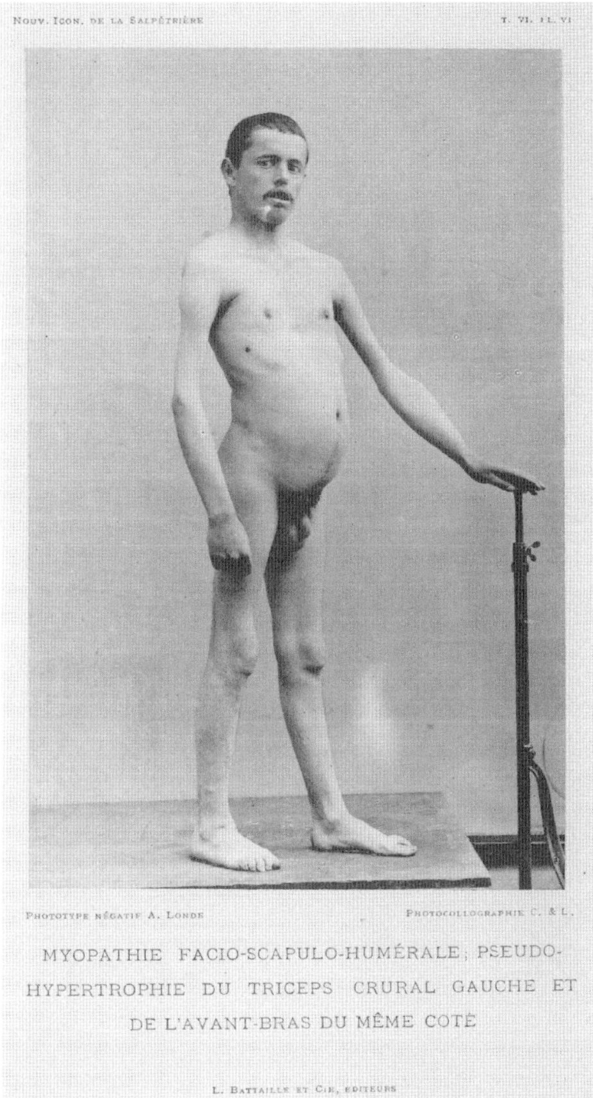

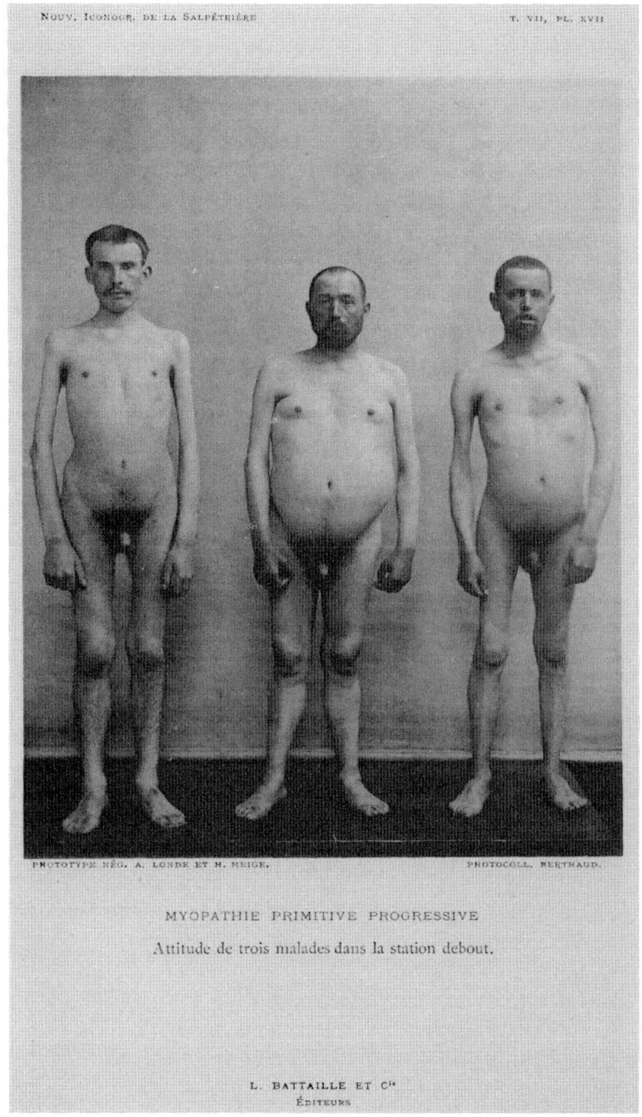

their manner of speaking and laughing was simply "sad."[97] In describing Bonnet's facial features specifically, Georges Guinon notes that his lips resembled the "rim of a chamber pot." Moreover, his inability to fully close his eyelids progressively worsened. In December 1889 the gap was four to five millimeters, but four years later it was approximately one centimeter.[98] Richer's sculptural intervention may have been prompted by the fact that representations of "the myopathic facies" were rare in art, and, according to Meige, "representations of limbs with muscle atrophy are better known."[99] We also learn that Charcot exhibited Bonnet regularly in his lessons "as the type of myopathic facies."[100] While Le Noir and Bezançon note that "these deformities render the physiognomy inexpressive," Meige adds that myopathy imparts "a silly air, an appearance of stupidity and imbecility," illustrating his comments with a drawing of Bonnet in profile (fig. 80).[101] The simple drawing (possibly by Meige) shows the head from a slightly lower vantage point, which emphasizes the protruding lips. It seems to have been copied from a photograph of Bonnet, itself used more than ten years later to illustrate a text on myopathy, in which his face appears less distorted and his open lips slightly less turned out (fig. 81).[102] He is seated, and his torso is visible to the waist. The emaciated upper arm, the shoulder blade that juts out over the back of the chair, and the convex belly all point to his condition. In contrast to the drawing, the bust and the photographs show the patient with the same look of shock or astonishment, not "stupidity." Richer makes evident in the sculpture the bags under the patient's eyes, which suggest fatigue. He cuts into the irises, animating the expression. He also sets the eyes in deep cavities and casts the gaze downward, lending the figure a pensive, even melancholic, air. The latter in particular complicates a reading of this work. By averting the sculpture's gaze, Richer has also diminished the patient's agency.

In the frontal photograph of the sculpture, it almost seems as if Richer has suppressed the deformity of Bonnet's body. His shoulders are almost even, with only a slight bulge on the contour of the figure's left shoulder alluding to his malady. But Albert Londe took a photograph of the sculpture in profile, probably at Richer's behest, that also illustrates the *Nouvelle Iconographie* (see fig. 66). Londe states in his seminal book on medical photography, published the year before, that it is the doctor's role to indicate the positions in which the patient should be shot by the camera.[103] The profile view is more indicative of Bonnet's pathology, revealing the projecting shoulder blade that is visible in the photograph of him sitting down. It illustrates Guinon and Souques's observation that the sternum is "strongly flattened" in this part of the chest in people with myopathy.[104] The photograph of Bonnet standing alone from the *Nouvelle Iconographie* makes this plain (see fig. 78).

While the photographs attest to the sculpture's resemblance to the patient, Richer has clearly regularized some of Bonnet's features: the eyes are straighter and more focused, the jawline stronger, the neck well defined, and the shoulders less sloped. That is, Richer's sculptural rendering of Bonnet appears generally less sickly, undermining its presumptive purpose—the representation of a pathology. At the same time, this attempt to beautify or idealize the sitter reinforces the link to traditional portraiture; antique portrait busts of men often showed bare-chested sitters. Also distracting from the realism and reminding us of the artist's hand are the locks of hair that seem to have been created from simple impressions of the sculptor's tool or finger and, even more so, the inscription underneath the left clavicle: "Bonnet / Myopathique / Juillet 1893" (see fig. 66). Deeper than a tattoo or an instance of hysterical dermographism, this incision seems particularly aggressive. The intrusion of these words on an otherwise realistic sculpture compels the viewer to see it as an artistic representation, as does its rough bottom edge, where the plaster's original soft texture is in evidence. Playing with the convention of indicating a sitter's identity on a bust's plinth, Richer's sculpture displays Bonnet's name on its very "skin." In the lantern slide of this work used by Richer at the École des beaux-arts, the sculpture is cut off just above the rough bottom edge, the beginning of the word "juillet" eliminated.[105] This omission would likely

Fig. 78 (opposite left)
Myopathie facio-scapulo-humérale; Pseudo-hypertrophie du triceps crural gauche et de l'avant-bras du même coté (*Facioscapulohumeral Muscular Dystrophy; Pseudohypertrophy of the Left Calf Muscles and the Forearm on the Same Side*). From *Nouvelle Iconographie de la Salpêtrière* 6 (1893): plate 6. Courtesy of the Wellcome Collection.

Fig. 79 (opposite)
Myopathie primitive progressive. Attitude de trois malades dans la station debout (*Muscular Dystrophy: Attitude of Three Patients in the Standing Position*). From *Nouvelle Iconographie de la Salpêtrière* 7 (1894): plate 17. Courtesy of the Wellcome Collection.

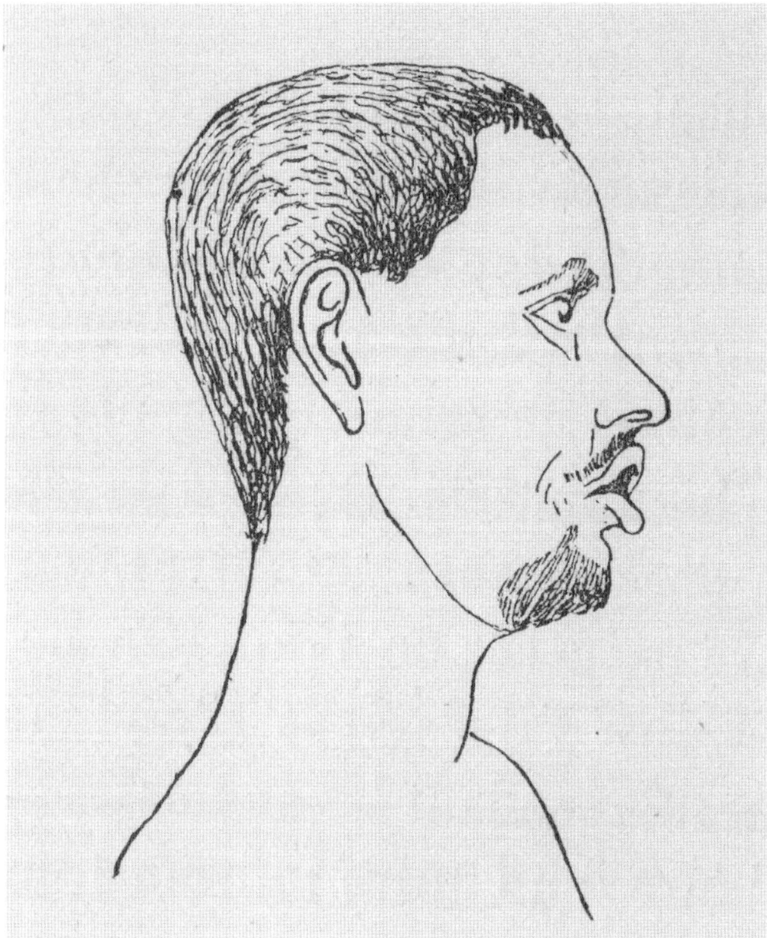

Fig. 80
Illustration from Henry Meige, "Les Amyotrophiques dans l'art," *Nouvelle Iconographie de la Salpêtrière* 7 (1894): 199, fig. 54. Courtesy of the Wellcome Collection.

have heightened the realism of the work in the projected image, making the incised words all the more jarring. Ludmilla Jordanova has written that portraits in the nineteenth century were often reproduced with not only the artist's signature but also the sitter's, "a further affirmation of who they were, of their particularity."[106] Here, Richer has appropriated the patient's proper name and inadvertently revealed the tension between individual and type, where Bonnet's surname is literally underlined by his illness. The individuality signaled by the proper name seems at odds with the work's didactic role as carrier of visual pathological symptoms.

Bonnet must have been at least somewhat aware, we can assume, of the powerful apparatus at the Salpêtrière for the dissemination of medical knowledge. Charcot regularly exhibited him in his lessons as a living specimen, and Bonnet was "presented" at a meeting of the Société anatomique by Guinon and Souques.[107] Moreover, as we have seen, he was also used as a case study in articles in the *Revue de médecine,* the *Nouvelle Iconographie de la Salpêtrière,* and the *Traité de médecine,* where his photograph and likeness illustrated several articles.[108] Even though his surname is visible on the sculpture itself in the *Nouvelle Iconographie* illustration, it was shortened to "Bonn" in Meige's article in order to preserve anonymity, as was the custom in the hospital's published case histories. In Richer's article in the same volume, he is called both "Bonn." and simply "B.," while in the study by Guinon from the year before, he is referred to as "Bon . . . Henri."[109] The ethical standards of the Salpêtrière became an issue in the nineteenth century because of the institution's practices involving the public exhibition of patients and its lax adherence to a policy of anonymity.[110] This volume of the *Nouvelle Iconographie* reveals some of those issues: not only is the patient's photograph available for comparison with an artistic representation, but the patient's full surname is also plainly inscribed *on* that artistic representation. At the same time, Richer's name is notably absent from the inscription on the sculpture, replaced by clinical notes: patient's name, diagnosis, and date. Richer here subverted standard artistic practice, as if his sculpture were simply an illustration of the case notes, a clinical object rather than an aesthetic one. After all, Meige calls Richer's sculptures "permanent clinical documents."[111] Indeed, Richer's signature seems altogether unnecessary. The factual data is the raison d'être for the work and testifies to Richer's role as both clinician and sculptor.

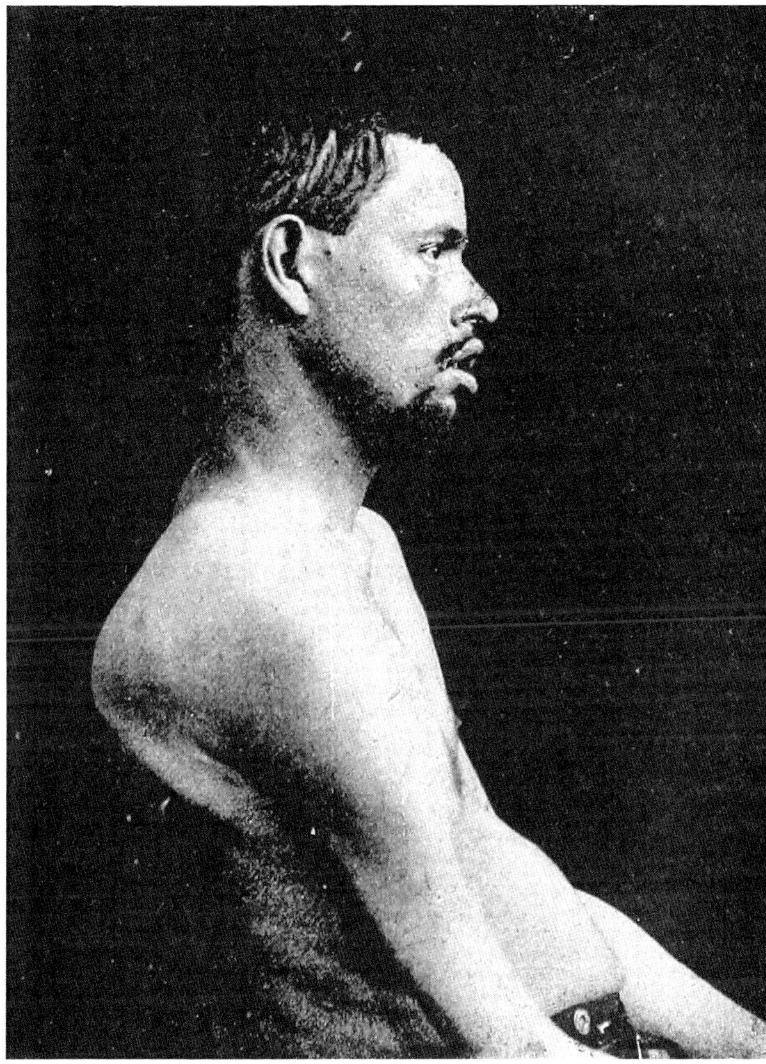

Fig. 81
Illustration from Émile Boix, "Myopathie primitive progressive," in *Traité de médecine*, edited by Bouchard and Brissaud, vol. 10 (Paris: Masson, 1905), 463, fig. 106. Courtesy of the Wellcome Collection.

Pathologizing the Nude

Richer's final work in this series on nervous pathology depicts a patient with juvenile hypothyroidism. The patient's name and age are inscribed on the plinth, along with the fact that the sculpture is one-third life-size (see fig. 67). *Infantilisme myxoedémateux* (*Juvenile Hypothyroidism*) (ca. 1898) shows a nineteen-year-old patient named René Aurillard (referred to as "O . . ." in published case histories). Meige states in an article from 1898 that it is "a faithful copy of a live model" from the Salpêtrière.[112] At the time, Aurillard was 1.03 meters (3 feet 5 inches) tall and weighed 23 kilos (50.6 pounds). The clinician writes that palpation of the patient's neck demonstrated that he had no thyroid.[113]

Juvenile hypothyroidism had only been identified clinically in 1873 and at first was thought to be a disorder that affected women exclusively.[114] By the end of the century, it was known that children, too, could have it, though it was considered rare.[115] Aurillard's physical and intellectual development stopped around his fourth birthday, when he began experiencing "nervous attacks" and pains in his limbs and abdomen.[116] His skin started to become thicker and more sensitive to the cold (thickened skin, a typical symptom of hypothyroidism, led Charcot to characterize the illness as "pachydermic").[117] When Aurillard entered the Salpêtrière in June 1897, his visage, "with . . . its effaced features, drowned, as it were, in a general puffiness, betrayed no glimmer of intelligence."[118] His spine had curved slightly in order to compensate for the significant shortening of his right leg, due in turn to the sharp inward angling of the knee. He had trouble walking because of his large belly, crooked leg, and deformed feet.[119] Additionally, his intelligence was developmentally arrested, according to Fulgence Raymond (1844–1910), who was in charge of his case. He could not read, spoke little, and had the ideas and tastes of a child. This "sad" young man often started crying uncontrollably for no discernible reason.[120]

Raymond began treating him by prescribing daily ingestion of one lobe of fresh mutton thyroid, though the frequency and amount changed often because Aurillard showed signs of intolerance.[121] After four months and the ingestion of sixty-one lobes, he had noticeably improved. His chronically low body temperature had normalized, his face had become less puffy, his hair had become finer, and his skin had "completely regenerated."[122] Many of his baby teeth had fallen out as well, and one adult incisor had emerged. He grew four centimeters, and X-ray studies showed that his bones, which had been stunted at the developmental stage of a three-year-old, had "aged" many years.[123] Moreover, "a remarkable transformation of intelligence and character" had taken place. Aurillard learned to read and had become happy and playful. "He makes fun of the hysterics who are around him," Raymond writes. "He copies their attacks."[124]

Meige's discussion of Richer's artwork begins with a repetition of Raymond's case notes regarding Aurillard, "a being who remained a child, past the age of childhood." He condescendingly asks, "Does he not have the face of a newborn still at the breast, with his big cheeks . . . , his little button nose, and his fleshy lips that still seem made for suckling?"[125] He comments that the body was covered in a layer of fat, which results in "the resemblance of the physique of childhood."[126] Richer is praised for the fact that his sculpture "corresponds exactly" to the symptoms of juvenile hypothyroidism.[127]

An article by Raymond from the same year that delineates the development and treatment of hypothyroidism includes before-and-after photographs of Aurillard (fig. 82).[128] In the "before" image, we see him standing almost frontally, facing the camera. His face does not look quite as childlike as the sculpture would suggest. While he has full cheeks and a round visage, he no longer resembles an infant. Raymond notes that he has a low forehead and that his skull appeared "stretched from the front to the back."[129] Just as he did with Henri Bonnet, Richer has given the sculpture of Aurillard thicker, more unruly hair, in keeping with Raymond's description of its abundance and stiffness.[130] The angle of the "before" photograph, however, dissimulates the large stomach and the "infiltration" of fat all over the body that Meige describes, whereas the sculpture highlights the belly.[131] In fact, judging from both *Juvenile Hypothyroidism* and the photograph, Meige's contention that fat hides the "muscles and bones" from view all over the body appears to be an exaggeration, since we can clearly see definition, especially in his arms and legs.

Meanwhile, other elements of Aurillard's condition have been replicated in the sculpture. Meige points out that the patient's sexual organs were the only part of his body that differed from the "typical sufferer" of juvenile hypothyroidism. Instead of being "miniscule," they are almost "normal" size. Richer, Meige writes, "wanting above all to be scrupulously faithful to natural reality, did not fail to render this anomaly."[132] The young man with the features of an infant is rendered as a "perfectly real image" of juvenile hypothyroidism, Meige recounts, but the dissonance between his overall childlike appearance and the adult size of his genitals effectively renders Aurillard

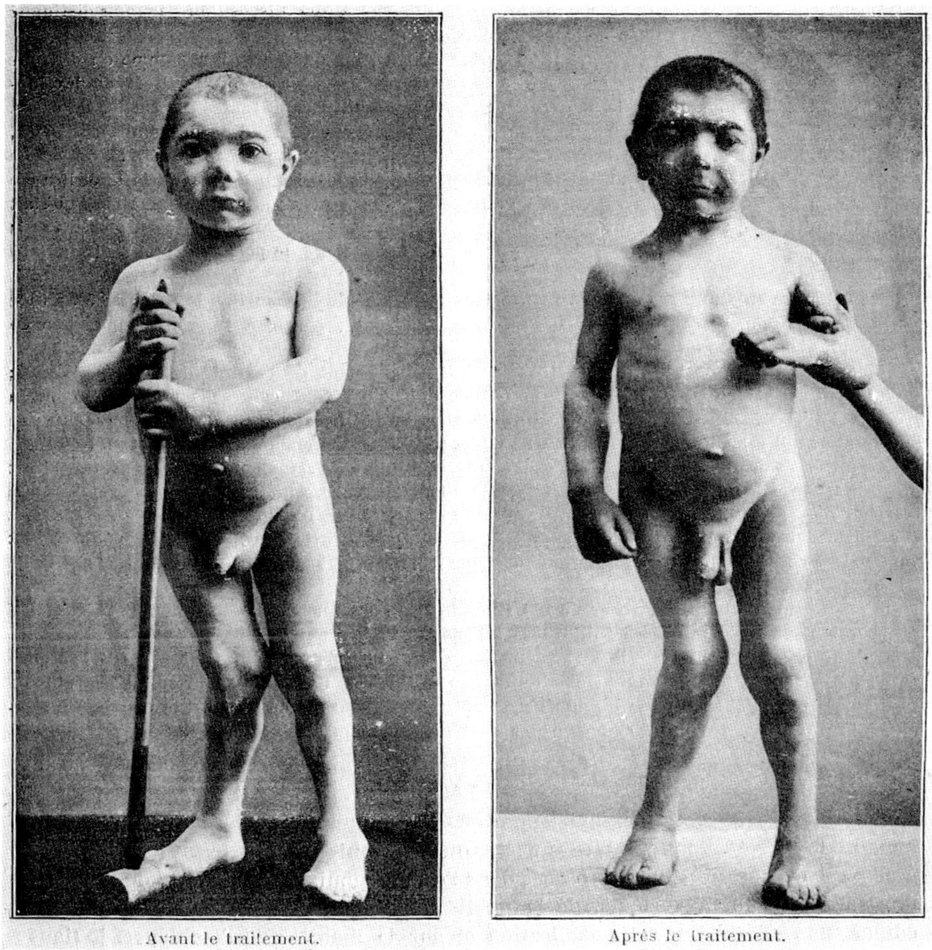

Fig. 82
Avant le traitement and *Après le traitement* (*Before Treatment* and *After Treatment*). From Fulgence Raymond, "Du myxoedème infantile et des autres formes de myxoedème. Pathogénie et traitement," *Revue internationale de thérapeutique et pharmacologie* 6, no. 1 (January 18, 1898): 47. Photo courtesy of the US National Library of Medicine.

monstrous.[133] As Richer recounts in an analysis of ancient sculptures of dwarfs in his book *L'Art et la médecine* (Art and medicine) (1902), the disproportionate size of the phallus makes evident their "satirical or caricatural intent."[134]

The pose of the young man in *Juvenile Hypothyroidism* was inspired by these same antique sculptures. In the "before" photograph, we can see that Aurillard needed to hold onto a stick—oddly, it appears to be a croquet bat—as his right knee and left clubfoot would have made it difficult for him to stand unsupported.[135] Walking was also difficult for him; his knees knocked into each other, and that physical discomfort is apparent in the abnormal position of his legs.[136] Those hands clasped tightly to the support in the photograph became fists in Richer's work, with Aurillard's arms parted to resemble a boxer's pose (fig. 83). Meige explains that this sculpture brings to mind the "supposedly legendary personages of which Art has given us numerous representations." It is in this context that he discusses the bizarre stance of the figure itself. In a casually patronizing tone that is jarring to today's sensibilities, he calls it reminiscent "of an artistic formula dear to antiquity, as the little child is represented in the pose of a pugilist. Now, it is known that the ancients had the custom of representing these Pygmies

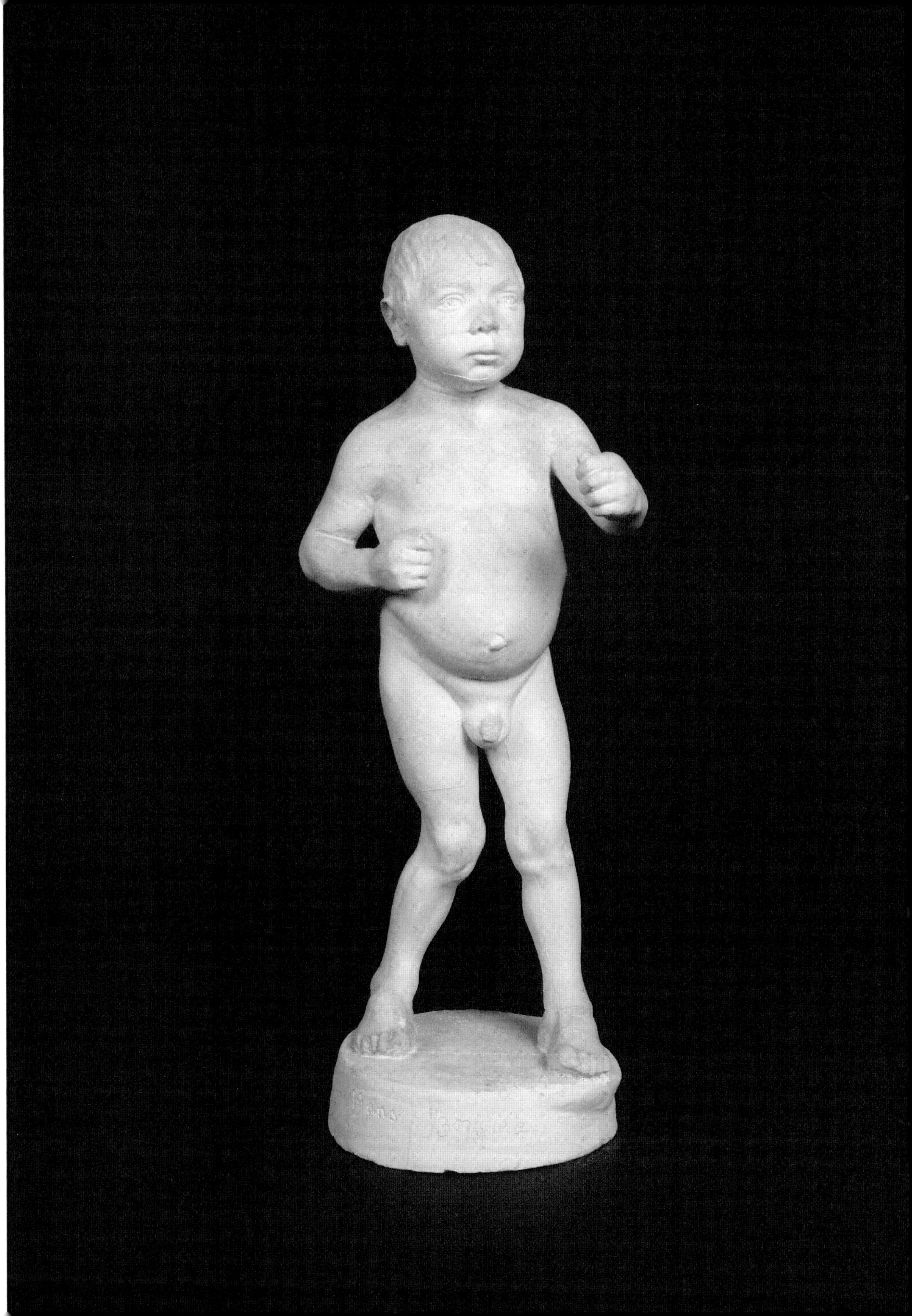

[*sic*] engaging in athletic exercises, wrestling, boxing, fighting each other or the cranes, their classical enemies. And these bellicose dwarfs appear to us . . . like portraits of this juvenile and hypothyroidal dwarf."[137]

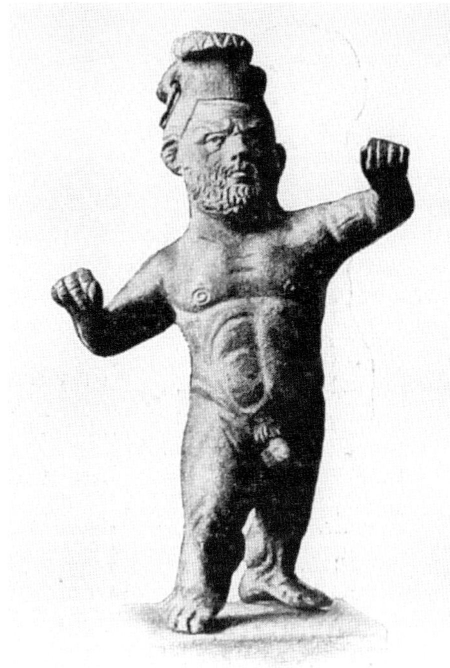

Fig. 83 (opposite)
Paul Richer, *Jeune atrophié* (*Atrophied Youth*), end of the nineteenth century [ca. 1898]. Plaster, 37.5 × 14.8 × 15 cm. Paris, Musée de l'Assistance Publique–Hôpitaux de Paris. Inv. AP 2352. Photo: AP-HP/musée–F. Marin.

Fig. 84
Pygmée (Bronze antique, musée du Louvre) (*Pygmy [Antique Bronze, Louvre Museum]*). From Paul Richer, *L'Art et la médecine* (Paris: Gaultier, Magnier, [1902]), fig. 123. Courtesy of the Wellcome Collection.

Richer's *L'Art et la médecine* seems to validate Meige's impression, as it includes a section on antique bronze sculptures of pygmies, who were figures of ridicule from an obscure comic tradition in ancient Greece and Rome. Among the illustrations is one that may well have served as a model for Aurillard's pose (fig. 84). In Greek mythology, the pygmies are a race of little people who fight with cranes each spring, as Meige mentions above.[138] Hercules finds them preparing to attack him and sweeps them up in his lion skin.[139] The sculpture in the illustration wears a headdress, with stylized striations denoting muscles on its chest and legs. Its hands are raised in fists, ready to fight. The posture of *Juvenile Hypothyroidism* appears to be a deliberate repositioning and recontextualization of Aurillard's hands to transform a gesture of grasping a support—probably copied from the aforementioned photograph of him—into the pugilist's pose of an antique sculpture. Richer mentions that nature itself was responsible for the "caricature of a man" in a person with dwarfism, which perhaps explains the gratuitous mockery inherent in this project.[140] Yet Meige concludes by calling Richer's sculpture "a photograph in three dimensions"—the strongest praise possible for an object that is meant to represent the "real" without personal interpretation.[141]

The Salpêtrière sculpture that is most well known today is often referred to as *La Parkinsonienne* (ca. 1895; fig. 85). It shows a woman with Parkinson's disease, which Charcot named after James Parkinson, who described this progressive condition that leads to constant shaking, rigid muscles, and slow movement in *An Essay on the Shaking Palsy* from 1817.[142] The sculpture, a "beautiful model of morbid morphology," portrays a patient called simply "Gell" in the clinical notes.[143] Richer and Meige write in an article from the 1895 volume of the *Nouvelle Iconographie* that she "[represents] the almost perfect clinical schema of Parkinson's disease" and that the sculpture "is a copy as faithful as possible to the patient in question."[144] Here it seems that the competing notions of "individual" and "type" have been reconciled: the patient's portrait is rendered faithfully *because* she exhibits the most typical symptoms of the disease. The authors explain that typical traits include an expressionless visage, forward inclination of the head and torso, a sunken chest, and flexed arms and legs. "In a word,"

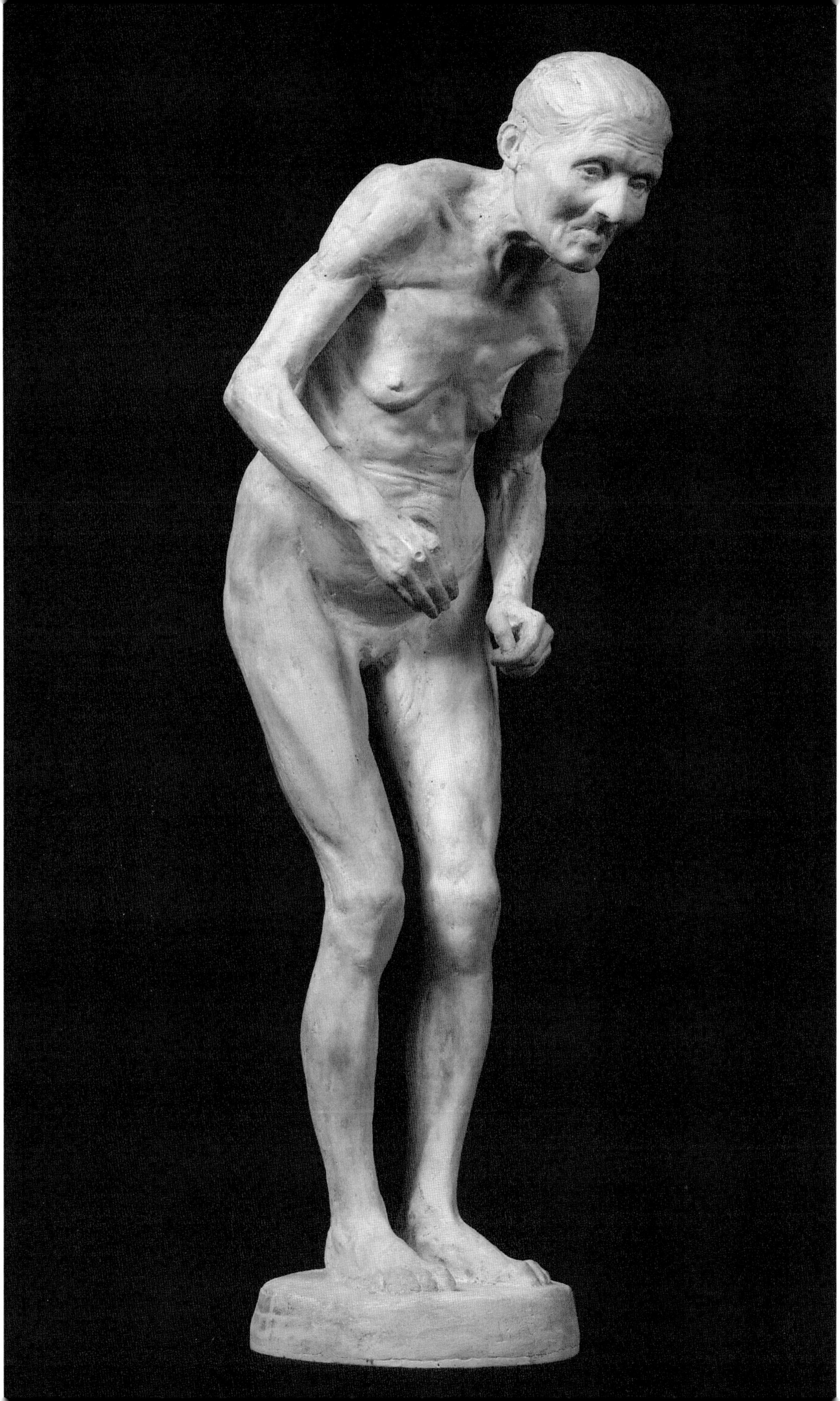

they conclude, she has "the look of an old person who has been welded together."[145] Charcot had also commented on this symptom, noting that people with Parkinson's disease resembled the "automatons that can be seen in exhibitions of animated wax figures."[146] Richer's sculpture is no automaton—the characteristic bodily tremors of Parkinson's cannot be replicated in inert matter. Yet the rigidity of plaster manages an apt suggestion of their rigid movements.[147]

Fig. 85 (opposite)
Paul Richer, *La Parkinsonienne*, ca. 1895. Plaster, 46 × 15.5 × 18 cm. Paris, École nationale supérieure des Beaux-Arts. Inv. MU11975–1. Photo © Beaux-Arts de Paris, Dist. RMN-Grand Palais / image Beaux-arts de Paris.

The ravages of the disease mar *La Parkinsonienne*'s body, which seems to have aged far beyond her almost sixty years. She exhibits a stooped posture, flexed limbs, and an expression of ingrained frustration. Richer and Meige write that in Parkinson's patients, the face below the eyes is "a blank mask in which life seems absent: neither pain, nor pleasure, the absence of all expression."[148] However, the deeply wrinkled brow, the heavy eyelids and downcast gaze, the hollow cheeks, and the pinched mouth contradict this idea of a "blank mask" (see fig. 85).[149] They conform more closely to the "permanent expression of mournfulness" that Charcot described as characteristic of Parkinson's in his standard work on the subject, "De la paralysie agitante" ("On the Shaking Palsy") from 1869.[150] Despite Richer and Meige's talk of a "blank mask" and their description of the sculpture as "the patient that we have chosen as the *type* of Parkinson's disease,"[151] there is an undeniable expression on the visage and a particular personality behind it. Artistic license has opened the door to empathy.

Richer and Meige reiterate the importance of studying the naked body, with the sculpture intended as proof. Given the fact that Parkinson's disease is easily diagnosed without disrobing the patient, according to the authors, some of the symptomatic changes to the body caused by the disease have been ignored, especially the realignment of the body's axes when standing.[152] The article includes a detailed analysis of each part of the sculpture's body, or, more specifically, the patient's body, as if they were one and the same. For example, they write that the "trilobate appearance" of the stomach under the navel is "a common problem in women who have had many children (this one had 11)" (see fig. 85).[153] Personal physical attributes, specific to Gell the individual, were replicated in a sculpture meant to represent a type. For Richer and his colleagues, clearly only the most perfect copy of the patient could prove the "truthfulness" of the representation of disease—even when the details were wholly irrelevant to the pathology.

As in the case of *Juvenile Hypothyroidism*, it is possible that Richer was working not from life but from a photograph as he sculpted *La Parkinsonienne*. He wrote in the preface to *Anatomie artistique* that he made all of the drawings for it "from life," yet it is known that he made them by copying photographs.[154] While this may have made the process of drawing the body easier, it would be an astonishing revelation about a clinician and, later, professor of anatomy. One can see a similar conflation of, or rather confusion over, art and life in the photographic comparison made in the article by Richer and Meige (figs. 68 and 86). The "type of Parkinson's disease" is illustrated in another set of images that shows a male patient by the name of "Oll . . ." (hereafter Oll), "who has often served in the past in the clinical lessons of . . . Charcot."[155] Albert Londe

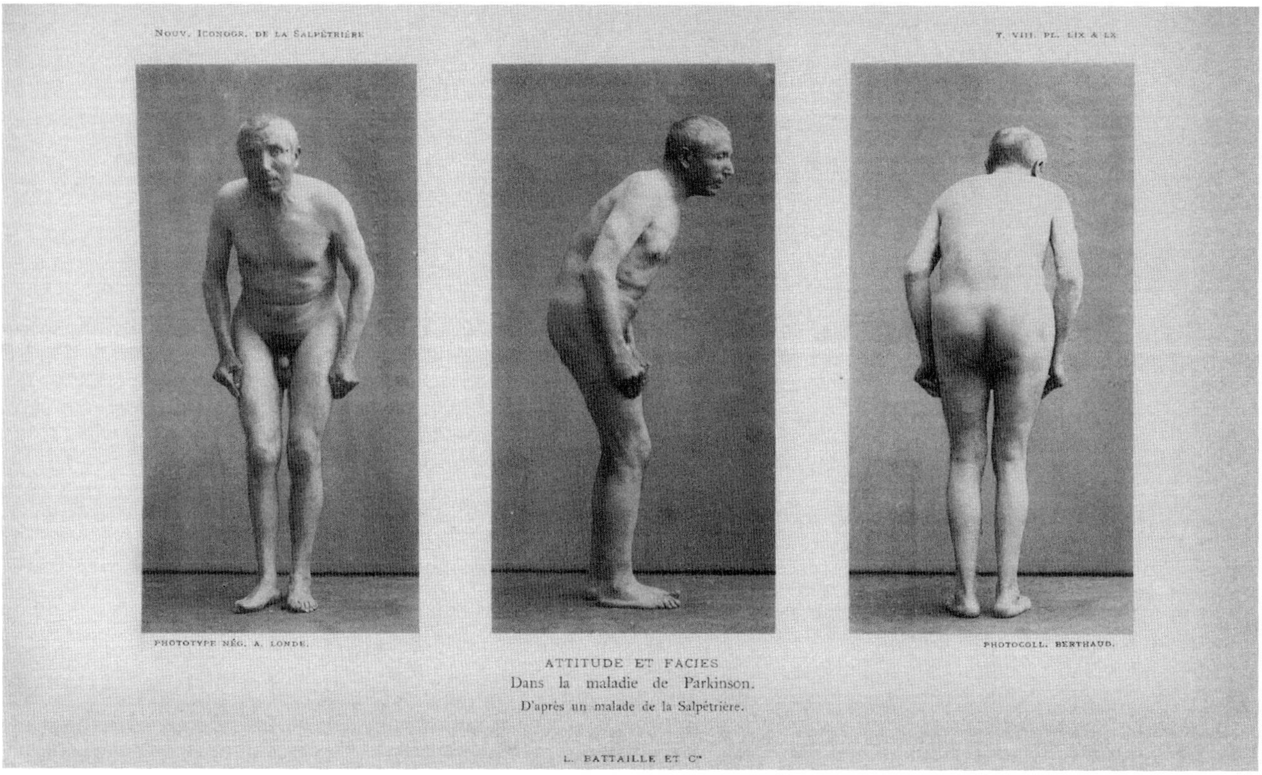

Fig. 86
Attitude et facies dans la maladie de Parkinson. D'après un malade de la Salpêtrière (Attitude and Facies of Parkinson's Disease: After a Patient at the Salpêtrière). From Paul Richer and Henry Meige, "Étude morphologique sur la Maladie de Parkinson," *Nouvelle Iconographie de la Salpêtrière* 8 (1895): plates 59–60 [*sic*]. Courtesy of the Wellcome Collection.

photographed Oll and *La Parkinsonienne* in the same three angles and under similar lighting conditions in order to facilitate their comparison. Richer and Meige conclude that "an identical morphology" is visible in both sets of images.[156] It is significant that at no point in their article do they mention that the sculpture is only forty-six centimeters (eighteen inches) tall. The comparison between the sculpture of Gell and the live patient Oll relies *entirely* on photographs that deceptively equalize their subjects' respective scale and on an absolute confidence in Richer's ability to render a sculpture that was identical to its model. The camera provided a vehicle through which to make an equivalence between patient and sculpture, and the latter was found to be a faithful copy. This test of the "scientific artwork" was meant to prove the objectivity of its creator and was also perhaps the ultimate test of realism.

The term "realism" is problematic in the discussion of these artworks, of course, as is the term "objectivity." As in the photograph of Richer with Oll—perhaps taken when Londe was preparing the aforementioned photographic comparison—the clinician's stance in the creation of these works is enigmatic (fig. 87).[157] Richer could never be perfectly "objective," nor did he want to be solely "artistic." Yet adjectives like "realistic" and "objective" belie the instability of representation and the oscillation between individual and type, portrait and specimen, embodied by these sculptures. Richer's works highlight the limitations of the language we use to understand and discuss medical imagery. To what degree are these objects "scientific" or "artistic," "realistic" or not? In the creation of these pathological portraits, which was more important:

the patient, the diagnosis, or the artistic tradition? Artistic and medical images have been characterized as "metaphor and fact," respectively, but those categories are difficult to separate in the case of the Salpêtrière sculptures.[158] They are testaments to the fact that neither art nor science has ever been a stable category—both have always been culturally determined and culturally determining.

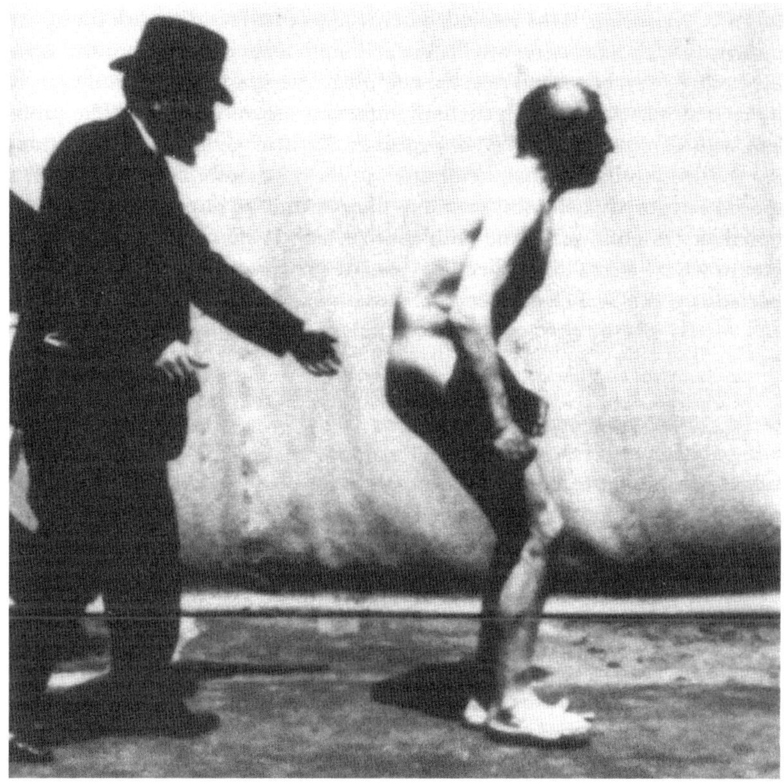

Fig. 87
Frame from one of Albert Londe's chronophotographic series for the analysis of pathological movement. From Lisa Cartwright, *Screening the Body: Tracing Medicine's Visual Culture* (Minneapolis: University of Minnesota Press, 1995), 49.

In *Objectivity*, Daston and Galison express an aspiration to "engage the curiosity of other scholars about topics that do not yet have a history, despite their leading role in creating modern science," including "the ways in which scientific experience is molded by image-making and image-reading" and "the mesh between the most concrete image-making practices and the most abstract epistemological goals."[159] The "scientific artworks" of Paul Richer, who combined his medical and artistic knowledge and skills to create "truthful" didactic representations of disease, do not fit easily into any of the paradigms identified by Daston and Galison. These sculptures of pathology illustrate the elasticity of the term "objectivity" at the Salpêtrière and highlight the role played by artistry in the creation of medical imagery. They are indeed scientific artworks.

Illness and Health, Science and Art

In his article on the sculpture of Aurillard, Meige sums up the importance of Richer's pathological portraits:

> The double merit, at once scientific and artistic, of figures of this genre renders them interesting for sculptors as well as clinicians. Indeed, the former rarely have occasion to contemplate the pathological nude, the revelation of which is often a surprise for them, and more of an education; the latter, to whom the knowledge of the anomalies of the human body are something familiar, often have the desire to be able to preserve the accurate representation of living, morbid types that pass under their eyes. Much better than a drawing, and even a photograph, a plastic work is able to satisfy one and the other.

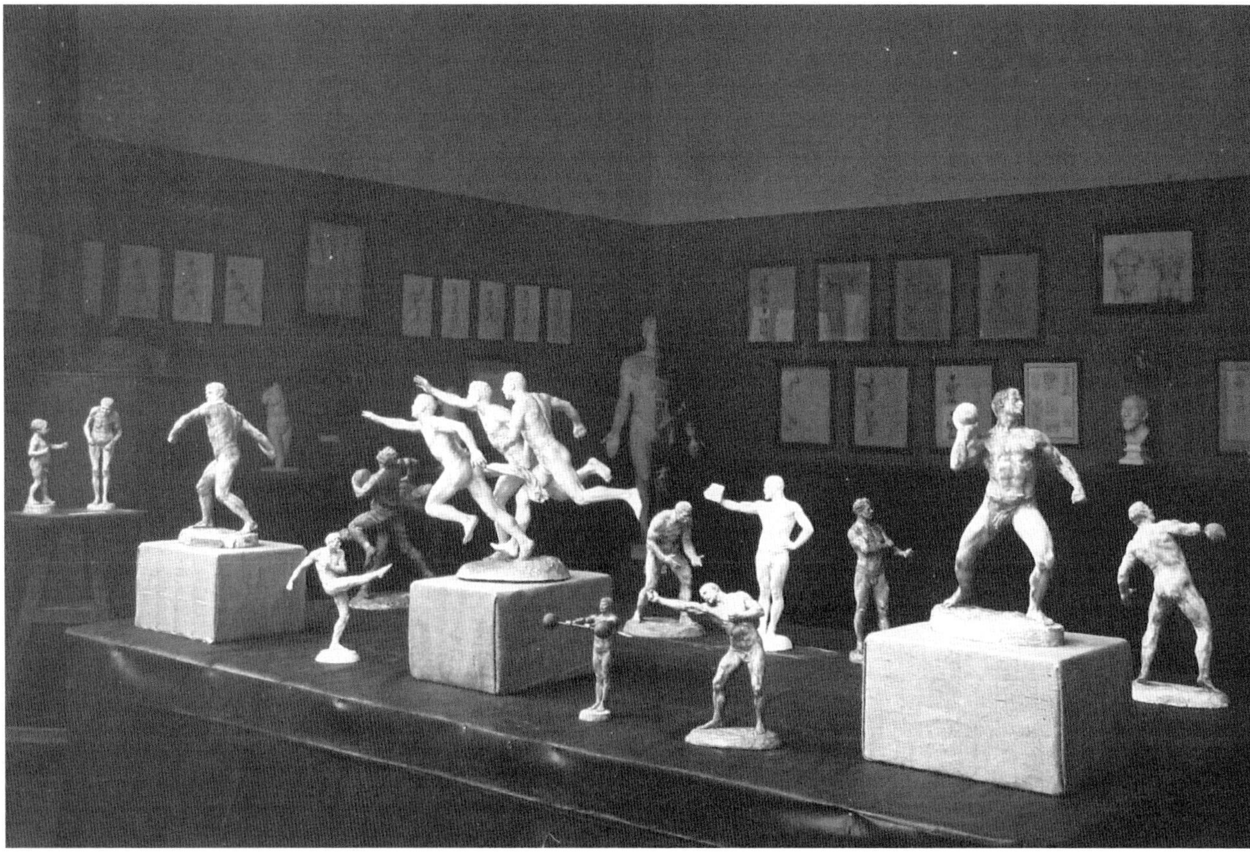

Fig. 88
Photograph of *Exposition École des beaux-arts*. Paris, Richer Family Archives. Courtesy of the Richer Family Archives.

He concludes, "the popularization of *these scientific artworks* presents a lively interest and a real utility."[160] In 1895 the Salpêtrière actually did attempt to market copies of Richer's sculptures of pathology, presumably to medical museums, under the title *Collection des plâtres de la Nouvelle Iconographie de la Salpêtrière*.[161] Yet more than ten years later, in rendering homage to Richer for being the first physician ever admitted to the Académie des beaux-arts, Raphaël Blanchard conceded that the sculptures were not well known.[162] In an undated photograph of the École des beaux-arts from the first half of the twentieth century, the anonymous athletes—runners, boxers, even a shot-putter—that Richer focused on in the second half of his career quite literally take center stage, crowding the platform in the middle of the room, while the small sculptures of pathology are isolated and relegated to the periphery (fig. 88).[163]

Richer delineated his ideas on the relationship of art and science, the artist and the *savant*, in an extraordinary series of articles in *La Nouvelle Revue* in 1897. Given that they were written while crafting his series of "scientific artworks," the texts shed significant light on his sculptural project. His "Dialogues sur l'art et la science" consist of a well-worn formula: a fictional conversation between an older teacher, Callias, and his younger pupil, Pamphile. The cynical Callias mourns the death of art at the hands of science. Invoking Victor Hugo's famous words from *Notre-Dame de Paris* (1831), Callias proclaims, "ceci tuera cela" (this will kill that).[164] For him, science is not only interested firmly in what is "real" but also allied with progress, industry, and the machine. For instance, he claims that the noble occupations of the harvester and sower—in a nod to Richer's own artistic output—are in danger from new agricultural practices.[165] Pamphile responds that there are strong affinities between the work of the artist and the scientist: these include creativity and the observation of nature. Science reveals as much about the scientist as art about the artist. He argues, "If [the scientist's] work belongs to everyone and becomes a part of our joint heritage, it is no less true that it comes from his mind and bears the stamp of his personality."[166] As examples, he likens Pasteur's inventiveness to that of the poet and states that Charcot was an artist "in the truest sense of the word."[167] Furthermore, Pamphile claims that science is "one of the essential conditions for art's very existence and its future progress."[168] Anatomy is a case in point: a deep understanding of the knowledge of the body provided by science allows the artist to manipulate it in his creations. Richer again obliquely insinuates his own work into the story when Pamphile notes the importance of a canon of proportions created through scientific means for the use of artists.[169]

Richer finishes the dialogues with a paean to humanity's inexorable evolution toward progress. Art cannot stay behind and simply imitate and repeat the past. Yet his generally bright view of the future is not without tinges of darkness:

> Science dominates the century and before it the ghosts of the past vanish. It continues its march fatally, irresistibly. Noble is its goal, lofty its aims; but, like a conqueror, it sometimes leaves behind grief and despair. The work of progress is not without sadness. Our age is the age of coal and iron. Coal's black smoke covers us with a veil that too often hides the sky from our eyes. But the dignity of man grows in suffering, and work will always bring to his head the divine halo which ennobles and glorifies. I do not know if the art that will be born from there will be gay, but it will surely be great.[170]

In this text Richer attempts to articulate the closeness of science and art and argues that the former is critical for the latter's advancement. As he prepared to apply for an influential role at the École, Richer argued that, if medical knowledge were used with artistic ends, "wouldn't the scientist become the greatest artist?"[171] When he assumed the prestigious title of professor of anatomy at the École des beaux-arts the following year, Richer's career itself would embody and extend the deep interconnectedness of medical science and art.

CODA

The Salpêtrière at the École des Beaux-Arts

If I am new among you, I am not exactly a stranger, because for a long time, I have been with you, so to speak, by the very nature of my tastes, my studies, and my work.

—PAUL RICHER, 1903

André Brouillet's *A Clinical Lesson at the Salpêtrière* was not the only image of Paul Richer to grace the walls of a Parisian exhibition. A year after Richer took up the post of professor of anatomy at the École des beaux-arts, Georges Leroux (1877–1957), one of his students and later winner of the Prix de Rome, depicted him in the act of demonstrating over a handsome cadaver in the right-hand panel of a triptych on *Les Études classiques de la peinture* (*Classic Studies of Painting*) (1904, location unknown; fig. 89).[1] Exhibited at the Salon des artistes français in 1904, Leroux's painting shows a female student being observed as she copies an antique bust at the Louvre in the left-hand panel, while in the center panel students at the Académie de la Grande Chaumière argue over the pose of a nude female model. The scene with Richer takes place in the École's amphitheater, with the body likely wheeled in for his demonstration.[2] Standing alongside the tools of his trade, Richer dispassionately discusses the body on the table below, his right hand positioned in a macabre echo of Michelangelo's God the Father leaning in toward an awakening Adam on the Sistine Chapel ceiling (ca. 1508–12). His left hand pinches a muscle on the arm of the cadaver, whose mutilated body recedes diagonally into the image, activating the space around it. One can just imagine the contrast of the vivid red of the flayed arm and the funereal suits of the men around the cadaver. Richer's distinctive profile is brightly illuminated against the background, as are the pates of the studious men standing around the body. Only the face of the sketching female student right beside the cadaver is in shadow, obscured by the brim of her hat. The pointed ends of the woman's light-colored scarf are like a pair of arrows drawing the eye down to the body that is the object of everyone's gaze—everyone except Richer, who looks out at his audience, unfazed. This painting by Leroux recalls the article by Mirbeau that begins *Pathology and Visual Culture*, in which the critic calls for a pendant to Rembrandt's celebrated painting of an anatomy lesson. Richer stands like a modern-day Doctor Tulp, teaching artists rather than surgeons.

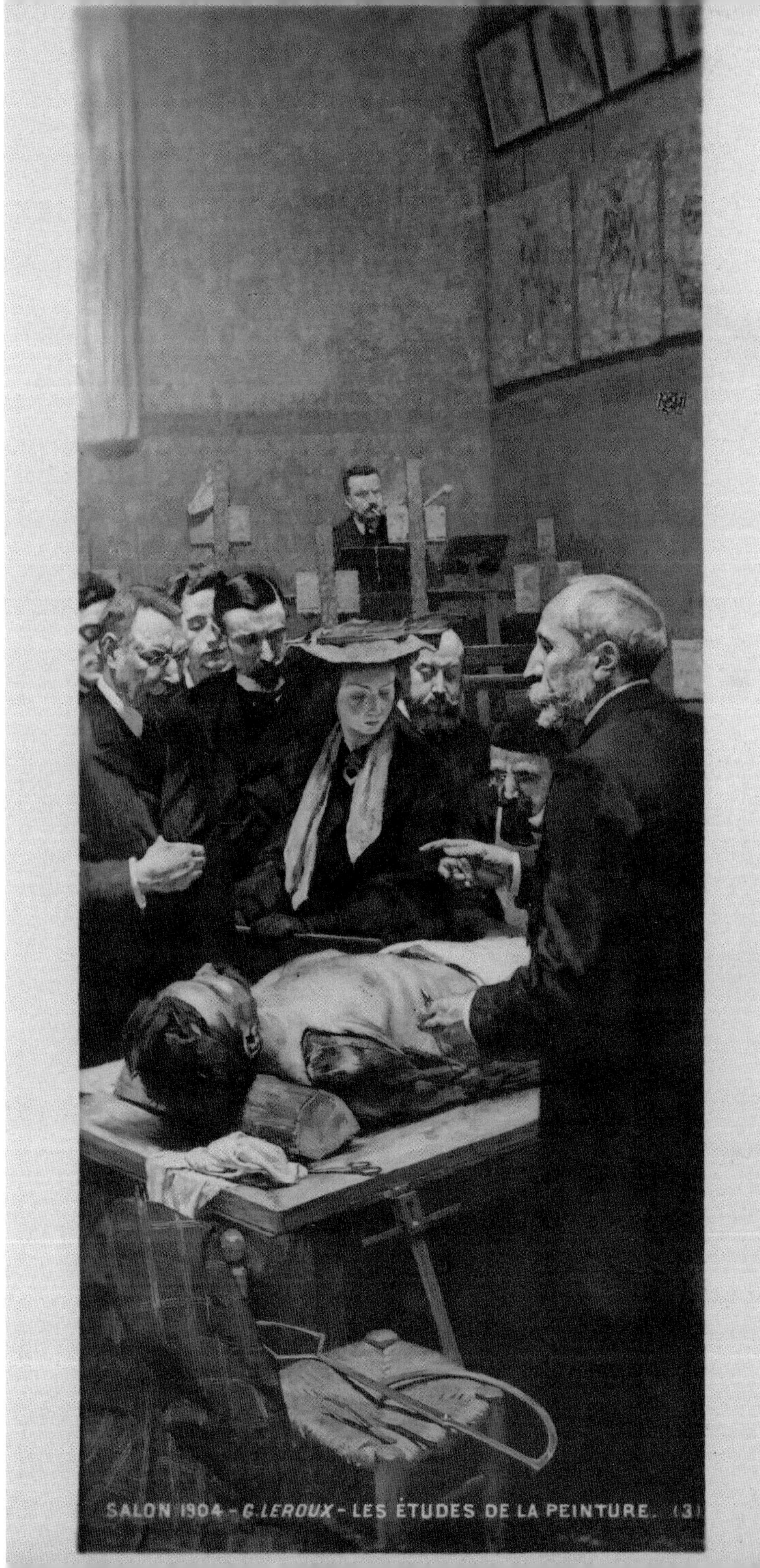

Fig. 89
Postcard of right-hand panel of Georges Leroux, *Les Études classiques de la peinture* (*Classic Studies of Painting*), 1904. Collection of Jacques Marie. Photo courtesy of Jacques Marie.

Richer seamlessly linked medicine and art at the start of the twentieth century, when his career took him from the thirteenth *arrondissement* of Paris to the sixth. In 1903, after a quarter century at the Salpêtrière, Richer moved to the most important school of fine arts in the Western world at the time. His "Dialogues sur l'art et la science" served as a statement to his suitability for the role and would lay the groundwork for his tenure there. "Who will give us a truly national art?" Richer wrote, adding, "Only the study of nature. What I would teach the young artist is not art, but science in its relation to the reality around us."[3] In other words, French art would be strengthened through the study of scientifically derived principles, like those set out in his books on artistic anatomy and the canon of proportions and, later, his three-dimensional study of the body's musculature, *L'Écorché vivant* (*Living Écorché*) (1906, Paris, École nationale supérieure des beaux-arts).[4] An "objective" understanding of the body ("nature") would guide artistic conceptions. This was Richer's endeavor both during *and* after his time at the Salpêtrière. As one writer put it, "his research on the 'abnormal' led him to devise the rigorous and truly scientific characteristics of the 'normal.'"[5]

While still at the Salpêtrière, Richer created at least fifteen sculptures of athletes undertaking strenuous movements.[6] This enterprise began shifting his focus from pathology to health. That is, he moved from the expression of what was conventionally considered ugly to what was conventionally considered beautiful. Richer claimed that the sculptures of both the athletes and the ill grew out of his most deeply ingrained belief: that art and science have the same goals and arise from the same source. In *L'Art et la médecine*, he reminds us that the Greek god Apollo "inspires the poet and fans genius. But he is also the divine doctor who gave his science to his son Asclepius in order to alleviate the ailments of the mortals who beseech him. He is the god of the Arts, he is the god of Medicine."[7]

The knowledge of anatomy that Richer had gained in a medical context served him in an artistic one. Richer felt that his work at the Salpêtrière was part of a larger commitment to the study of human anatomy, but it was at the École that Richer began to focus exclusively on the *healthy* body.[8] Like the artists of antiquity, who studied the athletic male body, Richer sculpted a series of anonymous sportsmen while obsessively photographing and measuring hundreds of healthy men and women.[9] He did so in an attempt to establish and codify the study of "living anatomy" during his twenty years at the École.[10] His practice seems to be evidence of a desire to distance himself from the sickly women at the Salpêtrière who started as patients under his care and ended up as corpses under his scalpel. Richer maintained, however, that at the École des beaux-arts he was simply continuing the research he had started at the hospital.

Igniting the Imagination

Continuity between depictions of the pathological (and primarily female) body at the Salpêtrière and the healthy (male) athlete at the École only makes sense if for Richer, as for Charcot and the other clinicians of the Salpêtrière School, there was no separation between the "scientific self" and the "artistic self." The connective tissue between the two is imagination. Even scientists committed to the purported transparency and veracity of the photograph, such as Duchenne de Boulogne and Étienne-Jules Marey, recognized it as essential to scientific practice. In his *Mécanisme de la physionomie humaine,* Duchenne recounted the moment when he saw the potential of controlled electric currents and it "ignited" his imagination.[11] Marey, in his discussion of chronophotography, insisted on the important role that the imagination played in helping the scientist "seek in a moving animal for positions hitherto unnoticed."[12] Richer himself suggests that "without imagination . . . creating new forms [and] inventing new circumstances," the two key scientific processes of observation and experimentation would founder.[13]

Imagination and creativity are essential conceptual tools for all scientists and artists, as they were to the Salpêtrière School. It is no wonder that some of the most important scientists and clinicians of the day, including Charcot and Louis Pasteur, had considered becoming artists in their youth.[14] As Richer wrote in *L'Art et la médecine,* it is "in practice [that] the union is made between Art and Science."[15] The scientific artworks produced at the Salpêtrière attest to its doctors' compulsion to create visual imagery and objects that would assist in working out symptoms and establishing clinical diagnoses. The curated albums of the Musée Charcot and the museum itself, along with Charcot's famous lectures and clinical discussions, were all productive spaces for the collective construction of knowledge. Collaborators included not only the clinicians at the hospital but also the French and foreign scientists, artists, writers, and other notables (Freud not least among them) who attended the lectures, visited the museum, paged through the albums, and witnessed the scientific artworks both at the hospital and in circulation.

The Salpêtrière presents a rich and complex case study because its clinicians saw art and medical science participating equally in the construction of knowledge, the results of which were disseminated in an increasingly global scientific network. This has also been the challenge of this project, and my language in this book has often reflected my struggle to come to grips with the "entwinement" of art and science at the Salpêtrière. Is the "intersection," "interconnectedness," or indeed "marriage" of art and medicine the right terminology to use? Does Charcot's language indicate a "slippage" between the two? And while I have both used and contested Daston and Galison's binaries—objectivity and subjectivity, the "scientific self" and "artistic self"—it seems to me that the clinicians working at the Salpêtrière redefined the relationship between the two through their scientific artworks. That there were scientists in France and elsewhere whose work pushed and pulled at these binaries in other ways is yet to be explored. William Viney, Felicity Callard, and Angela Woods have written about "forms of medical humanities research that can be open about shared confusions and unresolved complexities."[16] *Pathology and Visual Culture* has been my way of thinking through images and objects that occupy an intellectual space somewhere between the hospital and the Salon, between medical objectivity and individual artistry.

While Charcot and the Salpêtrière School seemed supremely confident about their theories and diagnoses in their lectures and texts, the images and objects they produced are much more equivocal. They demonstrate a desire both to understand and to convince that echoes Charcot and Richer's books on the possessed, deformed, and ill in art. They have an "affective force, whether or not it can be readily put into words."[17] They also reveal the pleasure these clinicians took in art making; as one of Charcot's obituaries put it, "one of his greatest joys was to reunite science and art on the same ground."[18] Scientists today continue to revel in the "beauty" of a "well-designed experiment" or "an elegant solution to a scientific problem."[19] Creativity is requisite in both art and medical science. The Salpêtrière's production makes that explicit but also shows that aesthetic and scientific experiments are not always wholly successful.

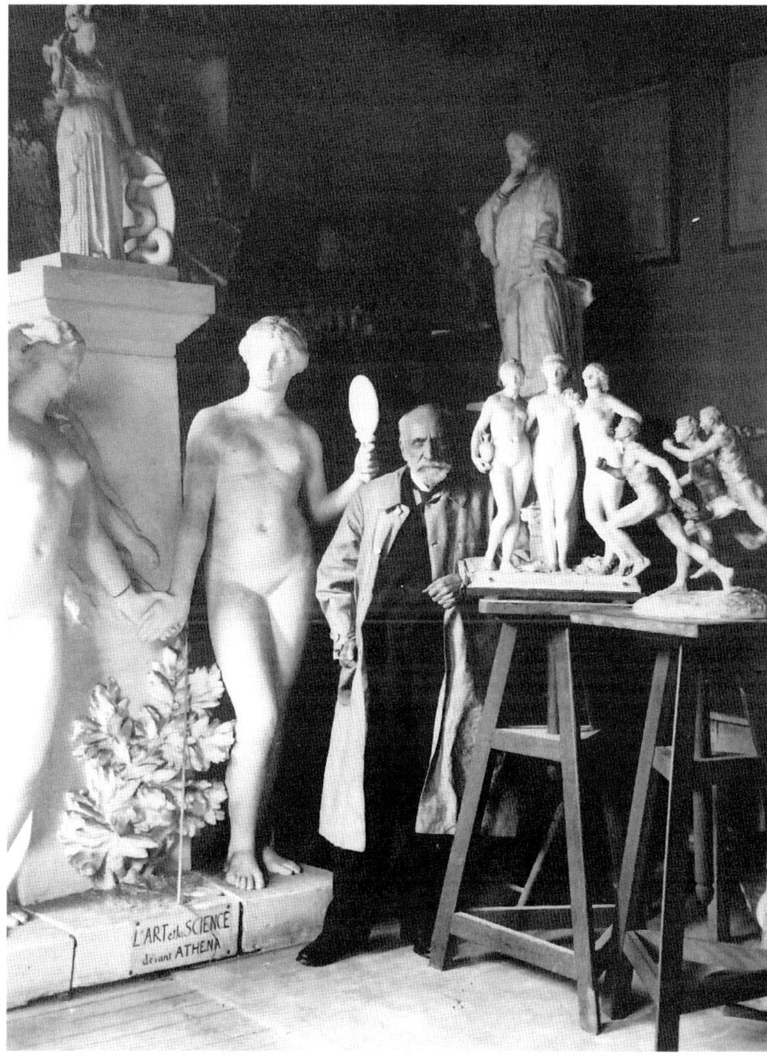

Fig. 90
Photograph of Paul Richer in his studio. Paris, Richer Family Archives. Photo courtesy of the Richer Family Archives.

Art and Science Before Athena

The painting by Leroux, which takes the doctor out of the hospital and into the École, highlights the importance of Paul Richer to this book and how his career exemplified the ways in which the Salpêtrière clinicians entwined medical science and art. Even after his retirement in 1922, when he passed the baton of professor of anatomy at the École to his former Salpêtrière colleague Henry Meige, Richer played a role in the arts as the Inspecteur général de l'Enseignement du dessin.[20] He also continued to sculpt, creating monuments and medals to the scientific heroes of the age.[21] And while one of the schematic diagrams of a figure walking down the stairs in his *Physiologie artistique de l'homme en mouvement* (1895) likely influenced Marcel Duchamp's important painting *Nude Descending a Staircase (No. 2)* (1912, Philadelphia, Philadelphia Museum of Art), Richer's contribution to the art of the twentieth century through his teachings at the École remains unstudied.[22]

One of his final works was a large-scale group that, he proudly claimed, symbolized his oeuvre: nude personifications of Art and Science standing before a severe

Athena, goddess of wisdom, war, art, and inspiration.[23] In this staid academic sculpture, a tightly coiffed Science raises a mirror to an Art who seems to admire her own flowing tresses; it shows "art and science walking hand in hand," precisely as Charcot had characterized Richer's work decades earlier.[24] Overlooking the two figures from a commanding position atop a central plinth, Athena holds a small statue of Nike bearing a laurel wreath to crown a victor. By holding hands, Art and Science signal that theirs is a joint victory. In a photograph of Richer in his atelier at the Institut de France taken a few years before his death, *L'Art et la science devant Athène* (*Art and Science Before Athena*) (1930, Chartres, musée des Beaux-Arts) towers over him. It is an apt summation of his career and a perfect portrait of the *savant-artiste* (fig. 90).

Notes

INTRODUCTION

1. Mirbeau, "Siècle de Charcot," 121 (originally published under the pseudonym Le Diable in *L'Événement*, May 29, 1885). All translations are the author's own unless otherwise indicated.
2. Dalligny, "Salon de 1887," 2. For a detailed discussion of this painting, see Hunter, *Face of Medicine*, esp. 166–241; Musée de l'Assistance Publique–Hôpitaux de Paris, *Leçon de Charcot*, 15–16; Walusinski, *Leçon clinique*. For more on Brouillet, see Bata et al., *André Brouillet*. For more on Charcot's lectures, see Munthe, *Story of San Michele*, 230; Babinski, "Eloge de J.-M. Charcot," 755.
3. For an overview of the history of hysteria, see Micale, *Approaching Hysteria*; Scull, *Hysteria*; Trillat, *Histoire de l'hystérie*. For a comprehensive discussion of sources that analyze hysteria from a variety of methodological approaches, see Micale, *Approaching Hysteria*, 33–107. For a feminist analysis of hysteria, see Beizer, *Ventriloquized Bodies*; Bronfen, *Knotted Subject*; Showalter, *Female Malady*, esp. 121–64. For a detailed history of the disorder in men, see Micale, *Hysterical Men*.
4. Goetz, Bonduelle, and Gelfand, *Charcot*, esp. 66–72. For more on the anatomoclinical method, see Foucault, *Birth of the Clinic*, esp. 124–48.
5. Wolff, "Courrier de Paris"; Ignotus, "Cabotinage." Illustrations—all by Daniel Vierge—include: *Service de l'électrothérapie à la Salpêtrière.—Électro-Diagnostique par le Dr Vigouroux* and *Service d'électrothérapie à la Salpêtrière.—Bain électrique.—Électrisation localisée*, in "Service de l'électrothérapie," 99 and 100, respectively, and *À la Salpêtrière: Un réfectoire* and *À la Salpêtrière: Un dortoir de femmes* in Guillemot, "À la Salpêtrière. II," 372 and 373, respectively. Alphonse and Léon Daudet, Jules Claretie, and Guy de Maupassant, among many others, discussed Charcot and the Salpêtrière in the popular press and based scenes in their novels on what they witnessed there: see Claretie, *Amours d'un interne*, and L. Daudet, *Morticoles*. See also Marquer, *Romans de la Salpêtrière*.
6. Paul Renouard, *Docteur Charcot*, cover of *La Revue illustrée* 4, no. 40 (August 1, 1887).
7. Baedeker, *Paris and Environs*, 259–60. For a history of the hospital, see Guillain and Mathieu, *Salpêtrière*.
8. Didi-Huberman, *Invention of Hysteria*, 77 (originally published in French in 1982).
9. The members of the audience include Jules Claretie, Paul Arène, Philippe Burty, and Victor Cornil. The painting was reproduced at the time with a key that named all the individuals; see, for example, "A Clinical Lesson at the Salpêtrière," 9556–57. For the full list, see Goetz, Bonduelle, and Gelfand, *Charcot*, 92–93.
10. Paul Richer, *Cahiers d'observations cliniques pendant les leçons de Charcot à la Salpêtrière*, 1882–83, Paris, École nationale supérieure des Beaux-Arts, inv. no. EBA 8142.

11. Ruiz-Gómez, "The Painter, the Psychiatrist"; Ruiz-Gómez and Liebrenz, "Ties that Bind."
12. Foucault, *Birth of the Clinic*, 88–89.
13. Souques, "Charcot intime," 697.
14. Freud, "Charcot," 12.
15. Ponsonhailhe, "Le Salon. Peinture. II," 49.
16. Fourcaud, "Art contemporain," 21, 23.
17. Fourcaud, "Peinture française," 156.
18. Brooks, *Realist Visions*, 3.
19. Charcot was both a clinician and a physician, but this book focuses on the clinical aspect of his practice. For more on the relationship of science and medicine during Charcot's time, see Bynum, *Science*.
20. Meige, "Sur une statuette," 136.
21. Meige, *Charcot artiste*, 13 (originally published in the *Nouvelle Iconographie de la Salpêtrière* 11 [1898]: 489–516).
22. Farge, *Allure of the Archives*, 42.
23. Gilles de la Tourette, "Jean-Martin Charcot," 241.
24. Capildeo, "Charcot in the 80s," 384.
25. Charcot and Dechambre, *De quelques marbres antiques*, 5 (originally published in the *Gazette hebdomadaire de médecine et de chirurgie*).
26. Ibid., 3.
27. Ibid., 6.
28. Ibid., 7.
29. Ibid., 7; emphasis removed.
30. Ibid., 9.
31. Ibid., 10.
32. Ibid., 11.
33. Richer quotes Charcot and Dechambre's article on Aesop at length in Richer, *L'Art et la médecine*, 190–93.
34. Ibid., 3–4.
35. Charcot and Richer, *Démoniaques dans l'art*, xi and 56. Given that Richer also repeats some of *Démoniaques dans l'art* verbatim in his *L'Art et la médecine*, it is possible that the ideas were his to begin with, even if they may have been shared with Charcot.
36. Ibid., 64. For the illustration, see Bourneville and Regnard, *Iconographie photographique de la Salpêtrière*, 1: plate 40.
37. Charcot, "Policlinique du mardi, 7 février 1888," 178.
38. Marie, "Éloge de J.-M. Charcot," 737.
39. Charcot, "Introduction. La Médecine empirique," xix.
40. Meige, "Charcot artiste," 505.
41. Charcot, "Foi qui guérit"; Goldstein, "Hysteria Diagnosis."
42. Levine, "Why Science Isn't Literature," 68.
43. Daston and Galison, *Objectivity*.
44. Ibid., 17.
45. Ibid., 37. Other works that have informed my thinking on objectivity include Daston, "Objectivity and the Escape from Perspective"; Daston and Lunbeck, *Histories of Scientific Observation*; Megill, *Rethinking Objectivity*; and Tauber, *Science and the Quest*.
46. Charcot, "Policlinique du mardi, 7 février 1888," 178; Daston and Galison, *Objectivity*, 4.
47. Daston and Galison, *Objectivity*, 372.
48. Burnett, "Objective Case," 134.
49. Charcot, "Policlinique du mardi, 7 février 1888," 178.
50. Daston and Galison, *Objectivity*, 381.
51. Richer, *Études cliniques*, 914–56.
52. Daston and Galison, *Objectivity*, 18.
53. Snyder, "Visualization and Visibility," 379–80; emphasis removed. See also Ellenbogen, *Reasoned and Unreasoned Images*.
54. T. Porter, "Objective Self," 645.
55. Kusch, "Objectivity and Historiography," 131.
56. Jones and Galison, "Introduction," 15.
57. Charcot and Richer, *Les Difformes et les malades*, iii.
58. Daston and Galison, *Objectivity*, 36–37.
59. Ibid., 38–39.
60. Richer, "Dialogues sur l'art et la science. III," 450.
61. J. Smith, review of *Objectivity*, 111. See also Elkins, "Art History and Images," 567.
62. Didi-Huberman, *Invention of Hysteria*, 4.
63. For example, Callen, *Spectacular Body*; Carroy, "L'hystérique, l'artiste et le savant"; Carroy-Thirard, "Hystérie, théâtre, littérature"; Eidenbenz, "Théâtre de l'objectivité," 105–6; Gordon, *Why the French*; Hunter, *Face of Medicine*; Marshall, *Performing Neurology*, esp. 213–40; McCarren, "Symptomatic Act"; Ruiz-Gómez, "Hysterical Reading"; Silverman, *Art Nouveau*. An exception is Blackshaw, who looks at the influence of the *Nouvelle Iconographie de la Salpêtrière*: Blackshaw, "Pathological Body."
64. Gordon, *Why the French*; Bonduelle and Gelfand, "Hysteria Behind the Scenes."
65. Callen, *Spectacular Body*; Ruiz-Gómez, "Hysterical Reading"; Silverman, *Art Nouveau*.

66. Bernheim, "Hypnotisme et suggestion." In much of the scholarship on Charcot, hysteria is linked with insanity or "madness," even though Charcot considered it a disease of the nervous system. For important studies on insanity, see Gilman, *Seeing the Insane*; Gilman, *Picturing Health and Illness.*
67. Goetz, Bonduelle, and Gelfand, *Charcot*, 100–119.
68. R. Porter, "Introduction," 2.
69. Garland-Thomson, *Staring*, 9, 11.
70. A. Daudet, "À la Salpêtrière," 16.
71. Farge, *Allure of the Archives*, 13.
72. Woloshyn, *Soaking Up the Rays*, 35–37.
73. Wallis, *Investigating the Body*, 33.
74. Jordanova, *Sexual Visions*, 2.
75. Callen, *Looking at Men*; Callen, "Masculinity and Muscularity."
76. Whitehead and Woods, "Introduction," 13. See also Johnstone, "Manifesto."
77. Viney, Callard, and Woods, "Critical Medical Humanities," 3.
78. Tucker, "Historian," 117.
79. Fitzgerald and Callard, "Entangling the Medical Humanities," 39; original emphasis.
80. Tucker, "Entwined Practices."
81. Hunter, *Face of Medicine*, 167.
82. Marshall, *Performing Neurology*.
83. Gelfand, *Charcot in Morocco*, 27.
84. Guillain, *J.-M. Charcot*, 24 (originally published in French in 1955).
85. Gelfand, *Charcot in Morocco*, 26.
86. Goetz, Bonduelle, and Gelfand, *Charcot*; Guillain, *J.-M. Charcot.*
87. Bogousslavsky, "Charcot and Art"; Goetz, "Visual Art"; Walusinski, "Albert Londe"; Walusinski, "Biographie de Paul Richer."
88. Bouchara, *Charcot*, 38, 55, and 104.
89. Wall label from *Charcot, une vie avec l'image*, May 12 to July 9, 2014, at the Pitié-Salpêtrière (visited July 3, 2014). This exhibition complemented the one organized by the Musée de l'Assistance Publique de Paris from September 17 to December 31, 1986; see Simon-Dhouailly, *Leçon de Charcot.*
90. Ballu, "Salon de 1887," n.p.; "A Clinical Lesson at 'La Salpêtrière,'" 9556; Gyp, "Au Salon"; H[ubert], "Salon de 1887," 284–85; Robida, "Au Salon."
91. Elkins takes this idea from Leo Steinberg, *Leonardo's Incessant Last Supper* (New York: Zone Books, 2011); Elkins, "Introduction to the Visual," 32.
92. Meige, "Sur une statuette," 140.

CHAPTER 1

1. Freud was in Paris from October 13, 1885 to February 28, 1886, and spent seventeen of those twenty weeks attending Charcot's lectures; Sulloway, *Freud*, 28.
2. Letter dated October 21, 1885; Freud, *Letters of Sigmund Freud*, 187.
3. Freud, "Report on My Studies," 8.
4. Freud and Breuer, *Studies in Hysteria*; Freud, *Five Lectures on Psycho-Analysis*, 20.
5. Letter dated November 24, 1885; Freud, *Letters of Sigmund Freud*, 196.
6. Freud, *Five Lectures on Psycho-Analysis*, 18; Gelfand, "'Mon cher Docteur Freud,'" 564–65; J. Miller, "Some Aspects of Charcot's Influence."
7. Meige, *Charcot artiste*, 20.
8. Clair, introduction to "Cabinet des antiques." For more on Freud's art collection, see Gamwell and Wells, *Sigmund Freud and Art*; Musée Rodin, *Passion à l'oeuvre.*
9. Printed reproductions of Brouillet's painting kept the image in the public consciousness even as the original languished in storage at a provincial museum (the Musée des beaux-arts de Nice) for almost seventy-five years, from about 1891 to 1965. Léon Daudet wrote in the 1920s that photographs of Brouillet's painting "courent les rues"; L. Daudet, "Professeur Charcot," 226.
10. Charcot is often and incorrectly described as a psychiatrist, probably because of Freud's incalculable impact on twentieth-century thought.
11. Ludmilla Jordanova, opening remarks at the Case Studies of Medical Portraiture Workshop, King's College London, June 2, 2011.
12. Fend, "Order and Affect"; Hunter, "'Effroyable réalisme'"; Hunter, *Face of Medicine*, 108–65; Tilles, "Histoire des bibliothèques médicales."
13. Charcot, *Oeuvres complètes*, 3:4.
14. "Hospice de la Salpétrière [*sic*].—Conférences cliniques de M. Charcot," 718.
15. "Hospice de la Salpêtrière.—M. Charcot," 913.
16. Didi-Huberman, *Invention of Hysteria.*
17. For some of the few published images, see Bouchara, *Charcot*; Gilman, *Seeing the Insane*, 195, 202, 203; Ruiz-Gómez, "Model Patient."
18. "Hospice de la Salpétrière [*sic*].—Conférences cliniques de M. Charcot," 719.

19. Delboeuf, "Visite à la Salpêtrière," 122–23.
20. Didi-Huberman, *Invention of Hysteria*, esp. 123–26; Hunter, "'Effroyable réalisme,'" 52–55; Hunter, *Face of Medicine*, esp. 169–71; Mayer, "Freud à Paris"; Mayer, *Sites of the Unconscious*, esp. 70–92; Simon-Dhouailly, *Leçon de Charcot*, 63–66; Tilles, "Histoire des bibliothèques médicales," 69–72; Trillat, "Espèce morbide."
21. The photograph could have been taken as early as 1888, when Richer sculpted the *Facies of Labio-Glosso-Laryngeal Paralysis* (see chapter 4), but it was published in 1894.
22. "Varia," 139.
23. A. Daudet, "À la Salpêtrière," 15.
24. Meige, *Charcot artiste*, 14; Guillain, *J.-M. Charcot*, 52. For a photograph of Charcot's study at the Salpêtrière, see Levillain, "Charcot et l'École," 111.
25. Brigo et al., "Jean-Martin Charcot's Medical Instruments." These chairs were still visible in the Bibliothèque Charcot until approximately 2011, when the library moved to a new location at the Salpêtrière.
26. "Hospice de la Salpêtrière.—M. Charcot." Henry Cros's work is discussed in more detail in chapter 3.
27. Guillemot, "À la Salpêtrière. II," 371.
28. Personal communication with the author; Véronique Leroux-Hugon, former librarian at the Bibliothèque Charcot, July 17, 2005.
29. A sculptor named Deniau is included in Lami, *Dictionnaire des sculpteurs*, 173.
30. Delboeuf, "Visite à la Salpêtrière," 263.
31. Guillemot, "À la Salpêtrière. II," 371. See also L. Daudet, *Devant la douleur*, 39.
32. Druick, "Framing *The Little Dancer*," 87, fig. 60.
33. Paris, "Exécution de Barré et Lebiez," 1.
34. Ibid., 1–2.
35. Guillemot, "À la Salpêtrière. II," 371.
36. Alberti, *Morbid Curiosities*, 72.
37. Inv. AP.2001.0.4.4.15, Paris, Musée de l'Assistance Publique–Hôpitaux de Paris (hereafter Musée de l'AP-HP). Ruiz-Gómez, "Of Sculptural and Corporal Remains."
38. Album AP 2003.7.2.1, Paris, Musée de l'AP-HP.
39. Inv. Morpho 18b, Paris, École nationale supérieure des beaux-arts (hereafter ENSBA). The annotation reads, in part, "la main est violacée." It is reproduced in Comar, *Figures du corps*, 386, cat. no. 314. This drawing is misattributed to Charcot in Bouchara, *Charcot*, 104. Two drawings by Richer of Bourdy's hysterical contractures, this time dated December 23, were included in Simon-Dhouailly, *Leçon de Charcot*, 78, cat. no. 163e and f (unillustrated).
40. Dias, "Corps en vitrine."
41. Delboeuf, "Visite à la Salpêtrière," 259. Charcot lent Wittmann to Dr. Jules Janet at the Hôtel Dieu in 1888, for example, as if she were just another specimen in this museum; Hustvedt, *Medical Muses*, 127.
42. Sappol, "'Morbid Curiosity.'"
43. Letter dated January 20, 1886; Freud, *Letters of Sigmund Freud*, 206. Charcot lived in the *hôtel* of the Prince de Chimay on the quai Malaquais until it was sold to house part of the École des beaux-arts; Pont-Calé, "Professeur Charcot," 3. He then moved to, and combined, 217 and 219 Boulevard Saint-Germain, which now houses the Maison de l'Amérique Latine. On the significance of the interior for Charcot, see Meige, *Charcot artiste*, 19–24; Silverman, *Art Nouveau*, 102–6.
44. Goetschy, "Femmes du monde artistes." For a discussion of Mme. Charcot in the context of the first Exhibition of the Arts of Woman in 1892, see Silverman, *Art Nouveau*, esp. 191–93. For more on the decorative arts in France at this time, see Jones, *Sculptors and Design Reform*.
45. Pons, "Hôtel de Varangeville." The sumptuous wood bookcases from Charcot's home would eventually form the basis of the Bibliothèque Charcot, donated by his son Jean-Baptiste Charcot to the Assistance Publique; Ricou, Leroux-Hugon, and Poirier, "Bibliothèque Charcot," 319; Ricou, Leroux-Hugon, and Poirier, *Bibliothèque Charcot*; Tilles, "Histoire des bibliothèques médicales," 60–65.
46. Arène, "Docteur Charcot"; Goetschy, "Femmes du monde artistes," 51; Chevallier and Hémard, *Catalogue des objets*.
47. L. Daudet, "Professeur Charcot," 209.
48. Guillain, *J.-M. Charcot*, 31.
49. This *boiserie* is now housed in the Metropolitan Museum of Art; see Pourfar, "Room from Jean-Martin Charcot's House," and "Boisierie from the Hotel de Varengeville" at https://www.metmuseum.org/art/collection/search/202996.

50. Meige, *Charcot artiste*, 20.
51. Ibid., 24.
52. Entry dated 26 May 1879; Goncourt and Goncourt, *Journal*, 21.
53. Goetschy, "Femmes du monde artistes," 43.
54. Ibid., 48.
55. Ibid. Meige makes the same comment in Meige, *Charcot artiste*, 23.
56. Levillain, "Charcot et l'École," 114; Meige, *Charcot artiste*, 23.
57. Goetschy, "Femmes du monde artistes," 51.
58. L. Daudet, *Devant la douleur*, 11.
59. Levillain, "Charcot et l'École," 114.
60. Meige, *Charcot artiste*, 19.
61. Guillemot, "À la Salpêtrière. 11," 371.
62. L. Daudet, *Devant la douleur*, 39; Delboeuf, "Visite à la Salpêtrière," 122.
63. Coutinho, Walusinski, and Teive, "Désiré Bourneville." This museum is no longer extant, and some of its contents are held by the Musée de l'Assistance Publique–Hôpitaux de Paris.
64. Tilles, "Histoire des bibliothèques médicales," 74. A photograph of this museum can be found in Simon-Dhouailly, *Leçon de Charcot*, 109, cat. 236.
65. Hooper-Greenhill, *Museums*, 123; Boëtsch, "From Cabinets of Curiosities," 78; Sappol, *Traffic of Dead Bodies*, 276.
66. Sappol, *Traffic of Dead Bodies*, 276.
67. Baudrillard, "System of Collecting"; Hunter, "'Effroyable réalisme.'"
68. Forty-seven album pages of photographs from the 1890s, not owned by the museum, were exhibited in 1984 at the Galerie Texbraun and in 2014 at the Galerie Baudoin-Lebon, Paris; see Autexier and Braunschweig, *De l'angoisse*.
69. Mossé, "Affection osseuse généralisée," 158. The caption to the drawing in the album reads "Salpetrière [*sic*] 1874 / Anne Marie, 64 ans. / carcin[ome] du sein gauche." An article penned by him in the next issue lists his title as "interne des hôpitaux"; Savard, "Fracture double verticale du bassin," 215–17.
70. Edwards and Hart, "Introduction," 12. See, for example, Album AP 2003.7.1.4, Paris, Musée de l'AP-HP.
71. Langford, *Suspended Conversations*, 11 and 41.
72. Ibid., 20.
73. Ibid., 41–42.
74. Callen, *Spectacular Body*, 53.
75. Freud, "Charcot," 12.
76. Meige, *Charcot artiste*, 12.
77. Souques, "Décès de M. Paul Richer," 708.
78. Barthes, "Rhetoric of the Image," 39.
79. Rawling, "Patient Photographs, Patient Voices," 257.
80. Gilman, *Picturing Health and Illness*, 16.
81. In Londe's book on medical photography, this patient is pictured with his hands on his chest; Londe, *Photographie médicale*, 1, plate 3.
82. Ibid., 82; Brauer, "Dangerous Doubles."
83. Londe, *Photographie médicale*, 79–80, fig. 23.
84. In 1903, Girard was still listed as a "marchand d'estampes français et etrangers" at 9, quai Voltaire in Bourcard, *À travers cinq siècles*, xxix.
85. Ruiz-Gómez, "Genius and Degeneracy."
86. Burckhardt, "Contribution à l'étude."
87. Emphasis removed.
88. "Editorial Notes." See also Sidlauskas, "Medical Portrait."
89. The collection of the George Eastman Museum has several of Thomas's cabinet cards with these stamps. Rachel E. Andrews (Assistant Collection Manager, Department of Photography, George Eastman Museum, Rochester, New York), personal communication with the author, May 17, 2017. As this photograph is glued down in the Musée Charcot album, it is impossible to determine if it too bears one of Thomas's promotional stamps.
90. Hallam, "Anatomy Display," 133.
91. Michel Foucault, *The Birth of the Clinic* (London: Tavistock Publications, 1976), 31; cited in Hooper-Greenhill, *Museums*, 167.
92. For more on the visualization of migraines, see Foxhall, *Migraine*, esp. 110–34.
93. One of these prints of a Salpêtrière patient with locomotor ataxia—an engraving by Paul Richer—was included in Charcot, *Leçons sur les maladies*, 2:473, plate 6. It illustrates an article in the same volume: "Luxations pathologiques," 365–76.
94. The caption under the images reads: "Porreau. Salpêtrière. / Paralysie Lab. gl. Laryng. / Atroph. Musculaire / Scl. Sym. des Cord. lateraux." The Musée de l'AP-HP has erroneously labeled this "Poireau." See also Duyckaerts et al., "Charcot identifies."
95. Ignotus, "Cabotinage."
96. Gombault, "Sclérose symétrique," 509.

97. Ibid., 510.
98. Ibid., 509.
99. I disagree with the curators of the Musée de l'Assistance Publique–Hôpitaux de Paris, who characterize the drawing as pencil and watercolor on paper. In my view, it is instead pen and black ink and gray wash, and this was confirmed by Freyda Spira (Robert L. Solley Curator of Prints and Drawings, Yale University Art Gallery), personal communication with the author, May 23, 2019.
100. Jordanova, *Sexual Visions*, 47; Hunter, "'Effroyable réalisme,'" 45.
101. *Contracture du membre inférieur droit*, illustrated in Richer, "Observation de contracture," 210, fig. 59.
102. Ibid., 211.
103. Mitchell, *What Do Pictures Want?*, 59.
104. "L'Oeuvre sculpturale." Paris, Richer Family archives.
105. Olivier Walusinski confirmed the date when Richer arrived at the Salpêtrière; personal communication with the author, April 26, 2017. For more on Richer's life and work, see Blanchard, *Hommage*; Jean-Baptiste Charcot, "Paul Richer"; Comar, "Leçon d'anatomie," esp. 56–60; Desprez, "Paul Richer"; "Le Docteur Paul Richer"; Le Gendre, "Richer"; Gilles de la Tourette, "Biographies médicales"; Meige, "Paul Richer et son oeuvre"; "Paul Richer," 65–76; Ruiz-Gómez, "Scientific Artworks"; Ruiz-Gómez, "Shaking the Tyranny"; Walusinski, "Biographie de Paul Richer"; Walusinski, "Keeping the Fire Burning," esp. 78–82; Walusinski, *Leçon clinique*, 74–80. Walusinski published his biography of Richer as this book was going to press: Walusinski, *Paul Richer*. Richer also published a catalogue raisonné of his work: Richer, *Notice sur les titres*.
106. "À côté du savoir médical un peu de talent artistique." This anecdote is taken from Richer's handwritten and unpublished memoirs. Paul Richer, "Notes biographiques" (ca. 1929). ENSBA, Inv. Ms. 837.
107. Richer, "Notes biographiques."
108. Meillet, *Des déformations permanentes*, plate 2 and "Explication des figures."
109. Desprez, "Paul Richer," 10. His drawings were etched in three plates.
110. "Dont les magnifiques gravures sont restées célèbres." Richer, "Notes biographiques." This anecdote is recounted in a slightly different form in other texts.
111. Richer placed third out of 223 students in the exam for the "Internat des Hôpitaux de Paris"; Walusinski, "Biographie de Paul Richer," 9. Qualifying for this internship signaled exceptional talent and put Richer in the company of the country's medical elite; Coury, *Enseignement de la médecine*, esp. 164–73.
112. Le Gendre, "Richer," 65; Desprez, "Paul Richer," 10. He may have received drawing instruction in medical school, as it was part of anatomy training for surgeons; Jean-François Minot (formerly Responsable des collections of the Musée de l'AP-HP), personal communication with author, June 14, 2013.
113. Cohen and Prendergast, *Spectacles of Realism*; Durey, "Réalisme"; Janson, "Realism in Sculpture"; Lenoir, *Histoire du réalisme*; Levine, *Realism and Representation*; Nochlin, *Realism*; Solomon-Godeau, "Realism Revisited"; Weinberg, *French Realism*; Weisberg, *European Realist Tradition*; Weisberg et al., *Illusions of Reality*, esp. Weisberg, "Reframing Naturalism"; Weisberg, *Realist Tradition*; Weisberg and Weisberg, *Realist Debate*.
114. Larroumet, *Salon de 1892*, 98.
115. Charcot, *Études pour servir*, plate 2.
116. I disagree with the curators of the Musée de l'Assistance publique-Hôpitaux de Paris, who characterize the drawing as pencil on paper. In my view, it is red chalk, and this was confirmed by Freyda Spira (Robert L. Solley Curator of Prints and Drawings, Yale University Art Gallery), personal communication with the author, May 23, 2019.
117. Richer, "Dialogues sur l'art et la science. II," 241 (this series of three articles was also published as Richer, *Dialogues sur l'art et la science*).
118. Prat, *Dessin français*, 505.
119. Meillet, *Des déformations permanentes*, plate 2, figures 5 and 6.
120. Misattributed to Charcot in Bouchara, *Charcot*, 38.
121. Charcot and Richer, *Mascaron grotesque*, 1 (originally published in the *Nouvelle Iconographie de la Salpêtrière* 1 [1888]: 87–92).
122. Ibid.; Ruskin, *Stones of Venice*, 3:121.
123. Charcot and Richer, *Mascaron grotesque*, 1.
124. Ibid., 5.
125. Richer, "Dialogues sur l'art et la science. II," 241.
126. Reproduced right side up in Bouchara, *Charcot*, 146.

127. There are two rather unskilled drawings of the nude body of another patient, Henri Morrison, included in this album and done by different hands; his case is detailed in Bouley, *Pathologie comparée*, 92–111.
128. For a summary of what was known about the illness in 1874, see ibid., 91.
129. Ibid., 115. The case notes that follow are taken from pages 111–19.
130. Ibid., 117.
131. Charcot's drawing cites an aneurysm as the cause of Moutarde's death.
132. Foucault, *Birth of the Clinic*, xi.
133. Charcot, "Introduction. La Médecine empirique," xxiii.
134. Duchenne, "Recherches sur la paralysie musculaire," 189n. Duchenne is here quoting the observation of M. Bergeron from the Hôpital Sainte-Eugénie, which, according to Duchenne, was presented to the Société médicale des hôpitaux on May 24, 1867, and then published in *Union médicale* (ibid., 19).
135. Ibid., 189n.
136. Ibid., 8, figs. 1 and 2. He states later in the article that the line drawings were made after his photographs; ibid., 19.
137. Ibid., 9.
138. Ibid., 6.
139. Murray, *Multiple Sclerosis*, 106–7.
140. Gilman, *Seeing the Insane*, 194–95.
141. Duchenne, "Recherches sur la paralysie musculaire," 189n. By this time, Duchenne had already published a text with photographs for the use of artists as well as physiologists: Duchenne, *Mécanisme de la physionomie humaine*. An article from 1894 by Paul Richer notes "les formes herculéennes" described by Duchenne; Richer, "De la station," 130.
142. Undated letter from Charcot to Jean-Baptiste Charcot, Charcot Family archives; quoted in Bouchara, *Charcot*, 12.
143. Souques, "Charcot intime," 697.
144. Many years later, Richer would use another painting presumed to be by Hals, the portrait of René Descartes, as the foundation of his scientific-artistic exercise in creating a portrait of Descartes from a cast of the skull presumed to be his; see Ruiz-Gómez, "Shaking the Tyranny," 243–44.
145. Reynolds is quoted without a reference in Liedtke, "Frans Hals," 32–33.
146. Slive, *Frans Hals*, 1:21.
147. Mantz, "Galerie Pourtalès"; Slive, *Frans Hals*, 3:19.
148. For a bibliography of their articles up to 1903, see "Oeuvre medico-artistique." A painting by Frans Hals the Younger (1618–1669) appears in Meige, "Peintres de la médecine," plate 48.
149. Charcot and Richer, *Les Difformes et les malades*, iii.
150. Richer, "Dialogues sur l'art et la science. III," 450.
151. Chu, *French Realism*.
152. Meige, *Charcot artiste*, 33–34.
153. Souques and Meige, "Jean-Martin Charcot," 333.
154. Meige, *Charcot artiste*, 15; original emphasis.
155. Charcot and Richer, *Démoniaques dans l'art*, xi and 56.
156. "Pathos, n.," and "pathology, n.," OED Online, March 2018, Oxford University Press, http://www.oed.com (both accessed May 4, 2018). My thanks to Andrew Graciano for this observation.
157. Hunter, *Face of Medicine*, 244.
158. Sappol, *Traffic of Dead Bodies*, 276.
159. Dias, "Corps en vitrine." See also Jordanova, "Museums: Representing the Real?"; Jordanova, "Objects of Knowledge."
160. Richer, Gilles de la Tourette, and Londe, "Avertissement," i.
161. Freud, "Autobiographical Study," 13.
162. Jordanova, "Portraiture, Beauty, Pain," 206.
163. Allart-Vallin-Charcot Archives, cited in Goetz, Bonduelle, and Gelfand, *Charcot*, 8.
164. Jordanova, *Sexual Visions*, 137.
165. Guillemot, "À la Salpêtrière. II," 371.
166. In 1906, the new Bibliothèque Charcot physically displaced the Musée Charcot, which was moved to the ground floor of the same building, the "division Parisot." For more on the dispersal of the Musée Charcot collection, see Ricou, Leroux-Hugon, and Poirier, *Bibliothèque Charcot*, 24–31.
167. Goetz, "Salpêtrière in the Wake."
168. L. Daudet, "Professeur Charcot," 242.

CHAPTER 2

1. Nochlin, *Courbet*, 113.
2. Ollendorf, *Salon de 1887*, 63; Ponsonhailhe, "Le Salon. Peinture. I," 444.
3. Levillain, "Charcot et l'École," 112.
4. Ponsonhailhe, "Le Salon. Peinture. I," 445.
5. Ponsonhailhe, "Le Salon. Peinture. II," 49.

6. Illustrated in Walusinski, *Leçon clinique*, 7.
7. Charcot, "Policlinique du mardi, 7 février 1888," 178.
8. Though the Salpêtrière is often touted as having the first photographic studio in a hospital setting, other hospitals installed them earlier; see Eidenbenz, "Théâtre de l'objectivité," 105–6; Dias, "Corps en vitrine."
9. "Hospice de la Salpêtrière.—M. Charcot."
10. Londe, "Service photographique," 282; Bernard and Gunthert, *Instant rêvé*, 75.
11. For the most complete biography of Londe, see Bernard and Gunthert, *Instant rêvé*.
12. Braun, *Picturing Time*, 85; Braun and Whitcombe, "Marey, Muybridge, and Londe," 222–23.
13. Londe, *Photographie médicale*, x. See also Londe, "Photographie en médecine."
14. Londe, "Photographie en médecine," 215–17.
15. Albert Londe, "L'Hystérie dans l'art" (unpublished manuscript), Paris, Bibliothèque Charcot, Cote IV-7.
16. Janssen quoted in Londe, *Photographie dans les arts*, 8.
17. He opened a second photography studio at the hospital in 1883 and the outdoor photography studio in 1893; Pichel, "Backstage of Hysteria."
18. "Plan du service photographique de la Salpêtrière," in Londe, *Photographie médicale*, 13. Claretie recounts the story of a hysteric who froze at a concert at the Théâtre de Châtelet after hearing a gong; Claretie, *Vie à Paris*, 129.
19. Charcot, *Oeuvres complètes*, 3:275–76.
20. For example, Baer, "Photography and Hysteria"; Miles, *Burning Mirror*, 154–55; O'Connor, "Camera Medica," 233.
21. Changeux and Régnier, "Préface," 11. There seem to be various editions published of each volume, based on the slightly different dates given in copies in libraries around the world. In this chapter, I illustrate the edition of Volume I held by the Bibliothèque Charcot, which is dated 1877. These are now digitized and available at https://patrimoine.sorbonne-universite.fr/en/collection/Fonds-Charcot. The *IPS* project probably died with the departures of Regnard in 1878 and Bourneville in 1879 for Bicêtre; Walusinski, "Albert Londe," 17.
22. Gelfand, "Neurologist or Psychiatrist?"; Goetz, Bonduelle, and Gelfand, *Charcot*, 208–13; Gauchet and Swain, *Vrai Charcot*.
23. Goetz, Bonduelle, and Gelfand, *Charcot*, 180.
24. Charcot and Marie, "Hysteria Mainly Hystero-Epilepsy," 628. Charcot's theories in the last decade of his life were fundamental to the development of scientific psychology and psychoanalysis; see Walusinski and Bogousslavsky, "Charcot, Janet." See also Foucault, *History of Sexuality*, 44.
25. Aragon and Breton, "Cinquantenaire de l'hystérie," 20.
26. Didi-Huberman, *Invention of Hysteria*.
27. Ibid., xi.
28. Ibid., 33.
29. Ibid., 61; emphases removed.
30. Ibid., 264.
31. De Marneffe, "Looking and Listening."
32. Ibid., 84.
33. Bourneville and Regnard, *Iconographie photographique de la Salpètrière* [*sic*], 2:ii.
34. Regnard and Bourneville, *Iconographie photographique de la Salpétrière* [*sic*].
35. The existence of this album came to my attention through an article by Michael Roth, who noted that it contained retouching instructions. However, he did not provide an inventory number for the album; Roth, "Hysterical Remembering," 22. I acted as a consultant on the Wellcome Collection's exhibition *Bedlam: The Asylum and Beyond*, which ran from September 25, 2016, to January 15, 2017; as a result, the Wellcome secured the loan of this album for the exhibition.
36. Gernsheim, "Medical Photography," 85.
37. Ibid., 88.
38. Gilman, *Face of Madness*.
39. Diamond, "On the Application of Photography," 19.
40. Ibid., 21.
41. Ibid., 20 and 24.
42. Phillips, "Photo-Logos," 155.
43. Morton, "Photography as an Authority," 181.
44. Hamilton, "The Beautiful and the Damned," 14.
45. E. Edwards, "Ordering Others," 55.
46. Duchenne, *Mécanisme de la physionomie humaine*, v. Duchenne's reliance on photography likely influenced Charcot; see Siegel, "Charcot and Duchenne."
47. Étienne-Jules Marey, *La Méthode graphique dans les sciences expérimentales et principalement en physiologie et en médecine*, 2nd ed. (Paris, 1885), v; quoted in Ellenbogen, *Reasoned and Unreasoned Images*, 4 and 223n4.

48. Wilder, "Visualizing Radiation," 349.
49. O'Connor, "Camera Medica," 238.
50. Gunthert, "Rétine du savant."
51. Sheehan, *Doctored*; Tucker, *Nature Exposed.*
52. Eidenbenz, "Théâtre de l'objectivité," 106.
53. Micale, *Approaching Hysteria*; Scull, *Hysteria*; Trillat, *Histoire de l'hystérie.*
54. Bourneville, "Préface," 1:iii–iv.
55. Pichel, "Backstage of Hysteria."
56. Sekula, "The Body and the Archive," 7; emphasis removed.
57. The only extended discussion of this volume that I have found is in Hustvedt, *Medical Muses*, 163–67.
58. The IPS Album is digitized and available at https://patrimoine.sorbonne-universite.fr/idurl/1/3437. The binding of this volume is Charcot's own design; Guillaume Delaunay (former conservateur des bibliothèques of the Bibliothèque Charcot), personal communication with the author, May 31, 2017.
59. Bourneville, "Préface," 1:iv.
60. Londe writes that at the time he arrived at the Salpêtrière in 1882, the wet collodion process was still in use; Londe, "Service photographique," 282.
61. Many pages also include the archives shelfmark of the album in pencil in a different hand, presumably written by an archivist.
62. Pichel contends that *most* of the photographs in the *IPS* were taken outside; Pichel, "Cuerpos patológicos," 47.
63. Hustvedt, *Medical Muses*, 165.
64. Bourneville and Regnard, *Iconographie photographique de la Salpétrière* [*sic*], 1:3.
65. Ibid., 1:11–13.
66. Delboeuf, "Visite à la Salpêtrière," 122.
67. Kriebel, "Theories of Photography," 42–43. For a discussion of the material practices of photography at the Salpêtrière, see Pichel, "Cuerpos patológicos."
68. Gunthert, "'Sans retouche.'" See also Fineman, *Faking It*, 60–64; Sheehan, *Doctored*, 68–73.
69. Gunthert, "'Sans retouche.'"
70. Fineman, *Faking It*, 61.
71. Périer, "Exposition universelle," esp. 194–96; Durieu, "Sur la retouche."
72. Duchenne, *Mécanisme de la physionomie humaine*, 65, vi. The second quotation is taken from the "Avertissement" in Duchenne's book in the Bibliothèque Charcot, which is not the same in some other editions; see https://patrimoine.sorbonne-universite.fr/idurl/1/3462.
73. Kemp, "'Perfect and Faithful Record,'" 143.
74. Tucker, *Nature Exposed*, 220.
75. Freund, *Photography and Society*, 64.
76. Baudelaire, "Modern Public and Photography," 291–98.
77. Alfred Lichtwark, *Die Amateurphotographie* (Halle, 1894); cited in Freund, *Photography and Society*, 65.
78. Johnson, *Complete Treatise*, 9.
79. Burrows and Colton, *Concise Instructions*, 38–39.
80. Bech, *Traité pratique de retouche*, 1.
81. Klary, *Art de retoucher*, xiii.
82. Johnson, *Complete Treatise*, 13.
83. Dommasch, "Development of Medical Photography," 169; Amirault, "Posing the Subject," 51–76; Sheehan, *Doctored*, 48–80.
84. Burns, "Early Medical Photography," 791.
85. Kemp, "'Perfect and Faithful Record,'" 137. See also Sidlauskas, "Inventing the Medical Portrait."
86. Sidlauskas, "Before and After."
87. Miles, *Burning Mirror*, 207–8. See also the discussion in Woloshyn, *Soaking Up the Rays*, esp. 90–136.
88. "Artifice, n.," OED Online, June 2020, Oxford University Press, https://www.oed.com (accessed June 11, 2020).
89. Barthes, *Camera Lucida*, 5.
90. Miles, *Burning Mirror*, 157.
91. "Éclaircir un peu le bas du vêtement et les mains / accentuer les yeux dans le sentiment du regard"; Album 646 FOSS 5, Paris, Archives de l'Assistance Publique–Hôpitaux de Paris (hereafter Archives de l'AP-HP).
92. Burrows and Colton, *Concise Instructions*, 4; original emphasis.
93. "Faire quelques plis dans la chemise"; Album 646 FOSS 5, Archives de l'AP-HP. Piquepé, *Traité pratique*, 54.
94. "Retoucher la figure pour enlever les points noirs / refaire un peu le linge et les mains"; Album 646 FOSS 5, Archives de l'AP-HP.
95. "Retoucher pour faire disparaître le double de la figure / éclaircir le bras et la main droite, donner quelques plis au linge"; Album 646 FOSS 5, Archives de l'AP-HP.
96. Ken, *Dissertations historiques, artistiques et scientifiques*, 146–47.
97. Didi-Huberman, *Invention of Hysteria*, 88.
98. Harvey, *Photography and Spirit*; Jolly, *Faces of the Living Dead.*
99. Bourneville and Regnard, *Iconographie photographique de la Salpétrière* [*sic*], 1:49.

100. Carroy-Thirard, "Possession, extase, hystérie"; Didi-Huberman, "Charcot, l'histoire et l'art."
101. Bourneville and Regnard, *Iconographie photographique de la Salpêtrière*, 2:202–25.
102. Regnard and Richer, "Études sur l'attaque hystéro-épileptique," 643.
103. "Bien retoucher la figure faire les cheveux / éclaircir la main"; Album 646 FOSS 5, Archives de l'AP-HP.
104. Young, *ABC of Retouching*, 45.
105. Ibid., 34–35; emphasis added.
106. Piquepé, *Traité pratique*, 41.
107. Johnson, *Complete Treatise*, 15.
108. Burrows and Colton, *Concise Instructions*, 21.
109. Bourneville and Regnard, *Iconographie photographique de la Salpêtrière* [*sic*], 1:67.
110. Johnson, *Complete Treatise*, 35.
111. "Retoucher les raies noires, la figure et remplir le carré de papier flou / par du dessin et du fond, <u>si c'est possible</u>"; Album 646 FOSS 5, Archives de l'AP-HP.
112. Johnson, *Complete Treatise*, 4.
113. B. A. Morel, *Traité des dégénérescences*.
114. Gilman, "Image of the Hysteric," 358.
115. Sontag, *On Photography*, 7.
116. Rawling, "'Annexed Photos.'"
117. Miles, *Burning Mirror*, 247.
118. Sontag, *On Photography*, 86.
119. Fineman, *Faking It*, 19. My discussion here is indebted to Fineman's insights.
120. Trachtenberg, "Photography," 18.
121. Vogel, "Photography and Truth," 264; original emphasis.
122. Larousse, *Grand Dictionnaire universel*, 15:908.
123. Henry Peach Robinson reiterates this dichotomy: "Truth and fact are not only two words, but, in art at least, they represent two things. A fact is anything done, or that exists—a reality. Truth is *conformity* to fact or reality—absence of falsehood. So that truth in art may exist without an absolute observance of facts." Robinson, *Pictorial Effect in Photography*, 78; original emphasis.
124. Ibid., 109.
125. Londe, *Photographie moderne*, 105; emphasis added.
126. Londe, *Photographie médicale*, 201.
127. Maehle, "Search for Objective Communication," 571–72.
128. Ibid.
129. Phillips, "Photo-Logos," 155.
130. O'Connor, "Camera Medica," 238; emphases removed.

CHAPTER 3

1. Charcot, "Physiologie pathologique."
2. Charcot and Gilles de la Tourette, "Hypnotism in the Hysterical," 606–10.
3. The loudest were the so-called Nancy School led by Hippolyte Bernheim; see Bernheim, "Hypnotisme et suggestion"; Goetz, Bonduelle, and Gelfand, *Charcot*, 310–11.
4. Théophraste, "Chronique scientifique."
5. Chayette, *Grand Musée anatomique*. The collection of the Spitzner Museum is now housed at the Université de Montpellier.
6. Centre culturel de la Communauté française de Belgique, *Cires anatomiques du XIXᵉ siècle*, 6.
7. Illustrated in Pinet, "Cires anatomiques," 52.
8. Ibid., 54.
9. The caption under the photograph states that the wax group is no longer extant; Blon et al., *Voir—La Collection Spitzner*, 43.
10. Peugniez, *J.-M. Charcot*, 5–6; emphasis removed.
11. Féré, "Description de quelques pièces," 202–3.
12. Papet, "Le Moulage sur nature," 93. The catalogue wrongly credits Paul Richer as the creator and dates the sculpture to 1895.
13. Tabes dorsalis is the slow degeneration of the nerves in the dorsal columns of the spinal cord, while locomotor ataxia is its most visible symptom. At the end of the nineteenth century and beginning of the twentieth, they were often used interchangeably. There is a single entry for both in *A Dictionary of Psychological Medicine*; Tuke, "Locomotor Ataxy." In 1918, they were used interchangeably in Maloney, *Locomotor Ataxia (Tabes Dorsalis)*. Locomotor ataxia was first described by Charcot's mentor and friend Duchenne de Boulogne; Duchenne, "De l'ataxie locomotrice progressive."
14. Mott, "Tabes," 43; Pierret, "Note sur la sclérose," 377.
15. Charcot and Richer, *Les Difformes et les malades*, iii.
16. Grootenboer, "Introduction," 6.
17. There is a tantalizing entry for Berthelot in one of the albums of the Musée Charcot, but the page where her image(s) would have appeared has been

cut out; see Album AP.2003.7.1.4, Musée de l'AP-HP.

18. Charcot quoted in *Transactions*, 128.

19. Charcot quoted in ibid., 130, caption under fig. 1.

20. The strong three-dimensionality of the *Ataxic Venus* is especially evident in photographs taken by the restorer Laurence Chicoineau; they are included in a report entitled "Rapport Technique de Restauration (restauration 9 et 10 mai 1995)" located in the Fonds Charcot, Musée de l'AP-HP. For the aversion to looking at (facial) disfigurement, see Biernoff, "Rhetoric of Disfigurement."

21. Charcot and Féré, "Affections osseuses."

22. Wittlich, "Closed Eyes."

23. Charcot and Richer, *Les Difformes et les malades*, 120–51. Didi-Huberman suggests erroneously that the *Ataxic Venus* was cast from a living patient; Didi-Huberman, *Invention of Hysteria*, 30.

24. *Transactions*, 130–32; *International Medical Congress*, 37, nos. 404–8. Féré discusses Berthelot's body in detail and includes an illustration of her while still alive in Féré, "Description de quelques pièces," 202–18.

25. Charcot quoted in *Transactions*, 128.

26. According to William Edwards, curator of the Gordon Museum, King's College London, this cast is no longer in the collection of Saint Thomas's Hospital; personal communication with the author, February 1, 2013. Charcot's donations of specimens to other British collections are noted in *Transactions*, 129. According to Féré, Charcot also gave ataxic specimens to the Hunterian Museum in London and a museum in Manchester as well as the Musée Dupuytren in Paris; Féré, "Description de quelques pièces," 202.

27. Letter from August 8, 1881, in the Allart-Vallin-Charcot Archives; quoted in Goetz, Bonduelle, and Gelfand, *Charcot*, 147.

28. Charcot quoted in Gelfand, *Charcot in Morocco*, 28n10.

29. Charcot quoted in *Transactions*, 129. The text of his lecture was also published in the *British Medical Journal*, giving it an even wider audience. Charcot, "Demonstration of Arthropathic Affections," 285. Charcot is in the front row of the composite group photograph of all the Congress participants created by Herbert Rose Barraud, attesting to his importance; see http://catalogue.wellcomelibrary.org/record=b1574994.

30. "Festivities of the Congress," 304.

31. Schnalke, "Casting Skin," 224.

32. Some of the literature from the 1890s mentions that the cast is unfinished; see Delboeuf, "Visite à la Salpêtrière," 123.

33. "Hospice de la Salpêtrière.—M. Charcot," 913, 913n2. A photograph from the *entre-deux-guerres* of Charcot's laboratory and casting studio is included in *Cent ans d'Assistance publique*, 105, fig. 314.

34. "Arrêté de nomination de M. Loreau, titre de modeleur de Bicêtre et de la Salpêtrière, 6 March 1880," from the Musée Charcot file in the Archives du musée de l'Assistance publique; quoted in Tilles, "Histoire des bibliothèques médicales," 70n195.

35. See figures 3 to 16 in that volume.

36. Bernard and Gunthert note that in 1882 Loreau probably recommended Londe for the job of "préparateur chimiste" at the hospital, his first post, after meeting him on the grounds of the hospital. Bernard and Gunthert, *Instant rêvé*, 89.

37. Charcot and Richer, "Contribution à l'étude," caption to plate 9. According to Londe, the casting studio at the Salpêtrière basically stopped running when Loreau left in 1884; Londe, "Service photographique," 282.

38. Bernard and Gunthert, *Instant rêvé*, 100; "Arrêté de nomination de M. Loreau, titre de modeleur de Bicêtre et de la Salpêtrière, 6 March 1880," from the Musée Charcot file in the Archives du musée de l'Assistance publique; quoted in Tilles, "Histoire des bibliothèques médicales," 70n195.

39. There is an erotics of touch in the casting process; see the discussion of Edouard Dantan's painting *Moulage sur le modèle vivant* (1887, Gothenburg, Konstmuseum) in Hunter, *Face of Medicine*, 147–49.

40. A. Daudet, *In the Land of Pain*, 14.

41. Schnalke, "Casting Skin," 216.

42. West, *Portraiture*, 21; Jordanova, "Portraiture, Beauty, Pain," 205; Biernoff, "Necessary Humanity."

43. Schnalke, "Casting Skin," 218.

44. Ibid.

45. The casts of hands that I discuss here are undated and could therefore have been made after Loreau left the Salpêtrière and Richer became head of the casting studio.

46. *Catalogue of Plaster Casts . . . Made for Sale for P. P. Caproni and Brothers* (Boston, 1901), 246–47; illustrated in Papet,

"À fleur de peau," 30, fig. 10. For an illustration of this cast hand from the Salpêtrière, see Ruiz-Gómez, "Hysterical Reading," 1010, fig. 18.

47. Cited in Panzanelli, "Introduction: Beyond the Pale," 2.

48. The sculptor Eleanor Crook suggested that the mold for the *Ataxic Venus* might have consisted of beef gelatin instead of plaster, a technique used at the time; since the gelatin is soluble in water, it would have been much easier to remove the wax cast from the mold. Personal communication with the author, July 6, 2017. For a detailed discussion of casting in plaster, wax, and gelatin, among other media, roughly contemporary to the making of the *Ataxic Venus*, see Lebrun et al., *Nouveau Manuel complet du mouleur*. A cast taken from a human body, either alive or dead, would have been a *moulage à creux*. It would have to have been taken before the cadaver's "refroidissement"; Drilhon and Tassery-Lahmi, "Technologie et mise en forme," 66. Clarke details the process of molding and casting an entire body in Clarke, *Molding and Casting*, 187–94. For the process of creating a pathological wax cast, see Noirot, "Jules Baretta." Most *mouleurs* would not have revealed the composition of their wax, or their exact methods, for fear of losing their livelihood; Schnalke, "Casting Skin," 224–25.

For more information on casting, especially in the nineteenth century, see Corpataux, *Corps à l'oeuvre*; Papet, *À fleur de peau*; Le Normand-Romain, "Moulage"; Le Normand-Romain, "Moulage sur nature"; Frederiksen and Marchand, *Plaster Casts*. For a theoretical discussion of casting and its artistic uses, especially in twentieth-century and contemporary art, see Didi-Huberman, *Empreinte*.

49. Hopwood, "Plastic Publishing in Embryology," 180.

50. *Courrier des médecins de Saint-Louis au Directeur de l'Assistance Publique*, June 1896 in the Archives de la bibliothèque Henri Feulard et du musée de l'hôpital Saint-Louis; quoted in Tilles, "Histoire des bibliothèques médicales," 140.

51. The Museo di Anatomia Patologica in Florence also has a life-size wax cast illustrating pathology as its centerpiece: the so-called *Leper* or *Man with Norwegian Scabies* (1851) by Luigi Calamai. For more, see Gabbriellini et al., "Collezione di cere," 51–70.

52. For more on wax sculpture, see S. Blondel, "Modeleurs en cire"; Breton, *Essai historique*; Gaborit and Ligot, *Sculptures en cire*; Lemire, *Artistes et mortels*; Panzanelli, *Ephemeral Bodies*, which includes the first English translation of the important essay by Julius von Schlosser, "The History of Portraiture in Wax" (1910–11). For more on anatomical waxes specifically, see Düring et al., *Encyclopaedia Anatomica*; Garnot, "Céroplastie médicale," 21–24; Pinet, "Cires anatomiques"; Schnalke, *Diseases in Wax*.

53. Panzanelli, "Introduction: The Body in Wax," 1. See also Freud, "'Uncanny.'"

54. Warner, *Phantasmagoria*, 24.

55. Ibid., 23.

56. For more on La Specola, see Lanza et al., *Cere anatomiche della Specola*.

57. Garnot, "Céroplastie médicale," 22.

58. Schnalke, "Casting Skin," 209.

59. Garnot, "Céroplastie médicale," 23.

60. Oursel, "*Buste de jeune fille*," 144; Schwartz, *Spectacular Realities*, 97.

61. Hunter, *Face of Medicine*, 152.

62. Papet calls the *Ataxic Venus* a "moulage retouché"; Papet, "Moulage sur nature," 93–94. Eleanor Crook suggests that this could have been done later, by another hand, to mend damage to the sculpture; personal communication with the author, July 6, 2017. This sculpture has visible dark patches all over that are likely dust—a thorough cleaning may reveal more nuances in the skin tone and more of the sculptor's marks.

63. Ballestriero, "Anatomical Models and Wax Venuses," 223–34; Didi-Huberman, *Ouvrir Vénus*; Ebenstein, *Anatomical Venus*; Jordanova, *Sexual Visions*, esp. 43–65; Stephens, "Venus in the Archive"; Stephens, *Anatomy as Spectacle*, 26–52.

64. Baudelaire, *Fleurs du mal*, 189; Reveillé-Parise, *Traité de la vieillesse*, 63.

65. Pick, *Faces of Degeneration*. The discovery that syphilis caused tabes dorsalis was made by Alfred Fournier in 1875; Mott, "Tabes," 11.

66. Ferrier, *On Tabes Dorsalis*, 46; Quétel, *History of Syphilis*, 134–35.

67. Jordanova, *Sexual Visions*, 47; Schnalke, "Casting Skin," 233.

68. Clark, *Painting of Modern Life*, 136–37.

69. W. Miller, "Epilogue," 152.

70. O'Shiel, "Kolnai's Disgust," 25; original emphasis.
71. W. Miller, *Anatomy of Disgust*, xi.
72. Reveillé-Parise, *Traité de la vieillesse*, 63; emphasis removed.
73. W. Miller, *Anatomy of Disgust*, 116.
74. Foucault, *History of Sexuality*, 70–71.
75. Sappol, *Traffic of Dead Bodies*, 276.
76. Lebrun et al., *Nouveau Manuel complet du mouleur*, 88.
77. Charcot and Richer, *Les Difformes et les malades*, 133.
78. Féré, "Description de quelques pièces," 203.
79. Richer, "Dialogues sur l'art et la science. 11," 238–39.
80. Panzanelli, "Introduction: The Body in Wax," 3; Héran et al., *Dernier Portrait*; Pointon, "Casts."
81. Hugh Honour, *L'Image du Noir dans l'art occidental*, vol. 2 (Paris: Gallimard, 1982), 24; cited in Édouard Papet, "Technique," 76. See also Lebrun et al., *Nouveau Manuel complet du mouleur*, esp. 78–83.
82. Balzac, *Chef-d'oeuvre inconnu* (1837) in Didi-Huberman, *Peinture incarnée*, 139.
83. Hoffmann, "Sleeping Beauties."
84. Charcot quoted in *Transactions*, 128.
85. De Marneffe, "Looking and Listening"; Mayer, *Sites of the Unconscious*, 16–17.
86. Papet, "Introduction," 13.
87. Goetz, Bonduelle, and Gelfand, *Charcot*, 290.
88. Ibid., 292.
89. Ibid., 293; Barnes, "Introduction," ix.
90. Entry dated December 31, 1893; Goncourt and Goncourt, *Journal*, 4:495.
91. A. Daudet, *In the Land of Pain*, 6.
92. Ibid., 21.
93. Ibid.
94. Ibid., 29.
95. Ibid., 15.
96. Scarry, *Body in Pain*, 4.
97. A. Daudet, *In the Land of Pain*, 5.
98. Féré, "Description de quelques pièces," 207. See also Mott, "Tabes," 64–65.
99. Ebenstein, *Anatomical Venus*, 49.
100. Delboeuf, "Visite à la Salpêtrière," 263.
101. Jordanova, *Sexual Visions*, 55.
102. De Ceglia, "Rotten Corpses," 437.
103. Arthur Kleinman quoted in Field et al., "Discussion," 354; original emphasis.
104. A. Daudet, *In the Land of Pain*, 43.
105. Biernoff, "Picturing Pain," 194.
106. Ibid., 200. See also Yamamoto-Wilson, *Pain, Pleasure and Perversity*, 195.
107. *Iconographie photographique de la Salpêtrière* 3: plates 38–40.
108. Kumar, "Between Life and Art," 257; Kumar is referring here to the sculpture by Fernández.
109. A. Daudet, *In the Land of Pain*, 24–25. Barnes also makes the comparison of the *Ataxic Venus* with Christ; Barnes, "Breaking the Mould."
110. Groebner, "Feeling for Images," 151.
111. "Patient, adj. and n.," OED Online, June 2017, Oxford University Press, http://www.oed.com (accessed July 5, 2017).
112. Jordanova, "Portraiture, Beauty, Pain," 199.
113. Panzanelli, "Introduction: Beyond the Pale," 2.
114. Graybill, "Proximate Violence."
115. H. Edwards, "Pain in Public," 93.
116. Charcot and Richer, *Les Difformes et les malades*, 139. For more on the artist, see Marquand, *Brothers of Giovanni della Robbia*, 101–30.
117. Charcot and Richer, *Les Difformes et les malades*, 139–40.
118. Panofsky, *Tomb Sculpture*, 80.
119. Ibid.
120. Panzanelli, "Introduction: Beyond the Pale"; Blühm, "In Living Colour," 11–60; Le Normand-Romain and Olivié, "Polychromie"; Papet, "Sculpture polychrome"; Syson, "Polychrome and Its Discontents."
121. B. Evans, *Jean-Léon Gérôme*, 93.
122. For a full list, see Ackerman, *Jean-Léon Gérôme*, 330–31, catalogue numbers 385–88.2. Ackerman illustrates two black-and-white photographs of the sculpture, both with and without polychromy, and notes that the sculpture was used as the model for the paintings (ibid., 390–91).
123. Geffroy, *Vie Artistique*, 289. See also Chevillot, "Réalisme optique et progrès esthétique."
124. Marcel Schwob, *Les Oeuvres complètes de Marcel Schwob (1867–1905)* (Paris: F. Bernouard, 1927), 270; quoted in Papet, "Sculpture polychrome," 22.
125. Bata, "Préface," 6.
126. Henri Trianon, "Sixième exposition de peinture par un groupe d'artistes," *Le Constitutionnel*, April 24, 1881, 2–3; reprinted in Berson, *New Painting*, 1:368.
127. Callen, *Spectacular Body*, 27–28. C[harles] E[phrussi], "Exposition des artistes indépendants," *La Chronique des arts et de la curiosité*, April 16, 1881, 127; quoted in Boggs et al., *Degas*, 343.

128. Elie de Mont, "L'Exposition du boulevard des Capucines," *La Civilisation*, April 21, 1881, 2; Comtesse Louise, "Lettres familières sur l'art: Salon de 1881," *La France nouvelle*, May 1–2, 1881, 2–3. Both are reprinted in Berson, *New Painting*, 1:362 and 1:356, respectively.
129. Joris-Karl Huysmans, *L'Art moderne. Certains* (Paris: Union générale d'éditions, 1976), 206; quoted in Papet, "Sculpture polychrome," 26.
130. Aicard, "M. Henry Cros," 67; Hawley, "Sculptures," 199; Héran, "Henry Cros," 103–18; D. Morel, "Henry Cros"; Olivié, "Henry Cros"; Testard, "Henry Cros."
131. A note to Charcot's speech thanking the Assistance Publique confirms that his claim that the museum was "très élégamment décoré" is in reference to the "décorations murales à la cire de M. Cros"; "Hospice de la Salpêtrière.—M. Charcot," 913n1.
132. Chevallier and Hémard, *Catalogue des objets d'art*, 30, no. 211; Héran, "Henry Cros," 114. *Pâte de verre* is an ancient technique using colored glass.
133. The caption incorrectly attributes this work to his brother, Charles, and misspells their surname as "Cross"; Goetschy, "Femmes du monde artistes," 42.
134. Entry dated May 26, 1879; Goncourt and Goncourt, *Journal*, 3:21.
135. Blondel, "Ciriers modernes," 231–32; Oulié, *Jean Charcot*, 37.
136. Oursel, "*Buste de jeune fille*," 141–46, cat. no. 28; Gonse, "Musée de Lille." The sculpture was intended for Alexandre Dumas fils; Boggs et al., *Degas*, 343.
137. Hunter, *Face of Medicine*, 173; Callen, *Spectacular Body*, 55.
138. Testard, "Henry Cros," 152.
139. Olivié, "*Prix du tournoi*," 215, cat. no. 57. See also Blondel, "Ciriers modernes," 230–31; Papet, "Henry Cros," 68.
140. Rodin quoted in Méryem, "Dessins d'Henry Cros," 174.
141. De Vergnes, *Antoine de Tounens*, 231.
142. Entry dated December 10, 1872; Goncourt and Goncourt, *Journal*, 2:923.
143. Cros and Henry, *Encaustique et les autres procédés*. As noted above, Cros also experimented with *pâte de verre*; Olivié, "Henry Cros," 213; Belfort, "Pâtes de verre," 176–87.
144. He won a gold medal at the 1900 Universal Exposition for his bas-relief *L'Histoire du feu*; Belfort, "Pâtes de verre," 186.
145. Aicard, "M. Henry Cros," 67.
146. Ibid.
147. Papet, "Moulage sur nature," 94.
148. Moscoso, *Pain*, 2.
149. Warner, *Phantasmagoria*, 41.
150. Guillemot, "À la Salpêtrière. II," 371. There is a common misconception, which began during Charcot's lifetime, that the *Ataxic Venus* shows a hysteric; see ibid., for example.
151. Fend, "Order and Affect," 80.
152. Brilliant, *Portraiture*, 8, 7.
153. Kumar, "Between Life and Art," 257.
154. Honoré de Balzac, *Le Chef-d'oeuvre inconnu* (1837), in Didi-Huberman, *Peinture incarnée*, 138.
155. Elkins, *Pictures of the Body*, 21.
156. Papet, "Moulage sur nature," 93; emphasis removed.
157. A. Daudet, *In the Land of Pain*, 15.

CHAPTER 4

1. The detail is from *Salon de 1887*, 170.
2. *L'Art du nu*, 123, cat. 123; Comar, *Figures du corps*, 155; Rouillé and Marbot, *Corps et son image*, 51.
3. Richer and Meige, "Étude morphologique," 363.
4. "Le Docteur Paul Richer," n.p.
5. Richer, "Notes biographiques."
6. Meige, "Sur une statuette," 140.
7. Ibid., 136.
8. Daston and Galison, *Objectivity*, 37.
9. Richer, "Dialogues sur l'art et la science. III," 450.
10. Blanchard, *Hommage*; Jean-Baptiste Charcot, "Paul Richer"; Comar, "Leçon d'anatomie," esp. 56–60; Desprez, "Paul Richer"; "Le Docteur Paul Richer," n.p.; Le Gendre, "Richer"; Gilles de la Tourette, "Biographies médicales"; Meige, "Paul Richer et son oeuvre," 123–26; "Paul Richer," 65–76; Ruiz-Gómez, "Scientific Artworks"; Ruiz-Gómez, "Shaking the Tyranny"; Walusinski, "Biographie de Paul Richer"; Walusinski, "Keeping the Fire Burning," esp. 78–82; Walusinski, *Leçon clinique*, 74–80. As noted above, Richer also published a catalogue raisonné of his work: Richer, *Notice sur les titres*.
11. Blanchard, *Hommage*, 14.
12. Ibid., 11. Richer's book was published in 1881 with an expanded second edition in 1885. Richer, *Études cliniques*.

13. Ruiz-Gómez, "Hysterical Reading."
14. In 1882, Charcot was awarded the Chair of Diseases of the Nervous System; it was at this time that he made Richer the head of his laboratory, which included the museum. Richer held the post until 1896. "Le Docteur Paul Richer," n.p.
15. Richer, *Feuilles d'autopsie*.
16. Charcot, "Policlinique du mardi 30 octobre 1888," 20–21; original emphasis.
17. Ibid., 22.
18. Ibid., 21–22.
19. Richer, *Anatomie artistique*, vii. Richer would later publish *Physiologie artistique de l'homme en mouvement* and six volumes of the *Nouvelle Anatomie artistique*. He also created an unpublished *Atlas physiologique* using chronophotographs by Albert Londe, which is in the collection of ENSBA. See also Callen, *Looking at Men*, esp. 53–54; Pichel, "From Facial Expressions."
20. Richer, *Anatomie artistique*, ix.
21. Epigraph by Topffer in ibid., half title.
22. Ibid., viii.
23. Ibid., xiii. Bernard and Comar argue that the term "après nature" for the drawings in the *Anatomie artistique* is still accurate as, for Richer, the photograph was "une transcription littérale du réel"; Bernard and Comar, catalogue entry for 130–32, in *Figures du corps*, 268.
24. Richer, "Dialogues sur l'art et la science. II," 243.
25. Richer, *Anatomie artistique*, xiii.
26. Ibid., xiv–xv.
27. Richer, "Anatomie vivant," 1089. It is worth highlighting that Richer's opening lesson to his art students is reprinted in a medical journal.
28. Callen, "Masculinity and Muscularity"; Poivert, "Variété et vérité."
29. For a list until 1896, see Richer, *Notice sur les titres*, 118–79.
30. Richer, *Canon des proportions*, 21. On page 11, as elsewhere, Richer highlights his distance from any particular artistic school and the "scientific" basis of his work as a mark of its veracity. This sculpture was obviously significant for Richer, as it appears on his *ex libris* (for example, in his personal copy of Richer, *Introduction à l'Étude de la figure humaine*, Paris, Richer Family archives). For more on Richer's canon, see Callen, "Man or Machine."
31. Gilles de la Tourette, "Biographies médicales."
32. Richer quoted in Omer, "Docteur Richer," 2. Paris, Richer Family archives.
33. "Un magnifique athlète"; Richer, "Notes biographiques."
34. Ibid.
35. "J'étais complètement ignorant de la technique"; ibid.
36. "Dix fois trop faible"; ibid.
37. "Si je n'y avais mis bon ordre, ma statue aurait bientôt été un véritable champ de blé"; ibid.
38. "'Comme il serait curieux que vous ne devinssiez un de nos bons sculpteurs!' et il me résuma son opinion sur mon oeuvre par cette simple phrase: 'c'est une très bonne préparation' voulant dire par-là qu'il n'y manquait que cette science du modelé qu'on enseignait alors dans les Écoles des Beaux-Arts"; ibid.
39. Mantz, "Le Salon VII," 2. Article located in Ms. 837, ENSBA.
40. Mantz, *Salon de 1889*, 93–94.
41. See ibid., 98. This figure was clearly important for Richer, as he reused it in a later relief sculpture entitled *Le Moisson*. My thanks to Olivier Walusinski for bringing this relief to my attention.
42. Ibid., 93–94.
43. "Chronique locale," n.p. Article located in Ms. 837, ENSBA.
44. Richer, "Notes biographiques." According to Prioux, Dalou was a member of the Salon jury that year; Prioux, *Deux médecins—Deux sculpteurs*, 20. Eschelbacher disagrees, writing that Dalou had not been a member of the jury of the Société des artistes français since 1884; Eschelbacher, "Gendering Modernity," 347n18.
45. Blanchard, *Hommage*, 14.
46. Richer, "Notes biographiques."
47. Albinson, "Dalou in England," 9; Hunisak, *Sculptor Jules Dalou*, esp. 174–205.
48. Dreyfous, *Dalou*, 1.
49. Caillaux, *Aimé-Jules Dalou*, 26–27.
50. Eschelbacher, "Gendering Modernity," 335; Dreyfous, *Dalou*, 278.
51. Hourticq, "Paul Richer," 147.
52. Eschelbacher, "Gendering Modernity," 344–45.
53. Richer, "Notes biographiques."
54. While both "realists" and "naturalists" were committed to depicting contemporary life, the latter were often less detached in their representations and often depicted the poor or rural life with a clear moral sentiment and political charge. However, at the time the terms

were used interchangeably. Becker and Weisberg, "Introducing Naturalism," esp. 13–14; Weisberg, "Realist Tradition," 3.
55. Eschelbacher, "Gendering Modernity," 345.
56. Desprez, "Paul Richer," 114; Comar, *Figures du corps*, 360, cat. 277.
57. Albinson, "Dalou in England," 12.
58. Ibid., 14.
59. Richer, "Notes biographiques."
60. Ibid.
61. Richer, "Art préhistorique," 458.
62. Ibid., 456.
63. *Vénus et Caïn*; Gindhart, "Art and Science."
64. Richer, "Art préhistorique," 458.
65. Richer, "Notes biographiques."
66. Richer, "Art préhistorique," 459, 461.
67. Ibid., 460.
68. Ibid., 461.
69. Gilles de la Tourette, "Biographies médicales."
70. Meige, "Facies"; Meige, "Amyotrophiques dans l'art."
71. Meige, "Facies," 379. As far as I know, there are only two extant copies of this sculpture, and both are in the collection of the Assistance Publique. The one in tinted plaster is inscribed on its proper left: "Paul Richer / 1888."
72. Ibid., 340. For illustrations of *alèzes*, see the catalogue by Natton, *Instruments et appareils*, 273–74.
73. Charcot, "Policlinique du mardi 28 février 1888"; Charcot, *Charcot the Clinician*, 164–86.
74. The photograph of the sculpture appears to be an uncropped print of the photograph used to illustrate the *Nouvelle Iconographie*. These photographs were found back-to-back in a box entitled "Photos de malades" that had not yet been inventoried at the Bibliothèque Charcot when I last visited.
75. Simon-Dhouailly, *Leçon de Charcot*, 65, cat. 125.
76. Charcot, "Policlinique du mardi 28 février 1888."
77. Ibid., 151.
78. Ibid., 152; original emphasis.
79. Richer, *Physiologie artistique*, 9.
80. Meige, "Facies," 379.
81. Chantoury-Lacombe, *Peindre les maux*, 336–37.
82. As far as I know, there are no extant copies of this sculpture. I have yet to find a reproduction that does not show it isolated.
83. Meige, "Amyotrophiques dans l'art."
84. Gould, *New Medical Dictionary*, 38; Meige, "Amyotrophiques dans l'art," 198.
85. Meige, "Amyotrophiques dans l'art," 200.
86. Ibid., 201.
87. [Jean-Martin] Charcot and A[médée] Dechambre, "De quelques marbres antiques concernant des études anatomiques," *Gazette hebdomadaire de médecine et de chirurgie* 4, no. 25 (1857); cited in Meige, "Amyotrophiques dans l'art," 198. See the introduction for a discussion of Charcot's article.
88. Meige, "Amyotrophiques dans l'art," 201.
89. Boix, "Myopathie primitive progressive," 446; Landouzy and Dejerine, "Contribution à l'étude," 478–81.
90. Le Noir and Bezançon, "Observation de myopathie progressive primitive," 307.
91. Guinon, "Deux types de myopathie progressive," 17.
92. Ibid., 17.
93. The photograph that includes Bonnet is mentioned in two articles in this volume and seems to serve as a general comparative illustration of myopathy. Richer, "De la station," 130n1; Meige, "Amyotrophiques dans l'art," 202.
94. Guinon and Souques, "Déformations thoraciques," 348–51.
95. Guinon, "Deux types de myopathie progressive," 17–18.
96. Richer, "De la station," 141.
97. Landouzy, "Note sur le facies myopathique," 420–21. One of the first descriptions of the myopathic facies is in Duchenne, *De l'électrisation localisée*, 518–19.
98. Guinon, "Deux types de myopathie progressive," 17.
99. Meige, "Amyotrophiques dans l'art," 203. Meige wrote extensively about Richer's artworks over the years. It seems likely that the two men were close and that the articles reveal Richer's thinking on the subjects as well.
100. Ibid., 202; Guinon, "Deux types de myopathie progressive," 16.
101. Le Noir and Bezançon, "Observation de myopathie progressive primitive," 309. Meige, "Amyotrophiques dans l'art," 198–204; emphasis removed. Meige confirms that the figure is a drawing of "Bonn" on page 201.
102. Boix, "Myopathie primitive progressive." This photograph seems to have been taken around the same time as those in

the *Nouvelle Iconographie*, even though it was published much later.

103. Londe, *Photographie médicale*, 68.
104. Guinon and Souques, "Déformations thoraciques," 349.
105. Illustrated in Comar, *Figures du corps*, 404.
106. Jordanova, *Defining Features*, 20.
107. Meige, "Amyotrophiques dans l'art," 202n1; Guinon and Souques, "Déformations thoraciques." Bonnet is not named in this article, but in "Deux types de myopathie progressive," Guinon notes that "Bonn" is the patient he presented to the meeting of the Société anatomique (17).
108. In addition to the others mentioned in this chapter, see Landouzy and Dejerine, "De la myopathie atrophique progressive"; Le Noir and Bezançon, "Observation de myopathie progressive primitive." The latter includes a portrait photograph of Bonnet as a fourteen-year-old boy as well.
109. Richer, "De la station," 130n2, 141; Guinon, "Deux types de myopathie progressive," 16. In Le Noir and Bezançon, he is referred to as "B . . . , Henri"; Le Noir and Bezançon, "Observation de myopathie progressive primitive."
110. Brouardel, *Secret médical*, esp. chapter 5; Ellenberger, "Charcot and the Salpêtrière School," 143.
111. Meige, "Paul Richer et son oeuvre," 124.
112. Meige, "Sur une statuette," 137.
113. Ibid., 138.
114. Raymond, "Du myxoedème infantile," 8; Benoît, *Contribution à l'étude*, 11.
115. Benoît, *Contribution à l'étude*, 14.
116. Raymond, "Du myxoedème infantile," 2. While Meige details the patient's case in his article in the *Nouvelle Iconographie*, the case notes here are taken from Raymond, "Du myxoedème infantile."
117. Charcot called it "cachexie pachydermique"; Benoît, *Contribution à l'étude*, 11.
118. Raymond, "Du myxoedème infantile," 2.
119. Ibid.
120. Ibid., 3.
121. Ibid., 4.
122. Ibid.
123. Meige, "Sur une statuette," 139.
124. Raymond, "Du myxoedème infantile," 4.
125. Meige and Allard, "Deux infantiles," 106.
126. Meige, "Sur une statuette," 139.
127. Ibid.
128. Raymond, "Du myxoedème infantile," 47.
129. Ibid., 2.
130. Ibid.
131. Meige, "Sur une statuette," 139.
132. Ibid., 140. Meige notes on the same page that an inguinal hernia makes Aurillard's genitals appear larger than they are.
133. Ibid.
134. Richer, *L'Art et la médecine*, 197.
135. Meige, "Sur une statuette," 139. Regarding another photograph in which a patient relies on an umbrella and a pedestal, Goetz, Bonduelle, and Gelfand note that the supports used "were likely objects found in the work studio of Charcot's neurological service"; Goetz, Bonduelle, and Gelfand, *Charcot*, 112, fig. 4–3.
136. Meige, "Sur une statuette," 138.
137. Ibid., 140.
138. They were first mentioned by Homer in the *Iliad*; W. Smith, *New Classical Dictionary*, 630.
139. *New Larousse Encyclopedia*, 172.
140. Richer, *L'Art et la médecine*, 198.
141. Meige, "Sur une statuette," 140.
142. Gould, *New Medical Dictionary*, 327; Charcot, *Charcot the Clinician*, 123; Walusinski, "Jean-Martin Charcot and Parkinson's Disease."
143. Richer and Meige, "Étude morphologique," 363.
144. Ibid.
145. Ibid., 364.
146. Charcot, "Policlinique du mardi 12 juin 1888," 332.
147. In one of his most famous clinical demonstrations, Charcot proved that one of the most conspicuous symptoms of Parkinson's, the uncontrolled trembling of the head, was a secondary symptom. In the Salpêtrière's amphitheater, he exhibited several patients with tremors, each wearing a headband to which he had affixed a long rod with a feather at the tip. As the audience watched, he asked his assistants to support the trunks of all the patients—and the feather on the head of the Parkinson's patient stopped moving because the tremor was not produced in the head or neck but was simply "overflow" from the body. Goetz, "Charcot and Parkinson's Disease," 24.
148. Richer and Meige, "Étude morphologique," 362.
149. Ibid. According to the case history, this patient also drooled, "ce qui donne au facies certaines analogies avec celui des malades atteints de paralysie gloss-labio-laryngée"; Richer and Meige, "Étude morphologique," 365.

150. Jean-Martin Charcot, *Oeuvres complètes. Leçons sur les maladies du système nerveux*, vol. 1 (Paris: Bureaux du progrès médical, 1886), 167; cited in Goetz, Bonduelle, and Gelfand, *Charcot*, 119.
151. Richer and Meige, "Étude morphologique," 369; emphasis added.
152. Ibid., 366–71.
153. Ibid., 370.
154. Comar, *Figures du corps*, 268.
155. Richer and Meige, "Étude morphologique," 369.
156. Ibid.
157. A series of chronophotographs of a man walking with assistance in *Figures du corps* might also be of Oll. See Comar, *Figures du corps*, 401–2, cat. 330.
158. McGrath, *Seeing Her Sex*, 18.
159. Daston and Galison, *Objectivity*, 6.
160. Meige, "Sur une statuette," 136–37; original emphasis.
161. Comar, *Figures du corps*, 404.
162. Blanchard, *Hommage*, 12. This was in contrast to his sculptures of laborers, which were cast in bronze editions for decades by Susse frères; Richer, "Notes biographiques." His *Écorché vivant* was also distributed for many years in 60 cm and 195 cm versions; advertisement by M. Barsanti, Paris, Richer Family archives.
163. This photograph was likely taken at the exhibition of Richer's work at the École des beaux-arts after his death. Philippe Richer, personal communication with the author, May 30, 2017.
164. Richer, "Dialogues sur l'art et la science. I," 42.
165. Ibid.
166. Ibid., 54.
167. Ibid., 43–44.
168. Ibid., 44.
169. Richer, "Dialogues sur l'art et la science. III," 443.
170. Ibid., 452.
171. Paul Richer, *Introduction à l'étude de la figure humaine* (Paris: Gaultier, Magnier, 1902), 20; cited in Comar, *Figures du* corps, 372.

CODA

1. For a brief biographical sketch of Leroux, see Aumasson and Pigallet, *Peintres de Pont-Aven*, 126.
2. Comar, *Figures du corps*, 256, cat. no. 108. ENSBA owns a study for the whole triptych: inv. no. EBA 7905, Paris, ENSBA; Brugerolles, "Paul Georges Leroux," 22. For an illustration of the table in the dissecting room (*laboratoire*), which was situated behind the amphitheater, see Lemaistre, *École des beaux-arts*, 129.
3. Richer, "Dialogues sur l'art et la science. III," 450.
4. Ruiz-Gómez, "Shaking the Tyranny."
5. R. Blondel, "Causerie médicale," n.p., Paris, Richer Family archives. This would also lead to Richer's association with eugenics; Brauer, "Dangerous Doubles"; Brauer, "Introduction."
6. See the advertisement by the Société d'édition artistique for the bronze editions of fifteen athletes by Richer from ca. 1900. See also Meige, "Sport dans l'art." Richer wrote about the representation of athletes too, possibly before he began sculpting them; Richer, "De la figuration artistique." All articles from Paris, Richer Family archives.
7. Richer, *L'Art et la médicine*, 3.
8. Opening lesson of November 25, 1903; quoted in Desprez, "Paul Richer," 40.
9. Callen, "Masculinity and Muscularity"; Comar, *Figures du corps*, 342–67; Mathon, "Corps modélisé"; Poivert, "Variété et vérité."
10. Ruiz-Gómez, "Shaking the Tyranny."
11. Duchenne, *Mécanisme de la physionomie humaine*, 14.
12. Marey, *Movement*, 304. See also Snyder, "Visualization and Visibility," 396; Jones and Galison, "Introduction."
13. Richer, *Physiologie artistique*, 7–8.
14. Hunter, *Face of Medicine*, 28.
15. Richer, *L'Art et la médicine*, 7.
16. Viney, Callard, and Woods, "Critical Medical Humanities," 5.
17. Elkins, *Domain of Images*, 52.
18. Joffroy, "Jean-Martin Charcot," 602.
19. Barker and Iacobuzio-Donahue, *Hidden Beauty*, 14.
20. Meige, "Docteur Paul Richer," 1–5. Paris, Richer Family archives.
21. Lacronique, *Médecins médailleurs*. Paris, Richer Family archives.
22. Richer, *Physiologie artistique*, fig. 114; Binet, "Paul Richer," 23; Comar, *Figures du corps*, 448–49.
23. Richer, "Notes biographiques"; Omer, "Docteur Richer," 2.
24. Undated letter from Charcot to Jean-Baptiste Charcot, Charcot Family archives; quoted in Bouchara, *Charcot*, 12.

Bibliography

PRIMARY SOURCES

Aicard, Jean. "M. Henry Cros—Les Cires." *La Renaissance littéraire et artistique* 1, no. 9 (June 22, 1872): 67.

Aragon, Louis, and André Breton. "Le Cinquantenaire de l'hystérie (1878–1928)." *La Révolution surréaliste* 4, no. 11 (March 15, 1928): 20–22.

Arène, Paul. "Le Docteur Charcot." *Gil Blas* 5, no. 1461 (November 18, 1883): 1–2.

Babinski, J[oseph]. "Eloge de J.-M. Charcot." *Revue neurologique* 1, no. 6 (June 1925): 746–56.

Baedeker, Karl. *Paris and Environs with Routes from London to Paris: Handbook for Travellers.* Leipzig: Karl Baedeker, 1894.

Ballu, Roger. "Salon de 1887." *L'Illustration*, April 30, 1887, n.p.

Baudelaire, Charles. *Les Fleurs du mal.* 1857. Paris: Librairie des Bibliophiles Parisiens, 1921.

———. "The Modern Public and Photography" [Salon of 1859]. In Charles Baudelaire, *Selected Writings on Art and Artists*, translated by P. E. Charvet, 291–98. Harmondsworth: Penguin, 1972.

Baudouin, A. "Quelques souvenirs de la Salpêtrière." *Paris médical*, no. 56 (1925): 517–20.

Baudouin, Marcel. *Guide médical à l'Exposition universelle internationale de 1889 à Paris.* Paris: Progrès médical / E. Lecrosnier & Babé, 1889.

Bech, M. *Traité pratique de retouche des clichés photographiques.* Paris, 1888.

Benoît, J. *Contribution à l'étude du myxoedème chez l'enfant et de ses formes frustres.* MD diss., Montpellier, 1903.

Bergert, Alphonse. "Académie des sciences." *Le Figaro*, January 21, 1913, 3.

Bernheim [Docteur]. "Hypnotisme et suggestion. Doctrine de la Salpêtrère et Doctrine de Nancy." *Supplément au journal Le Temps*, January 29, 1891, n.p.

Bertillon, Alphonse, and Arthur Chervin. *Anthropologie métrique.* Paris: Imprimerie nationale, 1909.

Blanchard, Raphaël. *Hommage à M. le Docteur Paul Richer à l'occasion de son élection à l'Académie des beaux-arts (22 juillet 1905).* Paris: Académie des beaux-arts, 1906.

Blondel, Raoul. "Causerie médicale. L'Art au service de la Science." *L'Écho de Paris*, June 3, 1925, n.p.

Blondel, Spire. "Les Ciriers modernes." *L'Artiste* 68, no. 1 (1898): 224–34.

———. "Les Modeleurs en cire." *Gazette des beaux-arts*, May 1, 1882, 493–504, and September 1, 1882, 259–72, 429–39.

Boix, Émile. "Myopathie primitive progressive." In *Traité de médecine*, vol. 10, edited by Charles Bouchard and Édouard Brissaud, 446–76. Paris: Masson, 1905.

Bonnetain, Paul. *Charlot s'amuse.* 1883. Paris: Flammarion, 2000.

Bouley, Paul. *Pathologie comparée. De l'ostéomalacie chez l'homme et les animaux domestiques.* MD diss., Paris, 1874.

Bourcard, Gustave. *À travers cinq siècles de gravures, 1350–1903. Les Estampes célèbres, rares ou curieuses.* Paris: Georges Rapilly, 1903.

Bourneville, [Désiré-Magloire]. "Préface." In *Iconographie photographique de la Salpétrière* [*sic*], by [Désiré-Magloire] Bourneville and P[aul] Regnard, vol. 1, iii–iv. Paris: Bureau du Progrès médical / Adrien Delahaye, 1877.

Bourneville, [Désiré-Magloire], and P[aul] Regnard. *Iconographie photographique de la Salpêtrière*. 3 vols. Paris: Bureau du Progrès médical / Adrien Delahaye, 1877–80.

Breton, Gaston le. *Essai historique sur la sculpture en cire*. Rouen: Espérance Cagniard, 1894.

Brouardel, P[aul]. *Le Secret médical*. Paris: Librairie J.-B. Baillière & fils, 1887.

Burckhardt, Gottlieb. "Contribution à l'étude de l'hystérie traumatique." *Revue médicale de la Suisse romande* 6 (1886): 735–46.

Burrows and Colton. *Concise Instructions in the Art of Retouching*. London: Marion, 1876.

Charcot, Jean-Baptiste. "Paul Richer." *Paris médical*, no. 92 (1934): 316–20.

Charcot, Jean-Martin. *Charcot the Clinician: The Tuesday Lessons; Excerpts from Nine Case Presentations on General Neurology Delivered at the Salpêtrière Hospital in 1887–88*. Translated, with commentary, by Christopher G. Goetz. New York: Raven Press, 1987.

———. "Demonstration of Arthropathic Affections of Locomotor Ataxia." *British Medical Journal*, August 13, 1881, 285.

———. *Études pour servir à l'histoire de l'affection décrite sous les noms de goutte asthénique primitive, nodosités des jointures, rhumatisme articulaire chronique (forme primitive), etc.* MD diss. Paris: Rignoux, 1853.

———. "La Foi qui guérit." 1892. In *Les Démoniaques dans l'art*, by J[ean-]M[artin] Charcot and Paul Richer, 111–23. Paris: Macula, 1984.

———. "Introduction. La Médecine empirique et la médecine scientifique parallèle entre les anciens et les modernes." 1867. In *Maladies des vieillards. Goutte et rhumatisme*, vol. 7, iii–xxxiii. Paris: Lecrosnier & Babé, 1890.

———. *Leçons sur les maladies du système nerveux faites à la Salpêtrière*. Vol. 2. Paris: Progrès médical / Adrien Delahaye, 1877.

———. *Oeuvres complètes*. Vols. 1–9. Paris: Bureaux du Progrès médical, 1888–94.

———. *Oeuvres complètes. Leçons sur les maladies du système nerveux*. Vol. 3. Paris: Aux Bureaux du Progrès médical / Lecrosnier & Babé, 1890.

———. "Physiologie pathologique.—Sur les divers états nerveux déterminés par l'hypnotisation chez les hystériques." *Comptes rendus hebdomadaires des séances de l'Académie des sciences* 94 (February 13, 1882): 403–5.

———. "Policlinique du mardi, 7 février 1888. Objet de la leçon: 1. Grande Hystérie ou Hystéro-Epilepsie; 2. Goître exophthamlique; 3. Hémichorée de Sydenham; 4. Paralysie faciale; 5. Dyspnée hystérique." In *Leçons du mardi à la Salpêtrière. Policlinique 1887–88. Notes de cours de MM. Blin, Charcot et Colin*, 173–97. Paris: Bureaux du Progrès médical / A. Delahaye & Emile Lecrosnier, 1887 [*sic*].

———. "Policlinique du mardi 12 juin 1888. Vingtième leçon. Objet: 1. Un cas complexe. Hystérie, Ataxie locomotrice, Vertige de Mônière chez une femme de 39 ans. 2. Un cas de maladie de Parkinson sans tremblement homme de 32 ans. 3. Un cas d'argyrie (coloration de la peau par l'argent) chez un ataxique." In *Leçons du mardi à la Salpêtrière. Policlinique 1878–1888. Notes de cours de MM. Blin, Charcot et H. Colin*, 321–43. Vol. 1. 2nd ed. Paris: Bureau du Progrès médical / Vve Babé, 1892.

———. "Policlinique du mardi 28 février 1888. Dixième leçon. Objet: 1. Sclérose latérale amyotrophique.—Paralysie labio-glosso-laryngée. 2. Astasie et Abasie, puis toux hystérique par accès réglés." In *Leçons du mardi à la Salpêtrière. Policlinique 1878–1888. Notes de cours de MM. Blin, Charcot et H. Colin*, 145–54. Vol. 1. 2nd ed. Paris: Bureau du Progrès médical / Vve Babé, 1892.

———. "Policlinique du mardi 30 octobre 1888. Deuxième leçon. 1er Malade: –Sur un même sujet: Sciatique avec déformation spéciale du tronc; à la suite d'un coup reçu sur le front, Neurasthénie et Hystérie. 2e Malade. –Chorée paralytique chez un enfant de huit ans; hérédité arthritique et névropathique." In *Leçons de mardi à la Salpêtrière. Policlinique 1888–1889. Notes de cours de MM. Blin, Charcot et Henri Colin*, 19–41. Paris: Progrès médical / E. Lecrosnier & Babé, 1889.

———. "Policlinique du mardi 31 janvier 1888. Huitième leçon. Objet: 1. Mal comitial. Automatisme ambulatoire. 2. Maladie de Parkinson (Paralysie agitante)." In *Leçons du mardi à la Salpêtrière. Policlinique 1887–1888. Notes de cours de MM. Blin, Charcot et H. Colin*, 112–27. Vol. 1. 2nd ed. Paris: Bureau du Progrès médical / Vve Babé, 1892.

Charcot, J[ean]-M[artin], and A. Dechambre. *De quelques marbres antiques concernant des études anatomiques*. Paris: Librairie de Victor Masson, 1857.

Charcot, J[ean]-M[artin], and Ch[arles] Féré. "Affections osseuses et articulaires du pied chez les tabetiques." *Archives de neurologie* 6, no. 18 (November 1883): 305–19.

Charcot, J[ean]-M[artin], and [Georges] Gilles de la Tourette. "Hypnotism in the Hysterical." In Tuke, *Dictionary of Psychological Medicine*, 1:606–10.

Charcot, J[ean]-M[artin], and A. Joffroy. "Deux cas d'atrophie musculaire progressive avec lésions de la substance grise et des faisceaux antérolatéraux de la moelle épinière." *Archives de physiologie normale et pathologique* 2 (1869): 354–67, 629–49, 744–60.

Charcot, [Jean-Martin], and Magnan. *Inversions du sens géneral et autres perversions sexuelles*. Paris: Bureaux du Progrès médical, 1883.

Charcot, J[ean]-M[artin], and Pierre Marie. "Hysteria Mainly Hystero-Epilepsy." In Tuke, *Dictionary of Psychological Medicine*, 1:627–41.

Charcot, [Jean-Martin], and Paul Richer. "Contribution à l'étude de l'hypnotisme chez les hystériques; du phénomène de l'hyperexcitabilité neuro-musculaire." *Archives de neurologie* 2 (1881): 173–215.

———. *Les Démoniaques dans l'art*. Paris: Adrien Delahaye & Émile Lecrosnier, 1887.

———. *Les Difformes et les malades dans l'art*. Paris: Lecrosnier & Babé, 1889.

———. *Le Mascaron grotesque de l'Église Santa Maria Formosa, à Venise et l'hémispasme glosso-labié hystérique*. Paris, 1888.

Chevallier, Paul, and René Hémard. *Catalogue des objets d'art et d'ameublement. . . . July 6–9, 1900*. Paris: Chevallier and Hémard, 1900.

"Chronique locale. Monluçon." *Le Centre*, June 9, 1889, n.p.

Claretie, Jules. *Les Amours d'un interne*. Paris: E. Dentu, 1881.

———. "Charcot, le consolateur." *Les Annales politiques et littéraires* 21, no. 1056 (1903): 179–80.

———. *La Vie à Paris, 1881*. Paris: Victor Havard, 1882.

"A Clinical Lesson at 'La Salpêtrière.'" *Scientific American Supplement* 23, no. 598 (June 18, 1887): 9556–57.

Cros, Henry, and Charles Henry. *L'Encaustique et les autres procédés de peinture chez les anciens. Histoire et technique*. Paris: J. Rouam, 1884.

Dalligny, Aug[uste]. "Le Salon de 1887. La Peinture." *Le Journal des arts* 9, no. 40 (June 3, 1887): 1–2.

Daudet, Alphonse. "À la Salpêtrière." *La Chronique medicale. Revue bi-mensuelle de médecine scientifique, littéraire et anecdotique* 5, no. 1 (January 1898): 15–18.

———. *In the Land of Pain*. Edited and translated by Julian Barnes. London: Jonathan Cape, 2002. Originally published as *La Doulou* (1930).

Daudet, Léon. *Devant la douleur. Souvenirs des milieux littéraires, politiques, artistiques et médicaux de 1880 à 1905*. Paris: Nouvelle Librairie nationale, 1915.

———. *Les Morticoles*. Paris: G. Charpentier & E. Fasquelle, 1894.

———. "Le Professeur Charcot ou le Césarisme de Faculté." In *Les Oeuvres dans les hommes*, 197–243. Paris: Nouvelle Librairie Nationale, 1922.

Delboeuf, J[oseph Rémi Léopold]. "Une visite à la Salpêtrière." *Revue de Belgique* 54 (1886): 121–47, 258–75.

Devillers, Hippolyte. "Salon de Paris." *La Jeune belgique*, 1887, 232–37.

Diamond, Hugh W. "On the Application of Photography to the Physiognomic and Mental Phenomena of Insanity." 1856. In *The Face of Madness: Hug W. Diamond and the Origin of Psychiatric Photography*, edited by Sander L. Gilman, 19–24. Secaucus, NJ: Citadel Press, 1976.

"Le Docteur Paul Richer." In *Figures contemporaines tirées de l'album Mariani*, vol. 6, n.p. Paris: Librairie Henri Floury, 1901.

Dreyfous, Maurice. *Dalou. Sa vie et son oeuvre*. Paris: Librairie Renouard, 1903.

Dubray, P. "Promenades au Salon." *L'Union médicale*, May 14, 1887, 753–59.

Duchenne (de Boulogne), G[uillaume]-B[enjamin]. "De l'ataxie locomotrice progressive, recherches sur une maladie caractérisée spécialement par les troubles généraux de la coordination des mouvements." *Archives générales de médecine*, 1858, 641–52.

———. "De l'atrophie musculaire progressive de l'enfance, et de son diagnostic éclairé par l'iconographie photographique." *Revue photographique des hôpitaux* 1 (1869): 41–45.

———. *De l'électrisation localisée et de son application à la physiologie, à la pathologie et à la thérapeutique*. 3rd ed. Paris: J. B. Baillière, 1872.

———. *Mécanisme de la physionomie humaine ou analyse électro-physiologique de l'expression des passions*. Paris: Jules Renouard, 1862.

———. "Recherches sur la paralysie musculaire pseudo-hypertrophique ou paralysie myo-sclérosique." *Archives générales de médecine*, 1868, 5–25, 179–209, 305–21, 421–43, 552–88.

Durieu, E[ugène]. "Sur la retouche des épreuves photographiques." *Bulletin de la Société française de la photographie*, October 1855, 297–304.

"Échoes. La Température." *Le Figaro*, April 19, 1928, 1.

"Editorial Notes." *Photographic Times and American Photographer* 25, no. 671 (July 27, 1894): 60.

Edwards, Henry Sutherland. *Old and New Paris: Its History, Its People, and Its Places*. Vol. 2. London: Cassell, 1894.

Esquirol, Jean-Étienne-Dominique. *Des maladies mentales considérées sous les rapports médical, hygiénique et médico-légal*. 1838. Paris: Frénésie Éditions, 1989.

Explication des ouvrages de peinture, sculpture, architecture, gravure et lithographie des artistes vivants exposés au Palais des Champs-Élysées le 1er mai 1889. 2nd ed. Paris: Paul Dupont, 1889.

Féré, Ch[arles]. "Description de quelques pièces relatives aux lésions osseuses et articulaires des ataxiques, conservées au musée anatomo-pathologique de la Salpêtrière." *Archives de neurologie* 4, no. 11 (September 1882): 202–18.

———. "Iconographie photographique de la Salpêtrière." *Archives de neurologie* 1, no. 4 (1881): 625–31.

———. "J.-M. Charcot et son oeuvre." *Revue des deux mondes*, 1894, 410–24.

Ferrier, David. *On Tabes Dorsalis: The Lumleian Lectures Delivered Before the Royal College of Physicians, London, March, 1906*. London: John Bale, Sons & Danielsson, 1906.

"The Festivities of the Congress." *British Medical Journal* 2 (August 13, 1881): 303–4.

Fourcaud, Louis de. "L'Art contemporain. École française." In *Revue de l'Exposition Universelle de 1889*, 1:20–26. Paris: Ludovic Baschet, 1889.

———. "La Peinture française. 11. Le dix-neuvième siècle." In *L'Art à l'Exposition Universelle de 1900*, edited by Jules Comte, 105–86. Paris: Librairie de l'art ancien et moderne, 1900.

Freud, Sigmund. "An Autobiographical Study." In *The Standard Edition of The Complete Psychological Works of Sigmund Freud*, edited and translated by James Strachey et al., vol. 20, *1925–1926*, 7–70. London: Hogarth Press and the Institute of Psycho-Analysis, 1959.

———. "Charcot." In *The Standard Edition of the Complete Psychological Works of Sigmund Freud*, edited and translated by James Strachey et al., vol. 3, *1893–1899*, 11–23. London: Hogarth Press and the Institute of Psycho-Analysis, 1962.

———. *Five Lectures on Psycho-Analysis*. 1910. Translated and edited by James Strachey. New York: W. W. Norton, 1989.

———. "On the History of the Psychoanalytic Movement." In *The Standard Edition of The Complete Psychological Works of Sigmund Freud*, edited and translated by James Strachey et al., vol. 14, *1914–1916*, 7–66. London: Hogarth Press and the Institute of Psycho-Analysis, 1957.

———. *The Letters of Sigmund Freud, 1873–1939*. Edited by Ernst L. Freud and translated by Tania and James Stern. London: Hogarth Press, 1961.

———. "Report on My Studies in Paris and Berlin." 1886. In *The Standard Edition of the Complete Psychological Works of Sigmund Freud*, edited and translated by James Strachey et al., vol. 1, *1886–1899*, 5–15. London: Hogarth Press and the Institute of Psycho-Analysis, 1966.

———. "The 'Uncanny.'" 1919. In *The Standard Edition of the Complete Psychological Works of Sigmund Freud*, edited and translated by James Strachey et al., vol. 17, *1917–1919*, 218–52. London: Hogarth Press and the Institute of Psycho-Analysis, 1955.

Freud, Sigmund, and Joseph Breuer. *Studies in Hysteria*. 1895. Translated by Nicola Luckhurst. New York: Penguin Books, 2004.

Geffroy, Gustave. *La Vie artistique*. 2nd ser. Paris: E. Dentu, 1893.

Gilles de la Tourette, Georges. "Biographies médicales. Les Médecins contemporains. Le Dr Paul Richer. Membre de l'Académie de Médecine." *Le Progrès médical*, July 2, 1898, 10.

———. "Jean-Martin Charcot." *Nouvelle Iconographie de la Salpêtrière* 6 (1893): 241–50.

Goetschy, Gustave. "Les Femmes du monde artistes. Madame Charcot." *Revue des arts décoratifs* 20, no. 1 (January 1900): 41–51.

Gombault, [Albert]. "Sclérose symétrique des cordons latéraux de la moëlle et des pyramides antérieures dans le bulbe. Atrophie des cellules des cornes antérieures de la moëlle. Atrophie musculaire progressive. Paralysie glosso-laryngée." *Archives de physiologie normale et pathologique* 4, no. 4 (1871–72): 509–18.

Goncourt, Edmond de, and Jules de Goncourt. *Journal: Mémoires de la vie littéraire*. Edited and annotated by Robert Ricatte. 4 vols. Paris: Fasquelle & Flammarion, 1956.

Gonse, Louis. "Musée de Lille. Le Musée Wicar. Objets d'art: La Tête de cire." *Gazette des beaux-arts*, March 1, 1878, 193–205.

Gould, George M. *A New Medical Dictionary: Including All the Words and Phrases Used in Medicine, with Their Proper Pronunciation and Definitions*. London: H. K. Lewis, 1890.

Guillemot, Maurice. "À la Salpêtrière." *Paris illustré*, September 24, 1887, 354–55.

———. "À la Salpêtrière. II." *Paris illustré*, October 1, 1887, 371–74.

Guinon, Georges. "Deux types de myopathie progressive du type Landouzy-Déjerine." *Nouvelle Iconographie de la Salpêtrière* 6 (1893): 8–20.

———. "Charcot intime." *Paris médical*, no. 56 (1925): 511–16.

Guinon, Georges, and A[chilles] Souques. "Déformations thoraciques dans la myopathie progressive primitive." *Bulletin de la Société anatomique de Paris*, June 1891, 348–51.

Gyp [Marie-Antoinette de Riqueti de Mirabeau, comtesse de Martel]. "Au Salon." *L'Univers illustré*, May 7, 1887, 298.

Hahn, G. "Charcot et son influence sur l'opinion publique." *Revue des questions scientifiques*, July 1894, 230–61, and October 1894, 353–79.

"Hospice de la Salpétrière [*sic*].—Conférences cliniques de M. Charcot." *Le Progrès médical* 3, no. 49 (December 4, 1875): 718–19.

"Hospice de la Salpêtrière.—M. Charcot." *Le Progrès médical* 7, no. 47 (November 2, 1879): 913.

Hourticq, Louis. "Paul Richer." *Bulletin de l'Académie des beaux-arts* 9, no. 18 (July 1933): 142–49.

H[ubert], É[douard]. "Salon de 1887. *Séance clinique de la Salpêtrière*. Tableau du M. A. Brouillet." *Le Monde illustré* 31, no. 1570 (April 30, 1887): 282, 284–85.

Ignotus [Félix Platel]. "Cabotinage." *Le Figaro* 29, no. 108 (April 18, 1883): 1.

———. "M. Charcot." In *Les Hommes de mon temps*, 377–88. Paris: Bureaux du Figaro, 1878.

International Medical Congress. Catalogue of Temporary Museum held at the Geological Society, Burlington House. Seventh Session. From August 2nd to August 9th, 1881. London, 1881.

Janet, Pierre. "J.-M. Charcot. Son oeuvre psychologique." *Revue philosophique* 39 (June 1895): 569–604.

Johnson, Robert. *A Complete Treatise on the Art of Retouching Photographic Negatives and Clear Directions How to Finish and Colour Photographs*. London: Marion, 1886.

Joffroy, A. "Jean-Martin Charcot." *Archives de médecine expérimentale et d'anatomie pathologique*, 1893, 577–606.

Ken, Alexandre. *Dissertations historiques, artistiques et scientifiques sur la photographie*. Paris: Librairie Nouvelle, 1864.

Klary, C. *L'Art de retoucher les négatifs photographiques*. Paris: Gauthier-Villars & fils, 1888.

Lacronique, R. *Médecins médailleurs. Le Dr Paul Richer et ses précurseurs*. Chalon-sur-Saône: E. Bertrand; Paris: Vve R. Serrure, 1905.

Lafenestre, G[eorge]. "Le Salon de 1887." *Revue des deux mondes*, June 1, 1887, 604–39.

Lami, Stanislas. *Dictionnaire des sculpteurs de l'École française au dix-neuvième siècle.* Vol. 10, *D–F.* Paris: Librairie ancienne Honoré Champion, 1916.

Landouzy, L[ouis]. "Note sur le facies myopathique et sa valeur dans la séméiotique de l'enfant et de l'adulte." *Bulletins et mémoires de la Société médicale des hôpitaux de Paris*, October 22, 1886, 419–28.

Landouzy, L[ouis], and J[oseph Jules] Dejerine. "Contribution à l'étude de la myopathie atrophique progressive (myopathie atrophique progressive, à type scapulo–huméral)." *Comptes rendus hebdomadaires des séances et mémoires de la Société de biologie* 3, no. 8 (1886): 478–81.

———. "De la myopathie atrophique progressive: Myopathie sans neuropathie débutant d'ordinaire dans l'enfance par la face." *Revue de médecine française* 5 (1885): 81–117, 253–366.

Larousse, Pierre. *Grand Dictionnaire universel du XIXe siècle, français, historique, géographique, mythologique, bibliographique, littéraire, artistique, scientifique, etc.* Paris, 1864–90.

Larroumet, Gustave. *Le Salon de 1892.* Paris: Boussod, Valadon, 1892.

Lebrun et al. *Nouveau Manuel complet du mouleur en plâtre, au ciment, à l'argile, à la cire, à la gélatine. . . .* Paris: Librairie encyclopédique de Roret, 1875.

Le Gendre, Paul. "Richer (Paul-Marie-Louis-Pierre)." *Les Biographies médicales. Notes pour servir à l'histoire de la médecine et des grands médecins* 9, no. 2 (February 1935): 65–76.

Lemaistre, Alexis. *L'École des beaux-arts. Dessinée et racontée par un élève.* Paris: Librairie Firmin-Didot, 1889.

Lenoir, Paul. *Histoire du réalisme et du naturalisme dans la poésie et dans l'art depuis l'antiquité jusqu'à nos jours.* Paris: Quantin, 1889.

Le Noir, P., and Paul Bezançon. "Observation de myopathie progressive primitive, type facio-scapulo-huméral de Landouzy-Dejerine." *Revue de médecine* 10, no. 4 (April 10, 1890): 307–14.

Levillain, F[ernand]. "Charcot et l'École de la Salpêtrière." *Revue encyclopédique* 4, no. 78 (March 1, 1894): 108–15.

Londe, Albert. *La Photographie dans les arts, les sciences et l'industrie. Conférence faite au Conservatoire national des Arts et Métiers le 18 mars 1888.* Paris: Gauthier-Villars & fils, 1888.

———. "La Photographie en médecine. Appareil photo-électrique." *La Nature*, no. 535 (September 1, 1883): 215–18.

———. "La Photographie et les falsifications." *La Nature*, no. 970 (January 2, 1892): 74–76.

———. *La Photographie médicale. Application aux sciences médicales et physiologiques.* Paris: Gauthier-Villars & fils, 1893.

———. *La Photographie moderne. Pratique et applications.* Paris: G. Masson, 1888.

———. "Sciences médicales. La Photographie en médecine." *Revue scientifique (Revue rose)* 49, no. 9 (February 27, 1892): 257–65.

———. "Le Service photographique de la Salpêtrière." *Archives de l'électricité médicale, expérimentales et cliniques* 7, no. 78 (June 15, 1899): 282–96.

Lorde, André de. *Théâtre d'épouvante.* Paris: Eugène Fasquelle, 1909.

Lubimoff, A[lexis]. *Le Professeur Charcot: Étude scientifico-biographique.* Translated by Comtesse Lydie Rostopchine. Paris: A. S. Souvorine, 1894.

Maloney, William J. M. A. *Locomotor Ataxia (Tabes Dorsalis): An Introduction to the Study and Treatment of Nervous Diseases, for Students and Practitioners.* New York: D. Appleton, 1918.

Mantz, Paul. "La Galerie Pourtalès." *Gazette des beaux-arts*, February 1, 1865, 97–117.

———. "Le Salon (Champs-Elysées) VI." *Le Temps* [Paris], June 18, 1890, 1–2.

———. *Salon de 1889.* Paris: Ludovic Baschet, 1889.

———. "Le Salon VII." *Le Temps* [Paris], June 24, 1888, 1–2.

Marey, Étienne-Jules, and G[eorges] Demeny. *Études de physiologie artistique faites au moyen de la chronophotographie.* Sér. 1, no. 1, *Des mouvements de l'homme.* Paris: Société d'éditions scientifiques, 1893.

Marey, É[tienne]-J[ules]. *Movement.* Translated by Eric Pritchard. New York: D. Appleton, 1895.

Marie, Pierre. "Éloge de J.-M. Charcot." *Revue neurologique* 1, no. 6 (June 1925): 731–45.

"M. Charcot à la Salpêtrière." *Les Annales politiques et littéraires* 3, no. 106 (July 5, 1885): 12–13.

Meige, Henry. "Les Amyotrophiques dans l'art." *Nouvelle Iconographie de la Salpêtrière* 7 (1894): 198–204.

———. "Charcot artiste." *Nouvelle Iconographie de la Salpêtrière* 11 (1898): 489–516.

———. *Charcot artiste.* Paris: Masson, 1925.

———. "Le Docteur Paul Richer." *Le Moniteur du dessin* 26, no. 282 (April 1922): 1–5.

———. "La Facies dans la paralysie glosso-labio laryngée [*sic*]." *Nouvelle Iconographie de la Salpêtrière* 7 (1894): 379–80.

———. "Paul Richer et son oeuvre." *La Presse médicale* 42, no. 6 (January 20, 1934): 123–26.

———. "Les Peintres de la médecine (Écoles flamande et hollandaise). Les Operations sur la tête. Suite et fin." *Nouvelle Iconographie de la Salpêtrière* 8 (1895): 291–322.

———. "Le Sport dans l'art. Les Statuettes athlétiques du Dr Richer." *La Vie au grand air* 3, no. 112 (November 4, 1900): 766–77.

———. "Sur une statuette représentant l'infantilisme myxoedémateux." *Nouvelle Iconographie de la Salpêtrière* 11 (1898): 136–40.

Meige, Henry, and Félix Allard. "Deux infantiles: Infantile myxoedèmateux et infantile de Lorain." *Nouvelle Iconographie de la Salpêtrière* 11 (1898): 105–13.

Meillet, Henri. *Des déformations permanentes de la main au point de vue de la séméiologie médicale.* MD diss. Paris: A. Parent, 1874.

Merson, Olivier. "Salon de 1887. II." *Le Monde illustré* 31, no. 1572 (May 14, 1887): 315, 318.

Méryem, Jean. "Les Dessins d'Henry Cros." *L'Art et les artistes* 15 (April–September 1912): 174–77.

Meurville. "Le Salon. XII. Deuxième partie. La Nature au salon." *Gazette de France,* May 28, 1887, n.p.

Mirbeau, Octave. "Le Siècle de Charcot." 1885. In *Chroniques du diable,* edited and annotated by Pierre Michel, 121–27. Paris: Diffusion les Belles Lettres, 1995.

Morel, B. A. *Traité des dégénérescences physiques, intellectuelles et morales de l'espèce humaine . . . Atlas de XII Planches.* Paris: J. B. Baillière, 1857.

Morton, [Reverend] H. J. "Photography as an Authority." *Philadelphia Photographer* 1 (1864): 180–83.

Mossé, A. "Affection osseuse généralisée à plusieurs parties du squelette. Fracture spontanée du fémur. Phlegmon orbitaire et fonte de l'oeil. Infection purulente." *Bulletin de la Société anatomique de Paris,* March 1878, 157–59.

Mott, F. W. "Tabes in Asylum and Hospital Practice." In *Archives of Neurology from the Pathological Laboratory of the London County Asylums, Claybury, Essex,* 2:1–327. London: Macmillan, 1903.

Munthe, Axel. *The Story of San Michele.* Hamburg: The Albatross, 1935.

Natton, P. *Instruments et appareils de l'art médical.* Paris: Grandrémy, 1900.

Nordau, Max. *Degeneration.* 1895. Lincoln: University of Nebraska Press, 1993.

"L'Oeuvre medico-artistique de la Nouvelle Iconographie de la Salpêtrière." *Nouvelle Iconographie de la Salpêtrière* 16 (1903): 413–29.

"L'Oeuvre sculpturale du Professeur Paul Richer, à Chartres." *La Dépêche d'Eure-et-Loir,* December 21, 1933, n.p.

Ollendorf, Gustave. *Salon de 1887. Cent planches en photogravures par Goupil & Cie.* Paris: Ludovic Baschet, 1887.

Omer, Georges. "Le Docteur Richer, de l'Académie de Médecine est aussi le sculpteur Paul Richer." *Paris-Soir,* March 6, 1931, 2.

Paris, Jean de. "Exécution de Barré et Lebiez." *Le Figaro,* September 8, 1878, 1–2.

"Paul Richer." *Les Biographies médicales* 9, no. 2 (February 1935): 65–76.

Périer, Paul. "Exposition universelle. Troisième article. Photographes français." *Bulletin de la Société française de la photographie,* July 1855, 187–200.

Peugniez, Paul. *J.-M. Charcot (1825–1893).* Amiens: Imprimerie Picarde, 1893.

Pierret, M. "Note sur la sclérose des cordons postérieurs dans l'ataxie locomotrice progressive." *Archives de physiologie normale et pathologique* 4, no. 3 (May 1872): 364–79.

Piquepé, Paul. *Traité pratique de la retouche des clichés photographiques.* Paris: Gauthier-Villars, 1881.

Ponsonhailhe, Charles. "Le Salon. Peinture. I." *L'Artiste* [Paris] 57 (June 1887): 411–45.

———. "Le Salon. Peinture. II." *L'Artiste* [Paris] 57 (July 1887): 19–49.

Pont-Calé. "Le Professeur Charcot." *Les Hommes d'aujourd'hui* 7, no. 343 (1890): 1–3.

Raymond, Fulgence. "Du myxoedème infantile et des autres formes de myxoedème. Pathogénie et traitement." *Revue internationale de thérapeutique et pharmacologie* 6, no. 1 (January 18, 1898): 1–14, and 6, no. 2 (February 16, 1898): 41–53.

Regnard, Paul, and [Désiré-Magloire] Bourneville. *Iconographie photographique de la Salpétrière* [*sic*]. *Service de M. Charcot.* [Paris?], 1875.

Regnard, P[aul], and P[aul] Richer. "Études sur l'attaque hystéro-épileptique faites à l'aide de la méthode graphique." *Revue mensuelle de médecine et de chirurgie* 2 (September 1878): 641–61.

Renouard, Paul. *Docteur Charcot. Revue illustrée* 4, no. 40 (August 1, 1887): cover.

"Retouching and Photographic Truth." *Photographic News*, January 19, 1872, 25–26.

Reveillé-Parise, J.-H. *Traité de la vieillesse hygiénique, médical et philosophique.* Paris: J.-B. Baillière, 1853.

Richer, Paul. *Anatomie artistique. Description des formes extérieures du corps humain au repos et dans les principaux mouvements.* Paris: Plon, 1890.

———. "L'Anatomie vivante. Leçon d'ouverture du Cours d'anatomie de l'École nationale des Beaux-Arts (November 9, 1908)." *Le Bulletin médical*, December 5, 1908, 1081–89.

———. "Anthropologie. Les Proportions du corps humain." *Revue scientifique (Revue rose)* 50, no. 18 (October 29, 1892): 558–64.

———. *L'Art et la médecine.* Paris: Gaultier, Magnier, [1902].

———. "L'Art préhistorique. À propos de la statue 'le Premier artiste' du Muséum." *L'Artiste*, 1891, 453–74.

———. *Canon des proportions du corps humain.* Paris: Librairie Ch. Delagrave, 1893.

———. "De la figuration artistique de la course." *La Revue de l'art ancien et moderne* 1, no. 4 (July 10, 1897): 304–20.

———. "De la station et de la marche chez les myopathiques." *Nouvelle Iconographie de la Salpêtrière* 7 (1894): 129–41.

———. *Dialogues sur l'art et la science.* Auxerre: Albert Lanier, 1897.

———. "Dialogues sur l'art et la science. I. Des rapports de l'art et la science." *La Nouvelle Revue*, July 1, 1897, 41–54.

———. "Dialogues sur l'art et la science. II. Le Vrai de l'art." *La Nouvelle Revue*, July 15, 1897, 228–41.

———. "Dialogues sur l'art et la science. III. L'Avenir de l'art." *La Nouvelle Revue*, August 1, 1897, 440–52.

———. *Documents inédits sur les démoniaques dans l'art.* Paris: Masson, 1896.

———. *Études cliniques sur la grande hystérie ou hystéro-épilepsie.* Paris: Adrien Delahaye & Emile Lecrosnier, 1881.

———. *Études cliniques sur la grande hystérie ou hystéro-épilepsie.* 2nd ed. Paris: Adrien Delahaye & Emile Lecrosnier, 1885.

———. *Feuilles d'autopsie pour l'étude des localisations cérébrales.* Paris: V. Adrien Delahaye / Bureaux du progrès médical, 1878.

———. *Introduction à l'Étude de la figure humaine.* Paris: Gaultier, Magnier, 1902.

———. "Notes biographiques." Unpublished manuscript. Inv. Ms. 837, École nationale supérieure des beaux-arts.

———. *Notice sur les titres et travaux scientifiques de M. le Dr Paul Richer.* Paris: L. Battaille, 1896.

———. *Nouvelle Anatomie artistique.* 6 vols. Paris: Plon-Nourrit, 1906–29.

———. "Observation de contracture. Hystérique guérie subitement après une durée de deux années." *Nouvelle Iconographie de la Salpêtrière* 2 (1889): 208–13.

———. *Physiologie artistique de l'homme en mouvement.* Paris: O. Doin, 1895.

Richer, Paul, [Georges] Gilles de la Tourette, and Albert Londe. "Avertissement." *Nouvelle Iconographie de la Salpêtrière* 1 (1888): i–iv.

Richer, Paul, and Henry Meige. "Étude morphologique sur la Maladie de Parkinson." *Nouvelle Iconographie de la Salpêtrière* 8 (1895): 361–71.

Robida, A[lbert]. "Au Salon." *La Caricature*, no. 390 (June 18, 1887): 1.

Robinson, Henry Peach. *Pictorial Effect in Photography: Being Hints on Composition and Chiaro-Oscuro for Photographers. To Which Is Added a Chapter on Combination Printing.* London: Piper and Carter, 1869.

Ruskin, John. *The Stones of Venice.* Vol. 3, *The Fall.* New York: Merrill and Baker, 1851.

Salon de 1887. Catalogue illustré. Peinture et sculpture. Paris: Ludovic Baschet, 1887.

Savard, P. "Fracture double verticale du bassin avec perforation de la vessie. Pas de lésions de l'urèthre." *Bulletin de la Société anatomique de Paris*, April 1878, 215–17.

"Service de l'électrothérapie, à la Salpêtrière." *Le Monde illustré* 31, no. 1585 (August 14, 1887): 99–102.

Smith, William. *A New Classical Dictionary of Biography, Mythology, and Geography*. London: John Murray, 1853.

Souques, A[chille]. "Charcot intime." *La Presse médicale*, no. 42 (May 27, 1925): 693–98.

———. "Décès de M. Paul Richer." *Bulletin de l'Académie de médecine*, December 19, 1933, 707–8.

Souques, Achilles, and Henry Meige. "Jean-Martin Charcot." *Les Biographies médicales*, May–June–July 1939, 329–36, 337–52.

Testard, Maurice. "Henry Cros." *L'Art décoratif*, no. 115 (April 1908): 149–55.

Théophraste. "Chronique scientifique." *Gazette de France*, May 30–31, 1887, n.p.

Transactions of the International Medical Congress. Seventh Session held in London, August 2nd to August 9th, 1881. Vol. 1. London: J. W. Kolckmann, 1881.

Tuke, Daniel Hack, ed. *A Dictionary of Psychological Medicine Giving the Definition, Etymology and Synonyms of the Terms Used in Medical Psychology with the Symptoms, Treatment, and Pathology of Insanity and the Law of Lunacy in Great Britain and Ireland*. 2 vols. London: J. & A. Churchill, 1892.

———. "Locomotor Ataxy, Tabes Dorsalis, Ataxie Locomotrice Progressive." In *A Dictionary of Psychological Medicine*, 2:750–51.

"Varia. Appréciation du *New York Medical Record* sur l'enseignement de M. Charcot à la Salpêtrière." *Le Progrès médical*, 2nd ser., vol. 1 (1885): 138–39.

Vogel, Hermann. *The Chemistry of Light and Photography*. New York: D. Appleton, 1875.

———. "Photography and Truth." *Philadelphia Photographer* 6 (1869): 262–64.

Wolff, Albert. "Courrier de Paris." *Le Figaro*, December 29, 1882, 1.

Young, Andrew. *The ABC of Retouching. With Examples and a Guide to the Anatomy of Expression*. London: Percy Lund, 1895.

SECONDARY SOURCES

Ackerman, Gerald. *Jean-Léon Gérôme. Monographie révisée. Catalogue raisonné mis à jour*. Courbevoie/Paris: ACR Édition, 2000.

Administration générale de l'Assistance Publique. *Cent ans d'Assistance Publique (1849–1949)*. Paris: Administration générale de l'Assistance Publique, 1949.

Alberti, Samuel J. M. M. *Morbid Curiosities: Medical Museums in Nineteenth-Century Britain*. Oxford: Oxford University Press, 2011.

Alberti, Samuel J. M. M., and Elizabeth Hallam, eds. *Medical Museums: Past, Present, Future*. London: Royal College of Surgeons, 2013.

Albinson, Cassandra. "Dalou in England: Portraits of Womanhood, 1871–1879." In *Dalou in England: Portraits of Womanhood, 1871–1879*, 9–16. New Haven: Yale Center for British Art, 2009. Exhibition catalog.

Amirault, Chris. "Posing the Subject of Early Medical Photography." *Discourse* 16, no. 2 (1993–94): 51–76.

L'Art du nu au XIXe siècle. Le Photographe et son modèle. Paris: Hazan/Bibliothèque nationale de France, 1997. Exhibition catalog.

Atkinson, Sarah, et al., eds. *The Edinburgh Companion to the Critical Medical Humanities*. Edinburgh: Edinburgh University Press, 2016.

Aumasson, Pascal, and Mathilde Pigallet. *Les Peintres de Pont-Aven et les Nabis*. Brest: Musée des beaux-arts de Brest, 2013. Exhibition catalog.

Autexier, Hughes, and François Braunschweig with Claude Léger. *De l'angoisse à l'extase*. Paris: Cimaise, 1984. Exhibition catalog.

Baer, Ulrich. "Photography and Hysteria: Towards a Poetics of the Flash." *Yale Journal of Criticism* 7, no. 1 (1994): 41–78.

Ballestriero, Roberta. "Anatomical Models and Wax Venuses: Art Masterpieces or Scientific Craft Works?" *Journal of Anatomy* 216, no. 2 (2010): 223–34.

Bann, Stephen. "The Photographic Album as a Cultural Accumulator." In *Art and the Early Photographic Album*, edited by Stephen Bann, 7–29. New Haven: Yale University Press, 2011.

Barker, Norman, and Christine Iacobuzio-Donahue, eds. *Hidden Beauty: Exploring the Aesthetics of Medical Science.* Atglen, PA: Schiffer Publishing, 2013.

Barnes, Julian. "Breaking the Mould." *The Telegraph,* December 15, 2001. http://www.telegraph.co.uk/culture/4727015/Breaking-the-mould.html.

———. "Introduction." In Alphonse Daudet, *In the Land of Pain,* edited and translated by Julian Barnes, v–xv. London: Jonathan Cape, 2002.

Barthes, Roland. *Camera Lucida: Reflections on Photography.* London: Jonathan Cape, 1982.

———. "Rhetoric of the Image." In *Image Music Text,* translated by Stephen Heath, 32–51. London: Fontana, 1977.

Bata, Philippe. "Préface." In Philippe Bata et al., *André Brouillet, 1857–1914,* 5–6. Poitiers: Musées de la Ville de Poitiers, 2000. Exhibition catalog.

Bata, Philippe, et al., *André Brouillet, 1857–1914.* Poitiers: Musées de la Ville de Poitiers, 2000. Exhibition catalog.

Baudrillard, Jean. "The System of Collecting." In *The Cultures of Collecting,* edited by John Elsner and Roger Cardinal, 7–24. London: Reaktion Books, 1994.

Becker, Edwin, and Gabriel P. Weisberg. "Introducing Naturalism." In Weisberg et al., *Illusions of Reality,* 13–16.

Beizer, Janet. *Ventriloquized Bodies: Narratives of Hysteria in Nineteenth-Century France.* Ithaca: Cornell University Press, 1994.

Belfort, Anne-Marie. "Pâtes de verre d'Henry Cros (1840–1907)." *Cahiers de la céramique du verre et des arts du feu,* no. 39 (1967): 176–87.

Bernard, Denis, and André Gunthert. *L'Instant rêvé. Albert Londe.* Nîmes: Jacqueline Chambon-Trois, 1993.

Berson, Ruth. *The New Painting: Impressionism 1874–1886.* Vol. 1. San Francisco: Fine Art Museums of San Francisco, 1996.

Biernoff, Suzannah. "A Necessary Humanity." In *War, Art and Surgery: The Work of Henry Tonks and Julia Midgley,* edited by Samuel J. M. M. Alberti, 120–27. London: Royal College of Surgeons of England, 2014.

———. "Picturing Pain." In *Encountering Pain: Hearing, Seeing, Speaking,* edited by Deborah Padfield and Joanna M. Zakrzewska, 190–213. London: UCL Press, 2021.

———. *Portraits of Violence: War and the Aesthetics of Disfigurement.* Ann Arbor: University of Michigan Press, 2017.

———. "The Rhetoric of Disfigurement in First World War Britain." *Social History of Medicine* 24, no. 3 (2011): 666–85.

Binet, J.-L. "Paul Richer et Elie Faure: Théoriciens de l'art et médecins." *Gazette médicale* 96, no. 28 (1989): 21–26.

Blackshaw, Gemma. "The Pathological Body: Modernist Strategising in Egon Schiele's Self-Portraiture." *Oxford Art Journal* 30, no. 3 (2007): 379–401.

Blon, Philippe, et al. *Voir—La Collection Spitzner.* Tressan: Antigone, 1998.

Blühm, Andreas. "In Living Colour: A Short History of Colour in Sculpture in the 19th Century." In *The Colour of Sculpture, 1840–1910,* edited by Andreas Blühm and Penelope Curtis, 11–60. Amsterdam: Van Gogh Museum, 1996. Exhibition catalog.

Boëtsch, Gilles. "From Cabinets of Curiosities to the Passion for the 'Savage.'" In *Human Zoos: The Invention of the Savage,* edited by Pascal Blanchard, Gilles Boëtsch, and Nanette Jacomijn Snoep, 78–97. Paris: Musée du Quai Branly / Actes Sud, 2011. Exhibition catalog.

Boggs, Jean Sutherland, et al. *Degas.* New York: Metropolitan Museum of Art, 1988. Exhibition catalog.

Bogousslavsky, Julien. "Charcot and Art: From a Hobby to Science." *European Neurology* 51, no. 2 (2004): 78–83.

Bonduelle, Michel. "Charcot et les Daudet." *La Presse médicale* 22, no. 32 (1993): 1641–48.

———. "Charcot intime." *Revue neurologique* 150, no. 8–9 (1994): 524–28.

Bonduelle, Michel, and Toby Gelfand. "Hysteria Behind the Scenes: Jane Avril at the Salpêtrière." *Journal of the History of the Neurosciences* 7, no. 1 (1998): 35–42.

Bouchara, Catherine. *Charcot, une vie avec l'image.* Paris: Philippe Rey, 2013.

Brais, Bernard. "The Making of a Famous Nineteenth Century Neurologist: Jean-Martin Charcot (1825–1893)." MPhil, Wellcome Unit for the History of Medicine, University College London, 1990.

Brauer, Fae. "'L'Art eugénique': Biopower and the Biocultures of Neo-Lamarckian

Eugenics." *L'Esprit créateur* 52, no. 2 (2012): 42–58.

———. "Dangerous Doubles: Degenerate and Regenerate Body Photography in the Eugenic Imagination." In *Image and Imagination*, edited by Martha Langford, 91–102. Toronto: McGill-Queen's University Press, 2005.

———. "Eroticizing Lamarckian Eugenics: The Body Stripped Bare During French Sexual Neoregulation." In Brauer and Callen, *Art, Sex and Eugenics*, 97–138.

———. "Flaunting Manliness: Republican Masculinity, Virilised Homosexuality and the Desirable Male Body." *Australian and New Zealand Journal of Art* 6, no. 1 (2005): 23–41.

———. "Introduction: Making Eugenic Bodies Delectable; Art, 'Biopower,' and 'Scientia Sexualis.'" In Brauer and Callen, *Art, Sex and Eugenics*, 1–34.

———. "The Stigmata of Abjection: Degenerate Limbs, Hysterical Skin, and the Tattooed Body." In *A History of Visual Culture: Western Civilisation from the 18th to the 21st Century*, edited by Jane Kromm and Susan Benforado Bakewell, 169–83. Oxford: Berg, 2010.

Brauer, Fae, and Anthea Callen, eds. *Art, Sex and Eugenics: Corpus Delecti*. Aldershot: Ashgate, 2008.

Braun, Marta. *Picturing Time: The Work of Etienne-Jules Marey (1830–1904)*. Chicago: University of Chicago Press, 1992.

Braun, Marta, and Elizabeth Whitcombe. "Marey, Muybridge, and Londe: The Photography of Pathological Locomotion." *History of Photography* 23, no. 2 (1999): 218–24.

Brigo, Francesco, et al. "Jean-Martin Charcot's Medical Instruments: Electrotherapeutic Devices in *La Leçon Clinique à la Salpêtrière*." *Journal of the History of the Neurosciences* (2020). https://www.tandfonline.com/doi/full/10.1080/0964704X.2020.1775391.

Brilliant, Richard. *Portraiture*. London: Reaktion, 1991.

Bronfen, Elisabeth. *The Knotted Subject: Hysteria and Its Discontents*. Princeton: Princeton University Press, 1998.

———. *Over Her Dead Body: Death, Femininity and the Aesthetic*. Manchester: Manchester University Press, 1992.

———. "The Sexuality of Seeing Sexuality." Review of *Sexual Visions*, by Ludmilla Jordanova, and *Sexuality: An Illustrated History*, by Sander Gilman. *Art History* 13, no. 4 (1990): 576–80.

Brooks, Peter. *Realist Visions*. New Haven: Yale University Press, 2005.

Brugerolles, Emmanuelle. "Paul Georges Leroux (Paris 1877–Paris 1957). *Études classiques de la peinture*." *La Revue des musées de France: Musée du Louvre*, no. 2 (2010): 22.

Burnett, D. Graham. "The Objective Case: A Review of *Objectivity*." Review of *Objectivity*, by Lorraine Daston and Peter Galison. *October* 133 (Summer 2010): 133–44.

Burns, Stanley B. "Early Medical Photography in America (1839–1883)." *New York State Journal of Medicine* 79, no. 5 (1979): 788–95.

Bynum, W. F. *Science and the Practice of Medicine in the Nineteenth Century*. Cambridge: Cambridge University Press, 1994.

Bynum, William F., and Roy Porter, eds. *Medicine and the Five Senses*. Cambridge: Cambridge University Press, 1993.

Caillaux, Henriette. *Aimé-Jules Dalou (1838–1902)*. Paris: Librairie Delagrave, 1935.

Callen, Anthea. "Doubles and Desire: Anatomies of Masculinity in the Later Nineteenth Century." *Art History* 26, no. 5 (2003): 669–99.

———. *Looking at Men: Art, Anatomy and the Modern Male Body*. New Haven: Yale University Press, 2018.

———. "Man or Machine: Ideals of the Labouring Male Body and the Aesthetics of Industrial Production in Early Twentieth-Century Europe." In Brauer and Callen, *Art, Sex and Eugenics*, 140–61.

———. "Masculinity and Muscularity: Dr Paul Richer and Modern Manhood." *Paragraph* 26, no. 1–2 (2003): 17–41.

———. *The Spectacular Body: Science, Method, and Meaning the Work of Degas*. New Haven: Yale University Press, 1995.

Capildeo, Rudy. "Charcot in the 80s." In *Historical Aspects of the Neurosciences: A Festschrift for Macdonald Critchley*, edited by F. Clifford Rose and W. F. Bynum, 383–96. New York: Raven Press, 1982.

Carroy, Jacqueline. "L'hystérique, l'artiste et le savant." In *L'Âme au corps: Arts et*

sciences, 1793–1993, by Jean Clair et al., 446–57. Paris: Éditions de la Réunion des musées nationaux, 1993. Exhibition catalog.
Carroy-Thirard, Jacqueline. "Figures de femmes hystériques dans la psychiatrie française au dix-neuvième siècle." *Psychanalyse à l'université* 4, no. 14 (1974): 313–24.
———. "Hystérie, théâtre, littérature au dix-neuvième siècle." *Psychanalyse à l'université* 7, no. 26 (1982): 299–317.
———. "Possession, extase, hystérie au dix-neuvième siècle." *Psychanalyse à l'université* 5, no. 19 (1980): 499–515.
Cartwright, Lisa. *Screening the Body: Tracing Medicine's Visual Culture*. Minneapolis: University of Minnesota Press, 1995.
Ceglia, Francesco Paolo de. "Rotten Corpses, a Disembowelled Woman, a Flayed Man: Images of the Body from the End of the 17th to the Beginning of the 19th Century; Florentine Wax Models in the First-Hand Accounts of Visitors." *Perspectives on Science* 14, no. 4 (2006): 417–56.
Centre culturel de la Communauté française de Belgique. *Cires anatomiques du XIXe siècle. Collection du Dr. Spitzner*. Paris: Centre culturel de la Communauté française de Belgique, 1980. Exhibition catalog.
Chadarevian, Soraya de, and Nick Hopwood, eds. *Model: The Third Dimension in Space*. Stanford: Stanford University Press, 2004.
Changeux, Jean-Pierre, and Gérard Régnier. "Préface." In Jean Clair et al., *L'Âme au corps: Arts et sciences, 1793–1993*, 11. Paris: Éditions de la Réunion des musées nationaux, 1993. Exhibition catalog.
Chantoury-Lacombe, Florence. *Peindre les maux. Arts visuels et pathologie, XIVe–XVIIe siècle*. Paris: Hermann, 2010.
Chayette, Hervé. *Grand Musée anatomique du Docteur Spitzner*. Paris: Nouveau Drouot, 1985.
Chevillot, Catherine. "Réalisme optique et progrès esthétique: La Fin d'un rêve." *Revue de l'art* 104, no. 1 (1994): 22–29.
Chu, Petra ten-Doesschate. *French Realism and the Dutch Masters: The Influence of Dutch Seventeenth-Century Painting on the Development of French Painting Between 1830 and 1870*. Utrecht: Haentjens Dekker & Gumbert, 1974.
Clair, Jean, ed. *Crime et châtiment*. Paris: Gallimard, 2010. Exhibition catalog.
———, ed. *Freud. Du regard à l'écoute*. Paris: Gallimard, 2018. Exhibition catalog.
———. Introduction to "Le Cabinet des antiques." In *Freud. Du regard à l'écoute*, edited by Jean Clair, 190. Paris: Gallimard, 2018. Exhibition catalog.
Clair, Jean, et al. *L'Âme au corps: Arts et sciences, 1793–1993*. Paris: Éditions de la Réunion des musées nationaux, 1993. Exhibition catalog.
Clark, T. J. *The Painting of Modern Life: Paris in the Art of Manet and His Followers*. Princeton: Princeton University Press, 1984.
Clarke, Carl Dame. *Molding and Casting for Moulage Workers, Sculptors, Artists, Physicians, Dentists, Criminologists, Craftsmen, Pattern Makers and Architectural Modelers*. Butler, MD: Standard Arts Press, 1972.
Cleaves, Tania. *See* Woloshyn, Tania.
Coakley, Sarah. "Introduction." In *Pain and Its Transformations: The Interface of Biology and Culture*, edited by Sarah Coakley and Kay Kaufman Shelemay, 1–16. Cambridge, MA: Harvard University Press, 2007.
Cohen, Kathleen. *Metamorphosis of a Death Symbol: The Transi Tomb in the Late Middle Ages and the Renaissance*. Berkeley: University of California Press, 1973.
Cohen, Margaret, and Christopher Prendergast, eds. *Spectacles of Realism: Body, Gender, Genre*. Minneapolis: University of Minnesota Press, 1995.
Comar, Philippe, ed. *Figures du corps. Une leçon d'anatomie à l'École des beaux-arts*. Paris: Beaux-Arts de Paris, 2008. Exhibition catalog.
———. "Une leçon d'anatomie à l'École des beaux-arts." In *Figures du corps. Une leçon d'anatomie à l'École des beaux-arts*, edited by Philippe Comar, 19–65. Paris: Beaux-Arts de Paris, 2008. Exhibition catalog.
———. *Mémoires de mon crâne. Réné Des-Cartes*. Paris: Gallimard, 1997.
Corpataux, Jean-François. *Le Corps à l'oeuvre*. Geneva: Librarie Droz, 2012.
Coury, Charles. *L'Enseignement de la médecine en France des origines à nos jours*. Paris: Expansion Scientifique Française, 1968.

Coutinho, Leo, Olivier Walusinski, and Helio A. Ghizoni Teive. "Désiré Bourneville: A Socialist in Charcot's Inner Circle." *European Neurology* 85, no. 1 (2022): 79–84.

Dagen, Philippe. "Le 'Premier Artiste.'" *Romantisme*, no. 84 (1994): 69–78.

Daston, Lorraine. "Objectivity and the Escape from Perspective." *Social Studies of Medicine* 22, no. 4 (1992): 597–618.

———, ed. *Things That Talk: Object Lessons from Art and Science*. New York: Zone Books, 2004.

Daston, Lorraine, and Peter Galison. "The Image of Objectivity." *Representations*, no. 40 (1992): 81–128.

———. *Objectivity*. New York: Zone Books, 2007.

Daston, Lorraine, and Elizabeth Lunbeck, eds. *Histories of Scientific Observation*. Chicago: University of Chicago Press, 2011.

Daston, Lorraine, and Katharine Park. *Wonders and the Order of Nature, 1150–750*. New York: Zone Books, 1998.

Daston, Lorraine, and H. Otto Sibum. "Introduction: Scientific Personae and Their Histories." *Science in Context* 16, no. 1–2 (2003): 1–8.

de Marneffe, Daphne. "Looking and Listening: The Construction of Clinical Knowledge in Charcot and Freud." *Signs* 17, no. 1 (1991): 71–111.

Desprez, Catherine. "Paul Richer: 1849–1933: Un médecin à l'École des Beaux-Arts." MD diss., Caen, 1987.

Dias, Nélia. "Le Corps en vitrine. Éléments pour une recherche sur les collections médicales." *Terrain* 18 (1992). https://terrain.revues.org/3033.

Di Bella, Maria Pia, and James Elkins, eds. *Representations of Pain in Art and Visual Culture*. New York: Routledge, 2013.

Didi-Huberman, Georges. "Charcot, l'histoire et l'art. Imitation de la croix et démon de l'imitation." In *Les Démoniaques dans l'art* [1887], by J[ean]-M[artin] Charcot and Paul Richer, 125–88. Paris: Macula, 1984.

———. *L'Empreinte*. Paris: Centre Georges Pompidou, 1993. Exhibition catalog.

———. "Esthétique et expérimentation chez Charcot." In *Doctrines, sciences ou pratiques sociales*, 1:121–38. Nancy: Presses Universitaires de Nancy, 1986.

———. *Invention of Hysteria: Charcot and the Photographic Iconography of the Salpêtrière*. Translated by Alisa Hartz. Cambridge, MA: MIT Press, 2003.

———. "Une notion du 'corps-cliché' au XIXe siècle." *Parachute*, no. 35 (1984): 8–14.

———. *Ouvrir Vénus. Nudité, rêve, cruauté*. Paris: Gallimard, 1999.

———. *La Peinture incarnée. Suivi de Le Chef-d'oeuvre inconnu par Honoré de Balzac*. Paris: Les Éditions de Minuit, 1985.

———. "Photography—Scientific and Pseudo-Scientific." In *A History of Photography: Social and Cultural Perspectives*, edited by Jean-Claude Lemagny and André Rouillé and translated by Janet Lloyd, 71–75. Cambridge: Cambridge University Press, 1987.

———. "Viscosities and Survivals: Art History Put to the Test by the Material." In Panzanelli, *Ephemeral Bodies*, 154–69.

Dommasch, H. S. "The Development of Medical Photography." *Journal of the Biological Photographic Association* 33, no. 4 (1965): 169–70.

Drilhon, France, and Anne Tassery-Lahmi. "Technologie et mise en forme." In Gaborit, Ligot, et al., *Sculptures en cire*, 59–71.

Druick, Douglas W. "Framing *The Little Dancer Aged Fourteen*." In Richard Kendall et al., *Degas and the Little Dancer*, 76–96. New Haven: Yale University Press, 1998. Exhibition catalog.

Durey, Philippe. "Le Réalisme." In *La Sculpture française au XIXe siècle*, 353–77. Paris: Éditions de la Réunion des musées nationaux, 1986. Exhibition catalog.

Duyckaerts, Charles, et al. "Charcot identifies and illustrates amyotrophic lateral sclerosis." *Free Neuropathology* 2, no. 12 (2021). https://doi.org/10.17879/freeneuropathology-2021-3323.

Düring, Monika, et al. *Encyclopaedia Anatomica: A Complete Collection of Anatomical Waxes*. Cologne: Taschen, 1999.

Ebenstein, Joanna. *The Anatomical Venus*. London: Thames & Hudson, 2016.

Edwards, Elizabeth. "Ordering Others: Photography, Anthropologies and Taxonomies." In *In Visible Light: Photography and Classification in Art, Science and the Everyday*, edited by Chrissie Iles and Russell Roberts, 54–68. Oxford: Museum of Modern Art Oxford, 1997. Exhibition catalog.

———. "Thinking Photography Beyond the Visual?" In *Photography: Theoretical*

Snapshots, edited by J. J. Long, Andrea Nobke, and Edward Welch, 31–48. New York: Routledge, 2009.

Edwards, Elizabeth, and Janice Hart. "Introduction: Photographs as Objects." In *Photographs Objects Histories: On the Materiality of Images*, edited by Elizabeth Edwards and Janice Hart, 1–15. London: Routledge, 2004.

———, eds. *Photographs Objects Histories: On the Materiality of Images*. London: Routledge, 2004.

Edwards, Holly. "Pain in Public." *Representations of Pain in Art and Visual Culture*, edited by Maria Pia Di Bella and James Elkins, 88–100. New York: Routledge, 2013.

Eidenbenz, Céline. "'L'Âme renversée': L'Arc hystérique et ses corps à rebours autour de 1900." In *Pulsion(s). Art et déraison*, by Laurence Brogniez et al., 53–89. Waterloo: La Renaissance du Livre, 2012. Exhibition catalog.

———. "Théâtre de l'objectivité. La Photographie chez les aliénistes au XIXe siècle." In *L'Évidence photographique. La Conception positiviste en question*, edited by Herbert Molderings and Gregor Wedekind, 103–29. Paris: Éditions des sciences de l'homme, 2009.

Elkins, James. "Art History and Images That Are Not Art." *Art Bulletin* 77, no. 4 (1995): 553–71.

———. *The Domain of Images*. Ithaca: Cornell University Press, 1999.

———. "An Introduction to the Visual as Argument." In *Theorizing Visual Studies: Writing Through the Discipline*, edited by James Elkins et al., 25–60. New York: Routledge, 2013.

———. *Pictures of the Body: Pain and Metamorphosis*. Stanford: Stanford University Press, 1999.

———. *What Photography Is*. New York: Routledge, 2011.

Ellenberger, Henri F. "Charcot and the Salpêtrière School." 1965. In *Beyond the Unconscious: Essays of Henri F. Ellenberger in the History of Psychiatry*, edited by Mark S. Micale and translated by Françoise Dubor and Mark S. Micale, 139–54. Princeton: Princeton University Press, 1993.

Ellenbogen, Josh. *Reasoned and Unreasoned Images: The Photography of Bertillon, Galton, and Marey*. University Park: Penn State University Press, 2012.

Emery, Alan E. H., and Marcia L. H. Emery. *Medicine and Art*. London: Royal Society of Medicine Press, 1988.

Endtz, L. J. "La Neurologie et l'illustration photographique du livre médical." *Revue neurologique* 139, no. 6–7 (1983): 439–44.

Eschelbacher, Andrew. "Gendering Modernity / Modernizing the Worker: Jules Dalou's *Monument to Labourers* and Industrial Virility." *Sculpture Journal* 23, no. 3 (2014): 331–48.

Evans, Bruce H. *Jean-Léon Gérôme*. With introduction and commentaries by Gerald M. Ackerman. Dayton: Dayton Art Institute, 1972. Exhibition catalog.

Evans, Martha Noel. *Fits and Starts: A Genealogy of Hysteria in Modern France*. Ithaca: Cornell University Press, 1991.

Farge, Arlette. *The Allure of the Archives*. Translated by Thomas Scott-Railton. New Haven: Yale University Press, 2013.

Fend, Mechthild. *Fleshing Out Surfaces: Skin in French Art and Medicine, 1650–1850*. Manchester: Manchester University Press, 2017.

———. "Order and Affect: The Museum of Dermatological Wax Moulages at the Hôpital Saint-Louis in Paris." In *The Agency of Display: Objects, Framings and Parerga*, edited by Johannes Grave, Christiane Holm, Valérie Kobi, and Caroline van Eck, 79–98. Dresden: Sandstein Verlag, 2018.

Fields, Howard L., et al. "Discussion: The Dislocation, Representation, and Communication of Pain." In *Pain and Its Transformations: The Interface of Biology and Culture*, edited by Sarah Coakley and Kay Kaufman Shelemay, 351–60. Cambridge, MA: Harvard University Press, 2007.

Fineman, Mia. *Faking It: Manipulated Photography Before Photoshop*. New York: Metropolitan Museum of Art; New Haven: Yale University Press, 2012. Exhibition catalog.

Fitzgerald, Des, and Felicity Callard. "Entangling the Medical Humanities." In Atkinson et al., *Edinburgh Companion*, 35–49.

Foucault, Michel. *The Birth of the Clinic: An Archaeology of Medical Perception*. 1963. Translated by A. M. Sheridan Smith. New York: Vintage Books, 1994.

———. *The History of Sexuality*. Vol. 1, *An Introduction*. Translated by Robert Hurley. New York: Vintage Books, 1990.

———. *Surveiller et punir. Naissance de la prison*. Paris: Gallimard, 1975.

Fox, Daniel, and Christopher Lawrence. *Photographing Medicine: Images and Power in Britain and America Since 1840*. New York: Greenwood Press, 1988.

Fox, Daniel M., and James Terry. "Photography and the Self Image of American Physicians, 1880–1920." *Bulletin of the History of Medicine* 52, no. 3 (1978): 435–57.

Foxhall, Katherine. *Migraine: A History*. Baltimore: Johns Hopkins University Press, 2019.

Frederiksen, Rune, and Eckart Marchand, eds. *Plaster Casts: Making, Collecting and Displaying from Classical Antiquity to the Present*. Berlin: De Gruyter, 2010.

Freund, Gisèle. *Photography and Society*. London: Gordon Fraser, 1980.

Gabbriellini, Chiara, et al. "La collezione di cere del Museo di Anatomia Patologica di Firenze. Note sulle vicende storiche, sulla tecnica esecutiva e sui restauri." *OPD Restauro*, no. 21 (2009): 51–70.

Gaborit, Jean-René, Jack Ligot, et al. *Sculptures en cire de l'ancienne Egypte à l'art abstrait*. Paris: Réunion des musées nationaux, 1987. Exhibition catalog.

Gamwell, Lynn, and Richard Wells, eds. *Sigmund Freud and Art: His Personal Collection of Antiquities*. London: Thames & Hudson, 1989. Exhibition catalog.

Garland-Thomson, Rosemarie. *Staring: How We Look*. Oxford: Oxford University Press, 2009.

Garnot, Nicolas Sainte Fare. "Céroplastie médicale: Art méconnu." In Gaborit, Ligot, et al., *Sculptures en cire*, 21–24.

Gasser, Jacques. *Photographie et médecine, 1840–1880*. Lausanne: Institut universitaire d'histoire de la médecine et de la santé publique, 1991.

Gauchet, Marcel, and Gladys Swain. *Le Vrai Charcot. Les Chemins imprévus de l'inconscient*. Paris: Calmann-Lévy, 1997.

Gelfand, Toby. *Charcot in Morocco*. Ottawa: University of Ottawa Press, 2012.

———. "Medical Nemesis, Paris, 1894: Léon Daudet's *Les Morticoles*." *Bulletin of the History of Medicine* 60, no. 2 (1986): 155–76.

———. "'Mon cher Docteur Freud': Charcot's Unpublished Correspondence to Freud, 1888–1893." *Bulletin of the History of Medicine* 62, no. 4 (1988): 563–88.

———. "Neurologist or Psychiatrist? The Public and Private Domains of Jean-Martin Charcot." *Journal of the History of the Behavioral Sciences* 36, no. 3 (2000): 215–29.

Gernsheim, Alison. "Medical Photography in the Nineteenth Century." *Medical and Biological Illustration* 11, no. 2 (1961): 85–92.

Gilman, Sander L. *The Case of Sigmund Freud*. Baltimore: Johns Hopkins University Press, 1993.

———. *Disease and Representation: Images of Illness from Madness to AIDS*. Ithaca: Cornell University Press, 1988.

———, ed. *The Face of Madness: Hugh W. Diamond and the Origin of Psychiatric Photography*. Secaucus, NJ: Citadel Press, 1976.

———, ed. *Hysteria Beyond Freud*. Berkeley: University of California Press, 1993.

———. "The Image of the Hysteric." In *Hysteria Beyond Freud*, edited by Sander L. Gilman et al., 345–452. Berkeley: University of California Press, 1993.

———. *Picturing Health and Illness: Images of Identity and Difference*. Baltimore: Johns Hopkins University Press, 1995.

———. *Seeing the Insane: A Cultural History of Madness and Art in the Western World, Showing How the Portrayal of Stereotypes Has Both Reflected and Shaped the Perception and Treatment of the Mentally Ill*. New York: John Wiley & Sons, 1982.

———. *Sexuality: An Illustrated History; Representing the Sexual in Medicine and Culture from the Middle Ages to the Age of AIDS*. New York: John Wiley & Sons, 1989.

Gindhart, Maria P. "The Art and Science of Late Nineteenth-Century Images of Human Prehistory at the National Museum of Natural History in Paris." PhD diss., University of Pennsylvania, 2002.

———. "A *pinacothèque préhistorique* for the Musée des Antiquités Nationales in Saint-Germain-en-Laye." *Journal of the History of Collections* 19, no. 1 (2007): 51–74.

Goetz, Christopher G. "Charcot and Parkinson's Disease." In *Parkinson's Disease and Clinical Management*, edited by Stewart A. Factor and William J. Weiner, 21–32. New York: Demos Medical Publishing, 2008.

———. "The Salpêtrière in the Wake of Charcot's Death." *Archives of Neurology* 45, no. 4 (1988): 444–47.

———. "Visual Art in the Neurologic Career of Jean-Martin Charcot." *Archives of Neurology* 48, no. 4 (1991): 421–25.

Goetz, Christopher G., and Michel Bonduelle. "Charcot as Therapeutic Interventionist and Treating Neurologist." *Historical Neurology* 45, no. 1 (1995): 2102–6.

Goetz, Christopher G., Michel Bonduelle, and Toby Gelfand. *Charcot: Constructing Neurology*. New York: Oxford University Press, 1995.

Goldstein, Jan. *Console and Clarify: The French Psychiatric Profession in the Nineteenth Century*. Chicago: University of Chicago Press, 1987.

———. "The Hysteria Diagnosis and the Politics of Anticlericalism in Late Nineteenth-Century France." *Journal of Modern History* 54, no. 2 (1982): 209–39.

———. "The Uses of Male Hysteria: Medical and Literary Discourse in Nineteenth-Century France." *Representations*, no. 34 (Spring 1991): 134–65.

Gordon, Rae Beth. *Dances with Darwin, 1875–1910: Vernacular Modernity in France*. Aldershot: Ashgate, 2009.

———. *Why the French Love Jerry Lewis: From Cabaret to Early Cinema*. Stanford: Stanford University Press, 2001.

Graybill, Lela. "A Proximate Violence: Madame Tussaud's Chamber of Horrors." *Nineteenth-Century Art Worldwide* 9, no. 2 (2010). http://www.19thc-artworldwide.org/index.php/autumn10/a-proximate-violence.

Green-Lewis, Jennifer. *Framing the Victorians: Photography and the Culture of Realism*. Ithaca: Cornell University Press, 1996.

Groebner, Valentin. "A Feeling for Images: Medieval *Personae* in Contemporary Photojournalism." In *Representations of Pain in Art and Visual Culture*, edited by Maria Pia Di Bella and James Elkins, 150–56. New York: Routledge, 2013.

Grootenboer, Hanneke. "Introduction: On the Substance of Wax." *Oxford Art Journal* 36, no. 1 (2013): 1–12.

Guillain, George. *J.-M. Charcot: His Life—His Work*. Edited and translated by Pearce Bailey. London: Pitman Medical Publishing, 1959.

———. "La Physionomie de J.-M. Charcot. Son caractère, ses idées sur la littérature, les arts, la philosophie." *Médecine de France* 73 (1956): 3–8.

Guillain, Georges, and P. Mathieu. *La Salpêtrière*. Paris: Masson, 1925.

Gunthert, André. "La Conquête de l'instantané. Archéologie de l'imaginaire photographique en France (1841–1895)." PhD diss., École des hautes études en sciences sociales, 1999.

———. "La Rétine du savant." *Études photographiques* 7 (May 2000). http://journals.openedition.org/etudesphotographiques/205.

———. "'Sans retouche': Histoire d'un mythe photographique." *Études photographiques* 22 (September 2008). http://etudesphotographiques.revues.org/index1004.html.

Gursel, Zeynep. "A Picture of Health." *Grey Room*, no. 72 (Summer 2018): 36–67.

Hagner, Michael. "Skulls, Brains, and Memorial Culture: On Cerebral Biographies of Scientists in the Nineteenth Century." *Science in Context* 16, no. 1–2 (2003): 195–218.

Hallam, Elizabeth. "Anatomical Bodies and Materials of Memory." In *Death Rites and Rights*, edited by Belinda Brooks-Gordon et al., 279–98. Oxford: Hart Publishing, 2007.

———. "Anatomy Display: Contemporary Debates and Collections in Scotland." In *Anatomy Acts: How We Come to Know Ourselves*, edited by Andrew Patrizio and Dawn Kemp, 119–35. Edinburgh: Birlinn, 2006.

———. *Anatomy Museum: Death and the Body Displayed*. London: Reaktion Books, 2016.

Hallam, Elizabeth, Jenny Hockey, and Glennys Howarth. *Beyond the Body: Death and Social Identity*. London: Routledge, 1999.

Hamilton, Peter. "The Beautiful and the Damned." In *The Beautiful and the Damned: The Creation of Identity in Nineteenth Century Photography*, by Peter Hamilton and Roger Hargreaves, 1–15. London: National Portrait Gallery, 2001. Exhibition catalog.

Hamilton, Peter, and Roger Hargreaves. *The Beautiful and the Damned: The Creation of Identity in Nineteenth*

Century Photography. London: National Portrait Gallery, 2001. Exhibition catalog.

Hammerschlag, Keren Rosa. *Frederic Leighton: Death, Mortality, Resurrection*. Farnham: Ashgate, 2015.

———. "The Gentleman Artist-Surgeon in Late Victorian Group Portraiture." *Visual Culture in Britain* 14, no. 2 (2013): 154–78.

———. "Identifying the Patient in George W. Lambert's *Chesham Street*." *Medical Humanities* 39, no. 1 (2013): 20–28.

———. "William Orpen (1878–1931): Looking at Bodies in Medicine and Art." *British Art Journal* 17, no. 1 (2016): 78–93.

Harris, James C. "A Clinical Lesson at the Salpêtrière." *Archives of General Psychiatry* 62, no. 5 (2005): 470–72.

Harvey, John. *Photography and Spirit*. London: Reaktion Books, 2007.

Haviland, Thomas N., and Lawrence Charles Parish. "A Brief Account of the Use of Wax Models in the Study of Medicine." *Journal of the History of Medicine* 25, no. 1 (1970): 52–74.

Hawley, Henry. "Sculptures by Jules Dalou, Henry Cros, and Medardo Rosso." *Bulletin of the Cleveland Museum of Art* 58, no. 7 (1971): 199–209.

Héran, Emmanuelle, et al. *Le Dernier Portrait*. Paris: Musée d'Orsay, 2002. Exhibition catalog.

———. "Henry Cros: Le Moyen Âge et la couleur." In *La Dame aux éventails. Nina de Callias, modèle de Manet*, edited by Luce Abélès, 103–18. Paris: Réunion des musées nationaux, 2000. Exhibition catalog.

Hoffmann, Kathryn A. "Sleeping Beauties in the Fairground." *Early Popular Visual Culture* 4, no. 2 (2006): 139–59.

Hooper-Greenhill, Eilean. *Museums and the Shaping of Knowledge*. London: Routledge, 1992.

Hopwood, Nick. "Plastic Publishing in Embryology." In Chadarevian and Hopwood, *Model*, 170–206.

Hunisak, John M. *The Sculptor Jules Dalou: Studies in His Style and Imagery*. New York: Garland, 1977.

Hunter, Mary. "'Effroyable réalisme': Wax, Femininity, and the Madness of Realist Fantasies." *RACAR* 33, no. 1–2 (2008): 43–58.

———. *The Face of Medicine: Visualising Medical Masculinities in Late Nineteenth-Century Paris*. Manchester: Manchester University Press, 2016.

———. "Intern, Orderly, Artist, Corpse: Emerging Masculinities in Henri Gervex's *Autopsy at Hôtel-Dieu*." *Oxford Art Journal* 38, no. 3 (2015): 405–26.

———. "The Sleep of Reason: Art, Medicine and Sexuality in Henri Gervex's *Avant l'opération*." *Object* 7 (2004–5): 43–61.

Hustvedt, Asti. *Medical Muses: Hysteria in Nineteenth-Century Paris*. London: Bloomsbury, 2011.

Janson, H. W. "Realism in Sculpture: Limits and Limitations." In *The European Realist Tradition*, edited by Gabriel P. Weisberg, 290–301. Bloomington: Indiana University Press, 1982.

Johnstone, Fiona. "Manifesto for a Visual Medical Humanities." *Medical Humanities* (blog), July 31, 2018. https://blogs.bmj.com/medical-humanities/2018/07/31/manifesto-for-a-visual-medical-humanities/.

Jolly, Martyn. *Faces of the Living Dead: The Belief in Spirit Photography*. London: British Library, 2006.

Jones, Caroline A., and Peter Galison. "Introduction: Picturing Science, Producing Art." In Jones and Galison, *Picturing Science, Producing Art*, 1–23.

———, eds. *Picturing Science, Producing Art*. New York: Routledge, 1998.

Jones, Claire. *Sculptors and Design Reform in France, 1848–1895: Sculpture and the Decorative Arts*. Farnham: Ashgate, 2014.

Jordanova, Ludmilla. *Defining Features: Scientific and Medical Portraits, 1660–2000*. London: Reaktion Books in association with the National Portrait Gallery, 2000.

———. "Material Models as Visual Culture." In Chadarevian and Hopwood, *Model*, 443–51.

———. "Medicine and the Visual Arts." In *Medicine, Health and the Arts: Approaches to the Medical Humanities*, edited by Victoria Bates et al., 41–63. Abingdon: Routledge, 2014.

———. "Museums: Representing the Real?" In *Realism and Representation: Essays on the Problem of Realism in Relation to Science, Literature, and Culture*, edited by George Levine, 255–78. Madison: University of Wisconsin Press, 1993.

———. *Nature Displayed: Gender, Science and Medicine 1760–1820*. London: Longman, 1999.

———. "Objects of Knowledge: A Historical Perspective on Museums." In *The New Museology*, edited by Peter Vergo, 22–40. London: Reaktion Books, 1989.

———. "Portraiture, Beauty, Pain." In *The Recovery of Beauty: Arts, Culture, Medicine*, edited by Corinne Saunders, Jane Macnaughton, and David Fuller, 199–216. Basingstoke: Palgrave, 2015.

———. "Science and Nationhood: Cultures of Imagined Communities." In *Imagining Nations*, edited by Geoffrey Cubitt, 192–211. Manchester: Manchester University Press, 1998.

———. *Sexual Visions: Images of Gender in Science and Medicine Between the Eighteenth and Twentieth Centuries*. New York: Harvester Wheatsheaf, 1989.

———. "Visualizing Identity." In *Identity*, edited by Giselle Walker and Elisabeth Leedham-Green, 127–56. Cambridge: Cambridge University Press, 2010.

Keller, Corey, ed. *Brought to Light: Photography and the Invisible, 1840–1900*. New Haven: San Francisco Museum of Modern Art in association with Yale University Press, 2008. Exhibition catalog.

Kelsey, Robin. *Archive Style: Photographs and Illustrations for U.S. Surveys, 1850–1890*. Berkeley: University of California Press, 2007.

Kemp, Martin. "'A Perfect and Faithful Record': Mind and Body in Medical Photography Before 1900." In *Beauty of Another Order: Photography in Science*, by Ann Thomas et al., 120–49. New Haven: Yale University Press, 1997. Exhibition catalog.

Koehler, Peter. "About Medicine and the Arts: Charcot and French Literature at the Fin-de-Siècle." *Journal of the History of the Neurosciences* 10, no. 1 (2001): 27–40.

Kriebel, Sabine T. "Theories of Photography: A Short History." In *Photography Theory*, edited by James Elkins, 3–49. New York: Routledge, 2007.

Kromm, Jane. *The Art of Frenzy: Public Madness in the Visual Culture of Europe, 1500–1850*. London: Continuum, 2002.

Kumar, Brinda. "Between Life and Art." In *Like Life: Sculpture, Color, and the Body*, edited by Luke Syson et al., 254–57. New York: Metropolitan Museum of Art and Yale University Press, 2018. Exhibition catalog.

Kusch, Martin. "Objectivity and Historiography." *Isis* 100, no. 1 (2009): 127–31.

Langford, Martha. *Suspended Conversations: The Afterlife of Memory in Photographic Albums*. Montreal and Kingston: McGill-Queen's University Press, 2001.

Lanza, Benedetto, et al. *Le cere anatomiche della Specola*. Florence: Arnaud Editore, 2007.

Larson, Barbara. *The Dark Side of Nature: Science, Society, and the Fantastic in the Work of Odilon Redon*. University Park: Penn State University Press, 2005.

Lemire, Michel. *Artistes et mortels*. Paris: Chabaud, 1990.

Le Normand-Romain, Antoinette. "Moulage." In *La Sculpture française au XIXe siècle*, 67–71. Paris: Éditions de la Réunion des musées nationaux, 1986. Exhibition catalog.

———. "Le Moulage sur nature: Objet de plaisir ou document de travail?" In *De Plâtre et d'or. Geoffroy Dechaume (1816–1892). Sculpteur romantique de Viollet-le-Duc*, edited by Association "Les Amis de L'Isle-Adam," 127–39. [Isle-Adam]: Val d'Oise Éditions, 1998. Exhibition catalog.

Le Normand-Romain, Antoinette, and Jean-Luc Olivié. "La Polychromie." In *La Sculpture française au XIXe siècle*, 149–59. Paris: Éditions de la Réunion des musées nationaux, 1986. Exhibition catalog.

Levine, George, ed. *Realism and Representation: Essays on the Problem of Realism in Relation to Science, Literature, and Culture*. Madison: University of Wisconsin Press, 1993.

———. "Why Science Isn't Literature: The Importance of Differences." In *Rethinking Objectivity*, edited by Alan Megill, 65–79. Durham: Duke University Press, 1994.

Liedtke, Walter. "Frans Hals: Style and Substance." *Metropolitan Museum of Art Bulletin*, Summer 2011, 5–48.

Maehle, Andreas-Holger. "The Search for Objective Communication: Medical Photography in the Nineteenth Century." In *Non-Verbal Communication in Science Prior to 1900*, edited by Renato G. Mazzolini, 563–86. Florence: Olschki, 1993.

Maerker, Anna. *Model Experts: Wax Anatomies and Enlightenment in Florence and Vienna, 1775–1815*. Manchester: Manchester University Press, 2011.

Marquand, Allan. *The Brothers of Giovanni della Robbia: Fra Mattia, Luca, Girolamo, Fra Ambrogio*. Princeton: Princeton University Press, 1928.

Marquer, Bertrand. *Les Romans de la Salpêtrière. Réception d'une scénographie clinique: Jean-Martin Charcot dans l'imaginaire fin-de-siècle*. Geneva: Droz, 2008.

Marshall, Jonathan W. *Performing Neurology: The Dramaturgy of Dr Jean-Martin Charcot*. New York: Palgrave Macmillan, 2016.

Mathon, Catherine. "Le Corps modélisé." In *L'Art du nu au XIXe siècle. Le Photographe et son modèle*, 152–63. Paris: Hazan / Bibliothèque nationale de France, 1997. Exhibition catalog.

Matlock, Jann. *Scenes of Seduction: Prostitution, Hysteria, and Reading Difference in Nineteenth-Century France*. New York: Columbia University Press, 1994.

Mayer, Andreas. "Freud à Paris: Souvenirs du musée Charcot." In *Freud. Du regard à l'écoute*, edited by Jean Clair, 51–59. Paris: Gallimard, 2018. Exhibition catalog.

———. *Sites of the Unconscious: Hypnosis and the Emergence of the Psychoanalytic Setting*. Chicago: University of Chicago Press, 2013.

McCarren, Felicia. "The 'Symptomatic Act' Circa 1900: Hysteria, Hypnosis, Electricity, Dance." *Critical Inquiry* 21, no. 4 (1995): 748–74.

McGrath, R. *Seeing Her Sex: Medical Archives and the Female Body*. Manchester: Manchester University Press, 2002.

Megill, Allan, ed. *Rethinking Objectivity*. Durham: Duke University Press, 1994.

Micale, Mark S. *Approaching Hysteria: Disease and Its Interpretations*. Princeton: Princeton University Press, 1995.

———. *Hysterical Men: The Hidden History of Male Nervous Illness*. Cambridge, MA: Harvard University Press, 2008.

———. "On the 'Disappearance' of Hysteria: A Study in the Clinical Deconstruction of a Diagnosis." *Isis* 84, no. 3 (1993): 496–526.

Miles, Melissa. *The Burning Mirror: Photography in an Ambivalent Light*. North Melbourne: Australian Scholarly Publishing, 2008.

Miller, Julian A., et al. "Some Aspects of Charcot's Influence on Freud." In *Freud: The Fusion of Science and Humanism*, edited by John E. Gedo and George H. Pollock, 115–32. Psychological Issues 9, no. 2–3, monograph 34–35. New York: International Universities Press, 1976.

Miller, William Ian. *The Anatomy of Disgust*. Cambridge, MA: Harvard University Press, 1997.

———. "Epilogue: Do I Disgust You? (Or, Rather, You Me?) Mes frères, mes soeurs, mes semblables?" In *Le Dégoût. Histoire, langage, esthétique et politique d'une émotion plurielle*, edited by Michel Delville, Andrew Norris, and Viktoria von Hoffmann, 149–61. Liège: Presses Universitaires de Liège, 2015.

Mitchell, W. J. T. "Method, Madness and Montage: Assemblages of Images and the Production of Knowledge." In *Image Operations: Visual Media and Political Conflict*, edited by Jens Eder and Charlotte Klonk, 79–85. Manchester: Manchester University Press, 2016.

———. *What Do Pictures Want? The Lives and Loves of Images*. Chicago: University of Chicago Press, 2005.

Morehead, Allison. "The *Musée de la folie*: Collecting and Exhibiting *chez les fous*." *Journal of the History of Collections* 23, no. 1 (2011): 101–26.

Morel, Dominique. "Henry Cros, *La Belle Viole* and *Circe, Flora, and Medea*." *Nineteenth-Century Art Worldwide* 16, no. 1 (2017). http://www.19thc-artworldwide.org/spring17/new-discovery-henry-cros-la-belle-viole-and-circe-flora-and-medea.

Moscoso, Javier. *Pain: A Cultural History*. Translated by Sarah Thomas and Paul House. Basingstoke: Palgrave Macmillan, 2012.

Murray, T. Jock. *Multiple Sclerosis: The History of a Disease*. New York: Demos, 2005.

Musée des Beaux-Arts de Rouen. *L'Écorché*. Rouen: Musée des Beaux-Arts de Rouen, 1977. Exhibition catalog.

Musée Rodin. *Passion à l'oeuvre. Rodin et Freud collectionneurs*. Paris: Nicolas Chaudun and Musée Rodin, 2008. Exhibition catalog.

New Larousse Encyclopedia of Mythology. Translated by Richard Aldington and Delano Ames. London: Hamlyn Publishing Group, 1959.

Nochlin, Linda. *Courbet*. London: Thames & Hudson, 2007.
———. *Realism*. Harmondsworth: Penguin Books, 1971.
Noirot, Fabien. "Jules Baretta et les secrets du moulage pathologique." *Histoire des sciences médicales* 48, no. 2 (2014): 203–8.
Nye, Robert A. *Crime, Madness, and Politics in Modern France. The Medical Concept of National Decline*. Princeton: Princeton University Press, 1984.
O'Connor, Erin. "Camera Medica." *History of Photography* 23, no. 3 (1999): 232–44.
———. *Raw Material: Producing Pathology in Victorian Culture*. Durham: Duke University Press, 2000.
Olivié, Jean-Luc. "Henry Cros." In Gaborit, Ligot, et al., *Sculptures en cire*, 213–14.
———. "*Le Prix du tournoi*." In Gaborit, Ligot, et al., *Sculptures en cire*, 215.
Ollerenshaw, Robert. "Medical Illustration: The Impact of Photography on Its History." *Journal of the Biological Photographic Association* 36, no. 1 (1968): 3–13.
O'Shiel, Daniel. "Kolnai's Disgust as Violation of Value." In *Le Dégoût. Histoire, langage, esthétique et politique d'une émotion plurielle*, edited by Michel Delville, Andrew Norris, and Viktoria von Hoffmann, 25–39. Liège: Presses Universitaires de Liège, 2015.
Oulié, Marthe. *Jean Charcot. L'Homme du "Pourquoi Pas?"* Paris: Gallimard, 1937.
Oursel, Hervé. "*Buste de jeune fille*." In Gaborit, Ligot, et al., *Sculptures en cire*, 141–46.
Palouzié, Hélène, and Caroline Ducourau. "De la collection Fontana à la collection Spitzner, l'aventure des cires anatomiques de Paris à Montpellier." *In Situ: Revue des patrimoines* 31 (2017). https://journals.openedition.org/insitu/14142.
Panofsky, Erwin. *Tomb Sculpture: Its Changing Aspects from Ancient Egypt to Bernini*. Edited by H. W. Janson. London: Thames & Hudson, 1964.
Panzanelli, Roberta, ed. *Ephemeral Bodies: Wax Sculpture and the Human Figure*. Los Angeles: Getty Research Institute, 2008.
———. "Introduction: Beyond the Pale; Polychromy and Western Art." In *The Color of Life: Polychromy in Sculpture from Antiquity to the Present*, edited by Roberta Panzanelli, 2–17. Los Angeles: J. Paul Getty Museum and the Getty Research Institute, 2008. Exhibition catalog.
———. "Introduction: The Body in Wax, the Body of Wax." In Panzanelli, *Ephemeral Bodies*, 1–11.
Papet, Édouard. "À fleur de peau: Le Moulage sur nature au XIXe siècle." In Papet, *À fleur de peau*, 16–44.
———, ed. *À fleur de peau. Le Moulage sur nature au XIXe siècle*. Paris: Éditions de la Réunion des musées nationaux, 2001. Exhibition catalog.
———, ed. *En couleurs. La Sculpture polychrome en France 1850–1910*. Paris: Hazan / Musée d'Orsay, 2018. Exhibition catalog.
———. "Henry Cros, *Le Prix du tournoi*, 1873." In *En couleurs. La Sculpture polychrome en France, 1850–1910*, edited by Édouard Papet, 68. Paris: Hazan / Musée d'Orsay, 2018. Exhibition catalog.
———. "Introduction." In Papet, *À fleur de peau*, 11–13.
———. "Le Moulage sur nature au service de la science." In Papet, *À fleur de peau*, 88–95.
———. "La Sculpture polychrome en France 1850–1910." In *En couleurs. La Sculpture polychrome en France 1850–1910*, edited by Édouard Papet, 17–32. Paris: Hazan / Musée d'Orsay, 2018. Exhibition catalog.
———. "Technique: 'Saisir la nature sur le fait.'" In Papet, *À fleur de peau*, 74–77.
Phillips, David. "Photo-Logos: Photography and Deconstruction." In *The Subjects of Art History: Historical Objects in Contemporary Perspectives*, edited by Mark A. Cheetham, Michael Ann Holly, and Keith Moxey, 155–79. Cambridge: Cambridge University Press, 1998.
Pichel, Beatriz. "The Backstage of Hysteria: Medicine in the Photographic Studio." *Remedia*, (2017). https://remedianetwork.wordpress.com/2017/01/16/the-backstage-of-hysteria-medicine-in-the-photographic-studio/.
———. "Cuerpos patológicos: Fotografía y medicina en el sigle XIX." *Alcores*, no. 19 (2015): 35–55.
———. "From Facial Expressions to Bodily Gestures: Passions, Photography and Movement in French 19th-Century Sciences." *History of the Human Sciences* 29, no. 1 (2015): 1–22.

Pick, Daniel. *Faces of Degeneration: A European Disorder, c. 1848–c. 1918.* Cambridge: Cambridge University Press, 1989.
Pinet, Hélène. "Cires anatomiques." In *Le Corps en morceaux*, edited by Anne Pingeot, 51–56. Paris: Réunion des musées nationaux, 1990. Exhibition catalog.
Pingeot, Anne, ed. *Le Corps en morceaux.* Paris: Réunion des musées nationaux, 1990. Exhibition catalog.
Pointon, Marcia. "Casts, Imprints, and the Deathliness of Things." *Art Bulletin* 96, no. 2 (2014): 170–95.
———. *Portrayal and the Search for Identity.* London: Reaktion, 2012.
Poirier, Jacques. "Joseph Babinski: Une personnalité complexe." *Bulletin de l'Académie nationale de médecine* 191, no. 7 (2007): 1343–53.
Poivert, Michel. "Variété et vérité du corps humain, l'esthétique de Paul Richer." In *L'Art du nu au XIX*[e] *siècle. Le photographe et son modèle*, 164–68. Paris: Hazan / Bibliothèque nationale de France, 1997. Exhibition catalog.
Pons, Bruno. "Hôtel de Varangeville." In *Le Faubourg Saint-Germain. La Rue Saint-Dominique. Hôtels et amateurs*, edited by Délégation à l'action artistique de la Ville de Paris [and] Société d'histoire et d'archéologie du VIIe arrondissement, 73–77. Paris: Musée Rodin, 1984. Exhibition catalog.
Porter, Roy. "Introduction." In *Patients and Practitioners: Lay Perceptions of Medicine in Pre-Industrial Society*, edited by Roy Porter, 1–22. Cambridge: Cambridge University Press, 1985.
Porter, Theodore. "The Objective Self." Review of *Objectivity*, by Lorraine Daston and Peter Galison. *Victorian Studies* 50, no. 4 (2008): 641–47.
Potts, Alex. "Colors of Sculpture." In *The Color of Life: Polychromy in Sculpture from Antiquity to the Present*, edited by Roberta Panzanelli, 78–97. Los Angeles: J. Paul Getty Museum and the Getty Research Institute, 2008. Exhibition catalog.
Pourfar, Michael H. "A Room from Jean-Martin Charcot's House at the Metropolitan Museum of Art." *Neurology* 65, no. 10 (2005): 1590.
Prat, Louis-Antoine. *Le Dessin français au XIX*[e] *siècle.* Paris: Somogy Éditions d'Art, 2011.
Prioux, Roger. *Deux médecins—Deux sculpteurs—Paul Richer et Raymond Sabouraud.* [MD diss.] Paris: Librairie Arnette, 1948.
Quétel, Claude. *History of Syphilis.* Translated by Judith Braddock and Brian Pike. Cambridge: Polity Press, 1990.
Rawling, Katherine D. B. "'The Annexed Photos Were Taken Today': Photographing Patients in the Late-Nineteenth-Century Asylum." *Social History of Medicine* 34, no. 1 (2019): 256–84.
———. "Patient Photographs, Patient Voices: Recovering Patient Experience in the Nineteenth-Century Asylum." In *Voices in the History of Madness*, edited by Robert Ellis, Sarah Kendal, and Steven J. Taylor, 237–62. Basingstoke: Palgrave Macmillan, 2021.
———. "'She Sits All Day in the Attitude Depicted in the Photo': Photography and the Psychiatric Patient in the Late-Nineteenth Century." *Medical Humanities* 43, no. 2 (2017): 99–110.
Richardson, Ruth. *Death, Dissection and the Destitute.* London: Penguin Books, 1988.
Ricou, Philippe, Véronique Leroux-Hugon, and Jacques Poirier. "La Bibliothéque Charcot à la Salpêtrière." *Histoire des sciences médicales* 28, no. 4 (1994): 319–23.
———. *La Bibliothèque Charcot à la Salpêtrière.* Paris: Éditions Pradel, 1993.
Roth, Michael S. "Hysterical Remembering." *Modernism/Modernity* 3, no. 2 (1996): 1–30.
Rouillé, André, and Bernard Marbot. *Le Corps et son image. Photographies du dix-neuvième siècle.* Paris: Contrejour, 1986. Exhibition catalog.
Ruiz-Gómez, Natasha. "Genius and Degeneracy: Auguste Rodin and the *Monument to Balzac*." In *Medicine and Maladies: Representing Affliction in Nineteenth-Century France*, edited by Sophie Leroy, 217–50. Leiden: Brill, 2018.
———. "A Hysterical Reading of Rodin's *Gates of Hell*." *Art History* 36, no. 5 (2013): 994–1017.
———. "The Model Patient: Observation and Illustration at the Musée Charcot." In *Visualizing the Body in Art, Anatomy, and Medicine Since 1800: Models and Modeling*, edited by Andrew Graciano, 203–32. New York: Routledge, 2019.

———. "Morceaux d'Amphithéâtre: Science and the Sculpture of Auguste Rodin." PhD diss., University of Pennsylvania, 2006.

———. "Of Sculptural and Corporal Remains." In *The Making of Rodin*, edited by Nabila Abdel Nabi, Chloé Ariot, and Achim Borchardt-Hume, 46–53. London: Tate, 2021. Exhibition catalog.

———. "The Painter, the Psychiatrist and a Fashion for Hysteria." *Wellcome Stories*, March 2020. https://wellcomecollection.org/articles/Xl44UhIAACEANhux.

———. "The "Scientific Artworks" of Doctor Paul Richer." *Medical Humanities* 39, no. 1 (2013): 4–10.

———. "Shaking the Tyranny of the Cadaver: Doctor Paul Richer and the *Living Écorché*." In *Bodies Beyond Borders: Moving Anatomies, 1750–1950*, edited by Kaat Wils, Raf de Bont, and Sokhieng Au, 231–57. Leuven: University of Leuven Press, 2017.

Ruiz-Gómez, Natasha, and Michael Liebrenz. "The Ties that Bind Past and Present: Tony Robert-Fleury, Philippe Pinel and the Salpêtrière; How Successes Long Believed to Be Safe Are Threatening to Slip Through Our Fingers." *Forensic Science International: Mind and Law* 2 (2021). https://doi.org/10.1016/j.fiml.2021.100049.

Saban, Roger, and Sylvie Hugues. "Les Musées d'anatomie de l'Institut d'anatomie." *Histoire des sciences médicales* 33, no. 2 (1999): 161–82.

Salomone, G., and R. Arnone. "Charcot and His Drawings: Images from 'Les Leçons du Mardi à la Salpêtrière 1887–1888.'" *Italian Journal of Neurological Sciences* 15, no. 4 (1994): 203–11.

Sappol, Michael. "'Morbid Curiosity': The Decline and Fall of the Popular Anatomical Museum." *Common-place* 4, no. 1 (2004). https://commonplace.online/article/morbid-curiosity/.

———. *A Traffic of Dead Bodies: Anatomy and Embodied Social Identity in Nineteenth-Century America*. Princeton: Princeton University Press, 2002.

Saunders, Corinne, Jane Macnaughton, and David Fuller, eds. *The Recovery of Beauty: Arts, Culture, Medicine*. Basingstoke: Palgrave, 2015.

Scarry, Elaine. *The Body in Pain: The Making and Unmaking of the World*. New York: Oxford University Press, 1985.

Schnalke, Thomas. "Casting Skin: Meanings for Doctors, Artists, and Patients." In Chadarevian and Hopwood, *Model*, 207–41.

———. *Diseases in Wax: The History of the Medical Moulage*. Translated by Kathy Spatschek. Berlin: Quintessence Books, 1995.

Schwartz, Vanessa R. *Spectacular Realities: Early Mass Culture in Fin-de-Siècle Paris*. Berkeley: University of California Press, 1998.

Scull, Andrew. *Hysteria: The Biography*. Oxford: Oxford University Press, 2009.

Sekula, Allan. "The Body and the Archive." *October* 39 (Winter 1986): 3–64.

Sheehan, Tanya. *Doctored: The Medicine of Photography in Nineteenth-Century America*. University Park: Penn State University Press, 2011.

Shorto, Russell. *Descartes' Bones: A Skeletal History of the Conflict Between Faith and Reason*. New York: Doubleday, 2008.

Showalter, Elaine. *The Female Malady: Women, Madness, and English Culture, 1830–1980*. New York: Pantheon Books, 1985.

———. *Hystories: Hysterical Epidemics and Modern Culture*. London: Picador, 1997.

Sicard, Monique, Robert Pujade, and Daniel Wallach. *À Corps et à raison. Photographies médicales, 1840–1920*. Paris: Marval, 1995. Exhibition catalog.

Sidlauskas, Susan. "Before and After: The Aesthetic as Evidence in Nineteenth-Century Medical Photography." In *Before-and-After Photography: Histories and Contexts*, edited by Jordan Bear and Kate Palmer Albers, 15–41. London: Bloomsbury, 2017.

———. "Inventing the Medical Portrait: Photography at the 'Benevolent Asylum' of Holloway, c. 1885–1889." *Medical Humanities* 39, no. 1 (2013): 29–37.

———. "The Medical Portrait: Resisting the Shadow Archive." *Nonsite*, no. 26 (2018). https://nonsite.org/the-medical-portrait/.

Siebers, Tobin. *Disability Aesthetics*. Ann Arbor: University of Michigan Press, 2010.

Siegel, Irwin M. "Charcot and Duchenne: Of Mentors, Pupils, and Colleagues."

Perspectives in Biology and Medicine 43, no. 4 (2000): 541–47.
Signoret, J. L. "Variété historique: Une leçon clinique à la Salpêtrière (1887) par André Brouillet." *Revue neurologique* 139, no. 12 (1983): 687–701.
Silverman, Debora L. *Art Nouveau in Fin-de-Siècle France*. Berkeley: University of California Press, 1989.
Simier, Amélie, with Marine Kisiel. *Jules Dalou, le sculpteur de la République. Catalogue des sculptures de Jules Dalou conservées au Petit Palais*. Paris: Paris-Musées, 2013. Exhibition catalog.
Simon-Dhouailly, Nadine. *La Leçon de Charcot. Voyage dans une toile*. Paris: Musée de l'Assistance Publique, 1986. Exhibition catalog.
Slipp, Naomi, et al. *Teaching the Body: Artistic Anatomy in the American Academy, from Copley, Rimmer, and Eakins to Contemporary Artists*. Boston: Boston University Art Gallery at the Stone Gallery, 2013. Exhibition catalog.
Slive, Seymour. *Frans Hals*. 3 vols. London: Phaidon, 1970–74.
Smith, Joel. Review of *Objectivity*, by Lorraine Daston and Peter Galison. *Art Bulletin* 92, no. 1–2 (2010): 109–13.
Snyder, Joel. "Visualization and Visibility." In Jones and Galison, *Picturing Science, Producing Art*, 379–97.
Solomon-Godeau, Abigail. "Realism Revisited." In *Self and History: A Tribute to Linda Nochlin*, edited by Aruna D'Souza, 69–75. London: Thames & Hudson, 2001.
Sonolet, Jacqueline. *J-M Charcot et l'hystérie au XIXe siècle*. Paris: Beba, 1982. Exhibition catalog.
Sontag, Susan. *Illness as Metaphor*. New York: Farrar, Straus and Giroux, 1977.
———. *On Photography*. New York: Anchor Books, 1973.
———. *Regarding the Pain of Others*. New York: Picador, 2003.
Stafford, Barbara Maria. *Artful Science: Enlightenment Entertainment and the Eclipse of Visual Education*. Cambridge, MA: MIT Press, 1994.
———. *Body Criticism: Imaging the Unseen in Enlightenment Art and Medicine*. Cambridge, MA: MIT Press, 1991.
Steinberg, Leo. "Art and Science: Do They Need to be Yoked?" *Daedalus* 115, no. 3 (1986): 1–16.
Stephens, Elizabeth. *Anatomy as Spectacle: Public Exhibitions of the Body from 1700 to the Present*. Liverpool: Liverpool University Press, 2011.
———. "Venus in the Archive: Anatomical Waxworks of the Pregnant Body." *Australian Feminist Studies* 25, no. 64 (2010): 133–44.
Stewart, Susan. *On Longing: Narratives of the Miniature, the Gigantic, the Souvenir, the Collection*. Baltimore: Johns Hopkins University Press, 1984.
Sulloway, Frank J. *Freud, Biologist of the Mind: Beyond the Psychoanalytic Legend*. New York: Basic Books, 1979.
Syson, Luke, ed. *Like Life: Sculpture, Color, and the Body*. New York: Metropolitan Museum of Art and Yale University Press, 2018. Exhibition catalog.
———. "Polychrome and Its Discontents." In *Like Life: Sculpture, Color, and the Body*, edited by Luke Syson et al., 14–41. New York: Metropolitan Museum of Art and Yale University Press, 2018. Exhibition catalog.
Tauber, Alfred I. *Science and the Quest for Meaning*. Waco: Baylor University Press, 2009.
Thomas, Ann, et al. *Beauty of Another Order: Photography in Science*. New Haven: Yale University Press, 1997. Exhibition catalog.
Thuillier, Jean. *Monsieur Charcot de la Salpêtrière*. Paris: Robert Laffont, 1993.
Tilles, Gérard. "Histoire des bibliothèques médicales et des musées des hôpitaux de l'Assistance Publique à Paris. L'Exemple de l'Hôpital Saint-Louis." PhD diss., Université Paris XII, 1995.
Tilles, Gérard, and Daniel Wallach, eds. *Le Musée des moulages de l'hôpital Saint-Louis*. Paris: Doin and Assistance Publique-Hôpitaux de Paris, 1996.
———. *Les Musées de médecine*. Toulouse: Privat, 1999.
Trachtenberg, Alan. "Photography: The Emergence of a Keyword." In *Photography in Nineteenth-Century America*, edited by Martha A. Sandweiss, 17–47. Fort Worth: Amon Carter Museum; New York: Harry N. Abrams, 1991. Exhibition catalog.
Trillat, Étienne. "L'Espèce morbide comme l'un des Beaux-Arts. A propos de 'Charcot, un grand médecin de son siècle,' de Michel Bonduelle, Toby

Gelfand et Christopher G. Goetz." *L'Evolution psychiatrique* 62, no. 3 (1997): 559–64.
———. *Histoire de l'hystérie*. Paris: Seghers, 1986.
Tucker, Jennifer. "The Historian, the Picture, and the Archive." *Isis* 97, no. 1 (2006): 111–20.
———. *Nature Exposed: Photography as Eyewitness in Victorian Times*. Baltimore: Johns Hopkins University Press, 2005.
———. "Objectivity, Collective Sight, and Scientific Personae." Review of *Objectivity*, by Lorraine Daston and Peter Galison. *Victorian Studies* 50, no. 4 (2008): 648–57.
Tucker, Jennifer, in collaboration with Tina Campt. "Entwined Practices: Engagements with Photography in Historical Inquiry." *History and Theory* 48, no. 4 (2009): 1–8.
Vénus et Caïn. Figures de la préhistoire, 1830–1930. Paris: Éditions de la Réunion des musées nationaux, 2003. Exhibition catalog.
Vergnes, André de. *Antoine de Tounens (1825–1878). Le Conquistador français fondateur du Royaume d'Araucanie et de Patagonie*. Paris: La Rochelle, 1979.
Viney, William, Felicity Callard, and Angela Woods. "Critical Medical Humanities: Embracing Entanglement, Taking Risks." *Medical Humanities* 41, no. 1 (2015): 2–7.
Wagner, Corinna. *Pathological Bodies: Medicine and Political Culture*. Berkeley: University of California Press, 2013.
Wallis, Jennifer. *Investigating the Body in the Victorian Asylum: Doctors, Patients, and Practices*. Basingstoke: Palgrave Macmillan, 2017.
Walusinski, Olivier. "Albert Londe. Le Photographe de Jean-Martin Charcot à La Salpêtrière." *Histoire des sciences médicales*, no. 1 (September 2018): 16–27.
———. "Biographie de Paul Richer." Unpublished manuscript, 2016.
———. "Jean-Martin Charcot and Parkinson's Disease: Teaching and Teaching Materials." *History of Neurology* 174, no. 7–8 (2018): 491–505.
———. "Keeping the Fire Burning: Georges Gilles de la Tourette, Paul Richer, Charles Féré and Alfred Binet." In *Following Charcot: A Forgotten History of Neurology and Psychiatry*, edited by Julien Bogousslavsky, 71–90. Basel: Karger, 2011.
———. *Une leçon clinique à La Salpêtrière. André Brouillet (1857–1914). Une peinture de la neurologie autour de Charcot*. Brou: Oscitatio, 2021.
———. *Paul Richer (1849–1933): Un neurologue professeur à l'École des beaux-arts*. Brou: Oscitatio, 2023.
Walusinski, Olivier, and Julien Bogousslavsky. "Charcot, Janet and French Models of Psychopathology." *European Neurology* 83, no. 3 (2020): 333–40.
Warner, Marina. *Phantasmagoria: Spirit Visions, Metaphors, and Media into the Twenty-first Century*. Oxford: Oxford University Press, 2006.
———. "Waxworks and Wonderlands." In *Visual Display: Culture Beyond Appearances*, edited by Lynne Cooke and Peter Wollen, 179–201. Seattle: Bay Press, 1995.
Weinberg, Bernard. *French Realism: The Critical Reaction, 1830–1870*. New York: Modern Language Association of America; London: Oxford University Press, 1937.
Weisberg, Gabriel P. *The European Realist Tradition*. Bloomington: Indiana University Press, 1982.
———. "The Realist Tradition: Critical Theory and the Evolution of Social Themes." In *The Realist Tradition: French Painting and Drawing, 1830–1900*, 1–20. Cleveland: Cleveland Museum of Art in cooperation with Indiana University Press, 1980. Exhibition catalog.
———. *The Realist Tradition: French Painting and Drawing, 1830–1900*. Cleveland: The Cleveland Museum of Art in cooperation with Indiana University Press, 1980. Exhibition catalog.
———. "Reframing Naturalism." In Weisberg et al., *Illusions of Reality*, 18–29.
Weisberg, Gabriel P., et al. *Illusions of Reality: Naturalist Painting, Photography, Theatre and Cinema, 1875–1918*. Brussels: Mercatorfonds, 2010. Exhibition catalog.
Weisberg, Yvonne M. L., and Gabriel P. Weisberg. *The Realist Debate: A Bibliography of French Realist Painting, 1830–1885*. New York: Garland Publishing, 1984.
West, Shearer. *Portraiture*. Oxford: Oxford University Press, 2004.

Whitehead, Anne, and Angela Woods. "Introduction." In Atkinson et al., *Edinburgh Companion*, 1–31.

Wilder, Kelley. *Photography and Science*. London: Reaktion Books, 2009.

———. "Visualizing Radiation: The Photographs of Henri Becquerel." In *Histories of Scientific Observation*, edited by Lorraine Daston and Elizabeth Lunbeck, 349–68. Chicago: University of Chicago Press, 2011.

Wittlich, Petr. "Closed Eyes, Symbolism and the New Shapes of Suffering." In Jean Clair et al., *Lost Paradise: Symbolist Europe*, 235–41. Montreal: Montreal Museum of Fine Arts, 1995. Exhibition catalog.

Woloshyn, Tania Anne. "Patients Rebuilt: Dr Auguste Rollier's Heliotherapeutic Portraits, c.1903–1944." *Medical Humanities* 39, no. 1 (2013): 38–46.

———. *Soaking Up the Rays: Light Therapy and Visual Culture in Britain, c. 1890–1940*. Manchester: Manchester University Press, 2017.

Woodall, Joanna. "Introduction: Facing the Subject." In *Portraiture: Facing the Subject*, edited by Joanna Woodall, 1–25. Manchester: Manchester University Press, 1997.

Yamamoto-Wilson, John R. *Pain, Pleasure and Perversity: Discourses of Suffering in Seventeenth-Century England*. Farnham: Ashgate, 2013.

Index

Italicized page references indicate illustrations. Endnotes are referenced with "n" followed by the endnote number.